Third Edition

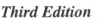

W9-BSJ-535

Basic Psychopharmacology for Mental Health Professionals

Richard S. Sinacola, Ph.D.
California State University – Los Angeles

Timothy Peters-Strickland, M.D.
Otuska Pharmaceutical Development and Commercialization, Inc. – Princeton

Joshua D. Wyner, Ph.D.
The Chicago School of Professional Psychology – Los Angeles

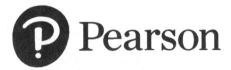

Director and Publisher: Kevin M. Davis
Portfolio Manager: Rebecca Fox-Gieg
Content Producer: Pamela D. Bennett
Portfolio Management Assistant: Maria Feliberty
Executive Field Marketing Manager: Krista Clark
Executive Product Marketing Manager: Christopher Barry
Procurement Specialist: Deidra Headlee
Cover Designer: Pearson CSC
Cover Photo: Miakievy/Getty Images
Full-Service Project Management: Pearson CSC, Freddie C. Domini and Rajakumar Venkatesan
Composition: Pearson CSC
Printer/Binder: LSC Communications, Inc.
Cover Printer: Phoenix Color/Hagerstown
Text Font: Times LT Pro 10/12

This text was previously published under the title *Basic Psychopharmacology for Counselors and Psychotherapists.*

Library of Congress Cataloging-in-Publication Data
Names: Sinacola, Richard S., author.
Title: Basic psychopharmacology for mental health professionals / Richard S.
    Sinacola, Ph.D., California State University -Los Angeles, Timothy
    Peters-Strickland, M.D., Otuska Pharmaceutical Development and
    Commercialization, Inc., Princeton, Joshua D. Wyner, Ph.D., The Chicago
    School of Professional Psychology, Los Angeles.
Other titles: Basic psychopharmacology for counselors and psychotherapists
Description: Third edition. | Hoboken : Pearson, [2020] | Revised edition of:
    Basic psychopharmacology for counselors and psychotherapists. c2012. |
    Includes bibliographical references and index.
Identifiers: LCCN 2018061200| ISBN 9780134893648 | ISBN 0134893646
Subjects: LCSH: Psychopharmacology.
Classification: LCC RM315 .S56 2020 | DDC 615.7/80835--dc23 LC record available at https://lccn.loc.gov/2018061200

34 2023

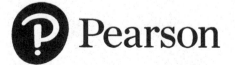

ISBN 10:   0-13-489364-6
ISBN 13: 978-0-13-489364-8

To my students, past and present, who always inspire me to do better.

R. S. Sinacola

To my loving family who help me grow and thrive: Howard, Alexia, and Alyssa.

T. Peters-Strickland

To my loving parents, Garret and Peggy, who taught me to be good, and to my amazing girls, Erin, Eliana, and Kayla, who push me to be better.

J. D. Wyner

ABOUT THE AUTHORS

Richard S. Sinacola, Ph.D., a licensed psychologist, is a Lecturer, Department of Psychology, California State University–Los Angeles. He is an Adjunct Full Professor and former Chair of Clinical Psychology at the Chicago School of Professional Psychology in Los Angeles, an Adjunct Professor of psychology and MFT at Brandman University, and an Adjunct Professor of theology and pastoral counseling at St. Clement Seminary. He maintains a private consulting and psychology practice in Pasadena and the Palm Springs area and currently serves as the APA curriculum consultant for Audio Digest Corporation in Glendale. He served as the former Director of Psychology Programs for Chapman University in Palm Desert and was the former Chair of Counseling and Addiction Studies at the University of Detroit Mercy. He has served on the editorial board of the Michigan Journal of Counseling and Development, and he is the past secretary of the Michigan Psychological Association. He holds degrees in psychology, counseling, clinical social work, and theology from the University of Detroit, Wayne State University, and St. Clement Seminary.

Timothy Peters-Strickland, M.D., is Vice President, Global Clinical Development, CNS and Digital Medicine, at Otsuka Pharmaceutical Development and Commercialization. He was former Medical Director in Neuroscience at Covance in Princeton and conducts clinical research in the mental health field. Dr. Peters-Strickland has held an appointment as a clinical instructor with the University of Southern California. He is a diplomate of the American Board of Psychiatry and Neurology with an added qualification in Addiction Psychiatry. Dr. Peters-Strickland obtained his medical degree from the University of Florida after obtaining a BA in Biochemistry from Florida State University. He completed his psychiatric residency at the University of Southern California.

Joshua D. Wyner, Ph.D., is an Associate Professor and Interim Department Chair of Marriage and Family Therapy at the Chicago School of Professional Psychology in Los Angeles. He maintains a private practice as a Licensed Marriage and Family Therapist in Los Angeles and serves as an outside supervisor for the Maple Counseling Center. He was the Psychophysiology Lab Manager for the USC Twin Project, a multi-decade longitudinal study that examines the genetics of psychopathology and related behaviors. He has also worked with USC's Optical Materials and Devices Laboratory, developing hardware for retinal prosthetics. Dr. Wyner holds degrees in Clinical Neuroscience, Electrical Engineering, and Marriage and Family Therapy from the University of Southern California.

PREFACE

Welcome to the third edition of *Basic Psychopharmacology for Mental Health Professionals (formally Basic Psychopharmacology for Counselors and Psychotherapists)*. With more psychotherapy patients taking psychotropic medications than ever before, counselors, psychologists, social workers, and family therapists need quick and accurate information. Finding this information is not easy because most textbooks on psychotropic medications are written by physicians for physicians. In the few cases that nonphysicians, usually biologically oriented Ph.D.'s, have attempted this endeavor, they have produced works that are more like physiological psychology texts, which are beyond the basic questions and interests of the student, counselor, or psychotherapist.

The third edition of *Basic Psychopharmacology for Mental Health Professionals,* like the first and second editions, is designed to provide basic yet comprehensive information for the typical graduate student in a mental health training program, as well as the practicing clinician in the field. Most graduate students have not taken undergraduate courses in physiological psychology, and their knowledge of the brain and neuronal functions is minimal. This textbook presents these and other topics in easy-to-understand language. In fact, the entire text continues to be written in a familiar style that invites the otherwise intimidated professional to learn more. The text is even written so the interested layperson can obtain a basic understanding of how these medications work. Medical jargon is kept to a minimum, and voluminous information on psychopathology is also omitted because we assume that clinicians and graduate students are familiar with the *Diagnostic and Statistical Manual of Mental Disorders,* 5th edition (DSM-5) and the criteria used in diagnostic determinations.

In addition to offering up-to-date information on the latest medications currently available for treating mental illness and other related conditions, this book will assist clinicians in working more effectively with their patients on medication and with the professionals prescribing them. The book is organized to address the most commonly presented types of pathology first.

What's New in the Third Edition

- Updated throughout to reflect DSM-5 criteria for diagnoses and appropriate considerations for psychopharmacology agents for those diagnoses
- Updated information on the latest medications used to treat a variety of mental health concerns
- Updated research on the newest medications, including novel applications of some of the older, well-known medications
- Updated tables in each treatment-related chapter that reflect the latest medications and their properties
- An updated comprehensive table of all psychopharmacology agents, located in the appendix
- An additional clinical case example providing the reader with two typical case examples in each treatment-related chapter
- The addition of new diagnostic considerations and medications in Chapter 14, Treatment of Comorbidity and Other Disorders

Chapter Outlines for the Third Edition

- Chapter 1 gives students and their professors and practicing clinicians reasons why the study of psychopharmacology is so important for the mental health professional. Some ethical and spiritual considerations are also explored.
- Chapter 2 provides a basic explanation of the functions of the brain and neurological system, including the anatomy and function of neurons, the role of neurotransmitters and other neurochemicals involved in emotions and behavior, and the electrical and chemical communications between cells.
- Chapter 3 addresses issues related to psychopharmacology and pharmacokinetics, including methods of administering drugs; absorption, distribution, and elimination of drugs; therapeutic dose and therapeutic index; tolerance, withdrawal, and discontinuance of drugs; synergism and potentiation; placebo effects; and prescription and pharmaceutical terms.
- Chapter 4 provides the therapist with tools and techniques for taking a thorough history of the patient, including a patient history outline, a mental status outline, assessment and testing instruments, and an outline for an initial patient interview. Suggestions for additional assessment tools are available online.
- Chapters 5 through 12 address trade and generic medications and herbals used to treat common mental health conditions: unipolar depression, bipolar illness, anxiety and psychotic disorders, ADHD and attention disorders, and cognitive, sleep, and personality disorders.
- Chapter 11 concentrates solely on sleep disorders. It was included because many clinicians who deal with patients presenting with these concerns are unfamiliar with the medications used to treat insomnia.
- Chapter 13 addresses chemical dependency, co-occurring conditions, and the special medications used to treat this population. This topic is not addressed in most other texts.
- Chapter 14 provides typical medication regimens used to treat patients with comorbid conditions, including patients with chronic pain, eating disorders and obesity, impulse control problems, sexual compulsivity, gambling, and other intrusive behaviors.
- Chapters 15 through 19 present cases across the developmental continuum, including children and adolescents and early, middle, and older adults. Many of the cases are based on actual patients. The cases are used to demonstrate both the diagnostic process and the rationale for choosing one medication over another.
- Complete, easy-to-read tables of medications appear throughout the text and are combined into a master table in the Appendix.

This text serves as a basic introduction to psychopharmacology for the nonmedical provider. Although information on dosage and use was accurate at the time of writing, the clinician should not use this information as a guide for prescribing medications. All clinicians should consult their respective codes of ethics and their home state's scope of practice to ensure that discussing medications and their effects with patients is within the scope of their license to practice.

This text was developed to be a brief yet comprehensive overview of clinical psychopharmacology. It can be read easily in a weekend and will serve as a handy reference guide for mental health professionals from all disciplines. Combined, we authors have more than 62 years of clinical experience—one of us as a psychologist with a private practice and a professor teaching psychopharmacology in a graduate setting, one as a psychiatrist treating patients from all walks of life and conducting research in the application of pharmaceutical agents, and one as an educator of marriage and family therapy who also practices as a marriage and family therapist. We hope that the readers find this book informative as well as interesting.

ACKNOWLEDGMENTS

We wish to acknowledge the editors and staff at Pearson for their help and encouragement in completing this task. We would also like to thank the following reviewers for their time and feedback in making this book a worthwhile contribution to the field: Darlene Clark, Penn State University; Jacqueline Frock, Oklahoma City Community College; Joy-Del Snook, Lamar University; and Genevieve Weber, Hofstra University.

R. S. Sinacola, Ph.D.

Los Angeles, CA

T. Peters-Strickland, M.D.

Princeton, NJ

J. D. Wyner, Ph.D.

Los Angeles, CA

BRIEF CONTENTS

CONTENTS

CHAPTER | **1**

Why Study Psychopharmacology

REASONS FOR THE NONMEDICAL THERAPIST TO READ THIS BOOK

Over the years, various counseling and psychotherapy models have emerged, flourished, continued, or faded from use. Many of these theories or models offered the clinician options for maximizing the therapeutic progress of his/her clients. Many of them emphasized humanistic, psychoanalytic, existential, or behavioral techniques that downplayed the role of medication in the treatment of many conditions. In fact, except for those patients with serious psychopathology requiring inpatient hospitalization, most patients were not placed on medications. This did not concern most psychologists, social workers, counselors, and other psychotherapists, as their work with the nonpsychiatric population was stable and secure. Many clinicians were quite happy providing nonmedical care, leaving the medications to psychiatrists and primary care physicians.

Today, a vast majority of the patients seen in private practice settings and in community mental health agencies have been, are, or will be on psychotropic medications. Most therapists, however, have not received adequate education to keep pace with a changing treatment arena. In fact, most nonmedical therapists—namely, psychologists, social workers, professional counselors, marriage and family therapists, and even clergy—have never taken a course in psychopharmacology, or they have taken only a brief survey course and feel ill prepared to handle patients and clients on psychotropic medications (Barlow & Herbert, 1995; Sinacola, 1997). Even if they have taken a formal course in psychopharmacology, the course typically does not cover the rather complex approaches to psychopharmacology, such as dealing with treatment, medication-resistant depression, or the need for polypharmacy to fully address a condition.

Some therapists choose not to seek this information. They offer the argument that they work with cancer patients and do not need to know the etiology or how to treat the disease. This argument has some truth in it; however, it might not be a valid premise for choosing to be naïve on the topic. For example, it has been well documented that all therapists need to be aware of the role physical illness plays in mental illness. If any ethical or professional therapist or counselor feels that a physical condition might be a cause for a patient's mental condition, the therapist should immediately refer the patient to a physician for an evaluation. Amazingly, many do not. Although a physical condition may resolve quickly when it is physically treated, a mental illness often requires a combination of psychotherapy and medication. As a mental health *expert*, the clinician is expected to diagnose and treat various conditions and be aware of the best treatment for them. To limit treatment options by excluding medications, which represent a large part of the available protocol, is a disservice to the patient. Therapists who claim that medication would interfere with their approach are often lulled into a false sense of inclusiveness. They believe the only way to treat a patient is with nonmedical therapy, and if the patient is not responding, they believe he or she is resisting treatment. Many never even consider the possibility that the patient may need something more than the clinician can provide. Some pastoral or Christian counselors have taken the position along with some of their clients that taking medication is unnatural and not in God's plan of treatment for them (Sinacola, 2017). They fail to understand that most major religions in the Eastern and Judeo-Christian philosophies, with the exception of some Christian

Science congregations, utilize modern medicine. It is important to work closely with clients from religious backgrounds to help them formulate a healthy approach to medication while maintaining their spiritual beliefs and practices.

For years, nonmedical therapists have accused psychiatrists of being "pill pushers." Indeed, changes in coverage on certain mental health insurance plans have reduced the amount of time psychiatrists can spend with patients. Nonmedical therapists often cite the refusal of psychiatrists to spend any real therapeutic time with patients as evidence that psychiatrists either lack therapeutic skills or view everything as a medical issue. The reduction in time often leads to less social and medical history being taken from the patient, leading to hasty diagnostic conclusions. The sad truth here is also that many nonmedical practitioners feel uncomfortable talking to psychiatrists and other prescribers about medications. Many nonmedical practitioners choose to reduce every psychological concern to purely behavioral manifestations and are reluctant to even consider the role of biology or neurology. This choice is not new, even among medical therapists. When advising clients, some social workers and nurses have minimized the need for psychological testing because they do not perform these services. Many were reluctant to refer clients to psychologists for psychological testing because they feared that the psychologist might steal their client, even when information like IQ is critical in determining the cause of behavior or the need for placement or custody. Historically, psychologists and psychiatrists have waged turf wars over the issue of who is really in charge. In many states, both the physician and the psychologist share hospital privileges. In addition, some states and jurisdictions, such as Louisiana, New Mexico, Illinois, Iowa, and Guam, allow properly trained psychologists to prescribe psychotropic medications. For years, clinical nurse specialists and physician assistants have been prescribing medications.

Many nonmedical therapists agree that knowledge of psychotropic medications is necessary and attempt to gain this knowledge, yet they still feel that their knowledge is inadequate. They shy away from discussing medications with clients and defer to the case physician. These therapists may claim that they do not wish to practice medicine without a license. Many therapists, such as licensed psychologists, are aware that their scope of practice in many states allows them to discuss medication options with patients, but they are not necessarily the person who may ultimately prescribe them. Still, these therapists claim ignorance and defer any decisions to the physician, nurse practitioner, or physician's assistant. They may be unclear as to what role they should take with patients regarding their medications.

An analogy may apply here. Your washing machine (patient) is not working properly. You need to repair (treat) it. In most cases, you would call a repair technician who comes to your home, listens to the machine (therapy), and makes a recommendation. The technician has a basic understanding of how the machine works and the function of each part, but not a deep understanding of why the part works or how to design or correct design flaws. The technician cannot usually explain why a part failed—only that it did and that it must be replaced. The mechanical engineer (the physician), who knows what the part was designed to do and why it physically failed, may be able to offer an explanation here and also may be able to fix the part if it is taken to the factory (hospital). If the machine has to be redesigned, the engineer, not the mechanic, would attempt to do it. A therapist who has no knowledge of psychotropic medications is like the repair technician who listens to the machine and says, "Yep, you have a problem all right, and I think it's in the rinse agitator. Maybe you want to see an engineer."

In reality, most good repair facilities and retailers employ mechanical engineers, electrical engineers, and technicians who work together to repair machines (provide treatment). In the same way, therapists and physicians need to work together in the best interests of the patient.

Today, the model of the *medical home* calls upon primary care doctors and providers to work collaboratively with mental health therapists in the service of the patient. It is imperative to have open channels of communication with other providers in the patient's case, especially the primary care physician.

How do nonmedical therapists or counselors determine just what they need to know? Consider the following quiz:

1. **What is an SSRI?**
    If you answered "an antidepressant," you get one point. But do you know that SSRI stands for selective serotonin reuptake inhibitors? Do you know the primary neurotransmitter involved in their action? Do you know the major side effects? Can you name the six major drugs in this class by brand name? Would you recognize the chemical or generic names if you saw them in a medical record? If a client told you a doctor placed him on meds and he was having side effects A, B, and C, would you know that the side effects came from the SSRI?
2. **What is a neuroleptic?**
    If you answered "a medication for treating schizophrenia," you get another point. But do you know the primary neurotransmitter that is involved in their action? Do you know the side effects? Do you know which medications are major tranquilizers and which are minor ones? Do you know which medications are better for the negative symptoms of psychoticism?
3. **What is a SPARI?**
    If you answered an "SSRI on steroids," you would be half right. How are these new-generation serotonin medications different, and how does partial agonism affect the drug's effectiveness?
4. **What is a benzodiazepine?**
    If you answered "They are used to treat anxiety," you once again get a point. But do you know where they interact in the brain? Do you know what neurotransmitter or amino acid is involved? Are they habit forming? Can someone overdose on them?

If you were able to answer all of the preceding questions correctly, you do not need to read this book and could probably teach others about psychopharmacology. If you knew a few answers, consider reading further and you will not be disappointed. If you knew none of the answers, definitely read on.

This book will help the nonmedical therapist to increase his or her knowledge of medications and their proper use. Without complicating the picture with excessive biological terms and neurochemistry, it will give the counselor or psychotherapist the necessary information to work safely with a patient currently taking or considering medications. It will also offer helpful suggestions to therapists working directly with psychiatrists and other prescribers, allowing them to feel confident using language both can understand in the optimum treatment of the patient.

CHAPTER 2

Basic Neurobiology

This chapter will provide basic information on the purpose and function of the brain's neurological system with regard to mental health functioning.

Topics to be addressed include the following:

- Neurons
- Neural communication
- Electrical and chemical properties of neural transmission
- Neurotransmitters of emotion and behavior

As a counselor or psychotherapist, you need to understand how the brain works to control thinking, behavior, and overall health. Further knowledge in this area should assist you in comprehending your client's symptoms and disease process. The field of psychopharmacology is evolving rapidly and will continue to change with advances in medical research. New interventions to treat psychiatric illnesses should enhance the quality of life for your mental health clients.

This chapter provides some basic information on which to build an understanding of various medications, their mechanisms of action, and how they might be used in day-to-day practice. This chapter describes the anatomy of nerve cells or neurons, how they fit together, and the ways they communicate.

NEURONS

Because the brain is the most complex organ in the body, the discussion here will be limited to neurons in the central nervous system and the effect of drugs on them. Within the central nervous system, neurons transmit messages or communicate with each other, and as will be explored later, drugs can affect this transmission. In order to understand how the messages are transmitted, you must first understand how a neuron is structured.

A neuron has four basic parts: the soma, dendrites, axon, and terminal buttons (see Figure 2.1).

- The *soma*, or cell body, contains the vital parts of the cell, including the nucleus, mitochondria, and other substances in the cytoplasm (the space inside the neuron). A membrane defines the boundary of the cell.
- *Dendrites* are large and small branches of the neuron, similar to branches of a tree, which receive messages from other neurons through multiple molecular receptors.
- The *axon* is a long, slender tube that carries messages from the soma to its terminal buttons.
- *Terminal buttons* are found at the ends of the axon. They contain small sacs, or vesicles, that hold chemical messengers, or *neurotransmitters*. Terminal buttons deliver neurotransmitters to other neurons across a physical gap called a *synapse*. The neurotransmitters can cross the synapse between a terminal button of one neuron and a dendrite of another neuron or between a terminal button of one neuron and the soma of another neuron.

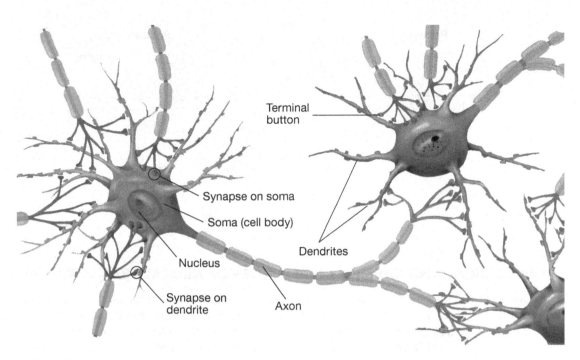

FIGURE 2.1   The Structure of a Neuron

NEURAL COMMUNICATION

Within the central nervous system, neuron communication is facilitated either electrically or chemically. This communication is facilitated electrically within the neuron and chemically between neurons.

All drugs and substances that can activate neurons in the brain or central nervous system and thus affect communication among neurons are classified as either endogenous or exogenous. *Endogenous* substances, such as endorphins, insulin, and adrenaline (also known as ephinephrine), come from within the body. *Exogenous* substances, such as caffeine, vitamins, herbs, and medications, are produced outside the body and introduced into the body in some manner.

Receptor sites on the postsynaptic membranes of dendrites are the most common targets of medications that can activate their respective cells. That action begins when a receptor is stimulated by a neurotransmitter. If enough receptors are stimulated at once, an electrical impulse (called an *action potential*) travels along the axon toward the terminal button. Because an electrical signal or impulse is unable to cross the synapse, the transmission of the signal across the synapse depends on chemical messengers, or neurotransmitters. After the electrical impulse reaches the terminal button, a neurotransmitter is released. It travels from the presynaptic membrane of the terminal button across the synapse to the postsynaptic membrane of another neuron's dendrites, where it might interact. The postsynaptic membrane of the dendrite contains numerous receptors that receive the chemical signal and, in turn, activate the postsynaptic cell, allowing it to transmit again (see Figure 2.2).

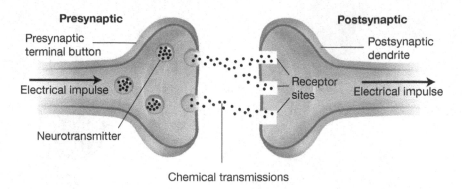

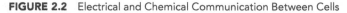

FIGURE 2.2   Electrical and Chemical Communication Between Cells

ELECTRICAL AND CHEMICAL PROPERTIES OF NEURAL TRANSMISSION

The electrical properties of a neuron are mediated by electrically charged particles called ions. In their resting state, most neurons are slightly negatively charged when compared to their surroundings, with the difference between intracellular (inside the cell) ion concentrations and extracellular (outside the cell) ion concentrations, known as the *resting potential*, typically averaging –70 millivolts (mV) (the outside is more negative than the inside). In this resting state, the extracellular spaces are populated primarily by sodium (Na^+) and chloride (Cl^-) ions, while the intracellular spaces are populated primarily by potassium (K^+). The *resting potential* of a neuron is the unexcited or relaxed state in which the average electrical difference between the inside and outside of the cell is about 70 millivolts (mV). Some drugs can directly affect various phases of the action potential, and it is therefore important to understand the process in more detail. This process can be broken down into four key phases: stimulation, rising phase, falling phase, and the refractory period.

Phase 1: Stimulation

For an action potential to occur, the membrane potential (the potential difference between the inside and outside of the cell) must be significantly reduced, usually to around –55mV (known as the *threshold potential*). Each time a receptor is activated by a neurotransmitter, it has the potential to either increase or decrease the membrane potential. Excitatory messages *depolarize* the cell, usually by allowing sodium (Na^+) to flow in; this reduces the membrane potential and increases the chance of reaching that threshold potential. Inhibitory messages *hyperpolarize* the cell, usually by allowing chloride (Cl^-) to flow in; this increases the membrane potential and decreases the chance of reaching the threshold potential. Neurons are constantly receiving both excitatory and inhibitory signals. Whether a message is or is not transmitted depends on the relative number of excitatory and inhibitory signals a neuron receives. For example, if the excitatory messengers outnumber the inhibitory messengers, an action potential (message) will be initiated along the axon.

All action potentials are the same size when they are generated, but not all behavioral responses are equal in magnitude. More significant, or stronger, environmental stimuli produce a higher number of action potentials (a higher rate of firing of action potentials). The higher the rate of firings of action potentials, the stronger we would expect the behavioral response. For example, a loud sound may generate 10 action potentials in a time period, whereas a soft sound may generate only 2 action potentials during the same period. Thus, the behavioral response to the loud sound is usually greater than the response to the soft sound. In short, the magnitude of an effect is typically related to the number of action potentials that occur in sequence rather than to any change in action potential strength.

Phase 2: Rising Phase

Once an action potential is triggered by reaching the threshold potential, *voltage-gated* sodium channels open and a positive feedback condition occurs known as *runaway*: As the cell lets in more sodium, more of these sodium channels open, and even more sodium enters the cell. The result is a rapid depolarization that typically continues until the cell reaches around +40mV (known as the *peak*). Certain drugs and toxins, such as the tetrodotoxin found in the puffer fish, can block these voltage-gated sodium channels and thus stop this rising phase and resultant action potential, leading to paralysis in severe cases.

As the depolarization continues, the cell begins to compensate by opening potassium (K^+) channels that allow potassium to flow *out* of the cell in order to hyperpolarize it (imagine a boat flooding with water $[Na^+]$ while the crew begins dumping buckets of water back out $[K^+]$). Because these potassium channels open more slowly, they typically are unable to match the speed of the sodium channels right away.

Phase 3: Peak and Falling Phase

Once the potassium channels fully open, they match the speed of the sodium channels such that the voltage no longer changes. In other words, for every sodium ion that enters the cell, a potassium ion leaves. This is called the *peak* of the action potential, and it usually occurs at around +40mV. At this point, the voltage-gated sodium channels do something special: They *inactivate*. This is a process unique to voltage-gated sodium channels and involves a small protein block that stops them from letting more sodium through even though they're still open (imagine a cork blocking the open channel). Once this inactivation occurs, the outgoing potassium flow is much greater than the incoming sodium, and the voltage rapidly drops. Certain drugs and toxins, such as the alpha toxins from a scorpion sting, can block this sodium inactivation, resulting in prolonged action potentials that do not have this traditional falling phase and in severe cases lead to ataxia (involuntary limb movement) and even muscle lock.

Phase 4: Undershoot and Refractory Period

Once this hyperpolarization is complete, the cell is typically at an even lower voltage than the –70mV resting potential discussed earlier. At this point, the cell has entered a *refractory period* during which it is nearly impossible to get another action potential started. This is because the cell is now almost entirely filled with sodium and has released most of its potassium stores into the extracellular space. During this time, *ion exchangers* move potassium back into the cell and sodium back out. This process can last nearly as long as the action potential itself and must be completed before another action potential can be stimulated. Once the cell has fully reset, the action potential is complete.

When the action potential reaches the nerve terminal, neurotransmitters are released by a process called *exocytosis*, the secretion of a substance by a cell (see Figure 2.3). At the end of the

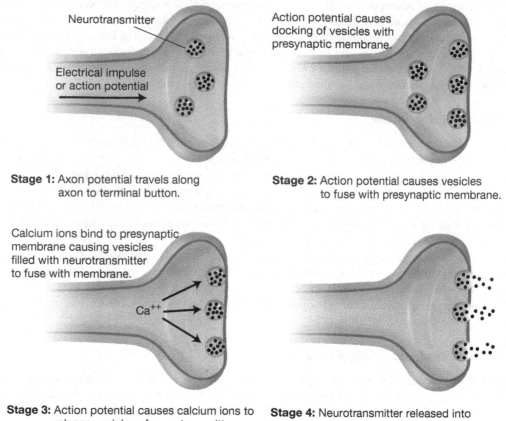

Stage 1: Axon potential travels along axon to terminal button.

Stage 2: Action potential causes vesicles to fuse with presynaptic membrane.

Stage 3: Action potential causes calcium ions to release vesicles of neurotransmitter into synapse.

Stage 4: Neurotransmitter released into synapse.

FIGURE 2.3   The Four Stages of Exocytosis

axon, the action potential causes calcium ions (Ca^{++}) in the terminal button to release the neurotransmitter into the synapse, which in turn causes *vesicles* (small packets of neurotransmitter) to bind to the cell wall. As these vesicles fuse, the neurotransmitter they contain diffuses across the synapse to interact with receptors on the postsynaptic membrane of the dendrites or soma. When receptors are activated, ion channels, or little gateways, open on the postsynaptic membrane, causing either depolarization or hyperpolarization. An excitatory signal leads to the process occurring again; an inhibitory effect decreases further signals. Remember that depolarization excites and hyperpolarization inhibits. The signaling is technically over only when the neurotransmitter is no longer present in the synapse. The primary method for removing neurotransmitter when some of the neurotransmitter is taken back into the terminal button in a process called *reuptake* (see Figure 2.4).

A neurotransmitter and its individual receptor site together act like a key fitting into a lock (see Figure 2.5). Receptors, located on the extracellular membrane, are specific types of protein structures made of amino acids. The structures make each receptor unique. By a process known as *signal transduction*, the first messenger or neurotransmitter binds to a receptor that transmits the message by changing the electrical characteristics of the cell, by starting a biochemical action

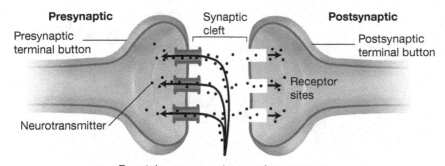

Reuptake pumps or transporters remove
the neurotransmitter from the synaptic cleft
via the terminal buttons. This terminates
the action potential.

FIGURE 2.4   The Process of Reuptake

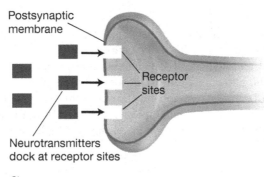

FIGURE 2.5   Receptor Sites

within the cell, or by both. (The second messenger will be explained later.) In general, a neurotransmitter may open an ion channel in either of two major ways. One direct way is through ligand-gated ion channel receptors (neurotransmitter and drugs are generally referred to as ligands). An ion channel opens when a ligand binds to the receptor site (see Figure 2.6). In turn, the influx of particular ions leads to either depolarization or hyperpolarization. For example, the acetylcholine receptor works in this manner. When two acetylcholine molecules occupy the two acetylcholine sites on a single receptor, a sodium channel is opened, resulting in an influx of sodium (Na^+) ions that causes depolarization.

The second way a neurotransmitter opens an ion channel is by inducing chemical changes within the cell. The majority of receptors that produce these effects are called G protein–linked receptors because they bind guanine nucleotides. For example, dopamine, glutamate, gamma-aminobutyric acid (GABA), and serotonin all facilitate neurotransmission by utilizing G protein–linked receptors.

After the first messenger or neurotransmitter interacts with the extracellular receptor, the chemical effects of the G proteins activate a second messenger within the cell. The best-known second messenger is cyclic adenosine monophosphate, or cyclic AMP. Thus, the neurotransmitter or first messenger binding to the receptor causes a cascade of chemical reactions in the postsynaptic neuron involving a second messenger. Cyclic AMP usually activates other molecules or

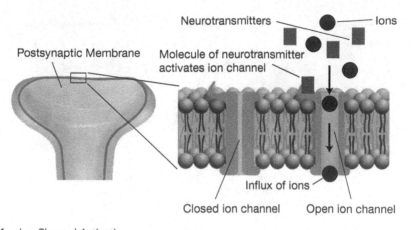

FIGURE 2.6   Ion Channel Activation

enzymes that in turn activate or inhibit other chemicals. The resulting substances are known as protein kinases. The protein kinases facilitate a change in the physical shape of other proteins that control the opening of an ion channel. The alteration in the physical shape of the protein permits the channel to open, allowing an influx of ions into the postsynaptic neuron. This ion influx causes either depolarization or hyperpolarization. The final results of this process vary but may include making other neurotransmitters, up- or down-regulating the number of receptors, sending further electrical charges, and so on. An increasingly complex cascade of effects occurs that alters cellular function.

NEUROTRANSMITTERS OF EMOTION AND BEHAVIOR

Three main neurotransmitters involved in emotion and behavior are the monoamines, comprised of two catecholamines (dopamine and norepinephrine) and one indolamine (serotonin). The category designation catecholamine or monoamine is based upon chemical structure. Other neurotransmitters that might be considered include three important amino acids: GABA, glycine, and glutamate. In addition, certain chains of amino acids known as neuropeptides, including substance P and endorphins, may play a role in emotion and behavior.

Dopamine and norepinephrine are closely related and synthesized from the same precursor substance known as tyrosine (see Figure 2.7). Tyrosine is an amino acid that comes from diet. Synthesized tyrosine can be purchased in a health food store; however, some believe tyrosine is not effective unless it is obtained from food. Dietary sources of tyrosine include meat, poultry, seafood, beans, tofu, and lentils. Tyrosine enters dopaminergic neurons by diffusion, where the cytoplasmic enzyme tyrosine hydroxylase converts it to L-DOPA. The L-DOPA is then converted by DOPA decarboxylase into dopamine. Some of the dopamine may be further converted by dopamine β-hydroxylase into norepinephrine.

The noradrenergic (or norepinephrine) pathways in the brain seem to be involved in the regulation of sleep–wake cycles, sustained attention, alertness, and biological responses to new stimuli. Noradrenaline is also thought to mediate anxiety, fear, and stress responses. Thus, noradrenergic abnormalities or drops in norepinephrine levels are thought to play a large role in mood and anxiety disorders.

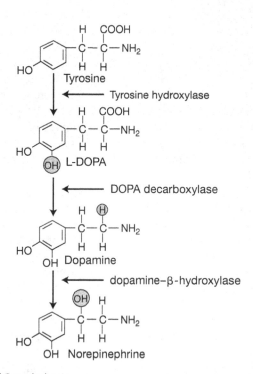

FIGURE 2.7   Synthesis of Catecholamines

Serotonin or 5-hydroxytryptamine (5-HTP) is synthesized from tryptophan in the diet (see Figure 2.8). Once again, synthesized tryptophan supplements have not been shown to be an effective way of obtaining serotonin. Dietary sources of tryptophan include bananas, sunflower seeds, and milk. Tryptophan is converted into 5-hydroxytryptophan by an enzyme called tryptophan hydroxylase. Then 5-hydroxytryptophan decarboxylase acts on 5-hydroxytryptophan to produce serotonin or 5-HTP.

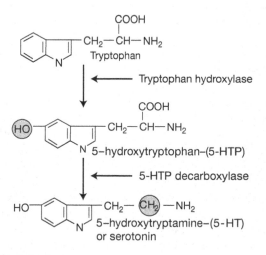

FIGURE 2.8   Synthesis of Indolamines

Scientists believe that serotonin plays a large role in brain functioning, including mood, anxiety, arousal, irritability, tranquility, cognition, appetite, sleep–wake cycles, and obsessions. Serotonergic abnormalities or drops in serotonin levels are associated with anxiety disorders, mood disorders, and even psychotic disorders. Explanations of neural activity might seem quite concrete and straightforward, but the systems are much more complex. Neurons have an extraordinary number of diverse interconnections. Because behavior is complicated, no one neurotransmitter should be considered in isolation; for example, an individual's depression might be caused by insufficient levels of serotonin, norepinephrine, dopamine, or, in some cases, all three. Most brain functions result from multiple influences of several different neurotransmitters trying to find their own delicate balance.

Drugs may alter behavior by interfering with or interrupting any of the processes that occur during neural communication. A drug that increases the availability or action of a neurotransmitter is called an *agonist*. Agonists are agents that bind to receptors and act. For example, fluoxetine (Prozac) increases the action of serotonin on the postsynaptic membrane. Conversely, a drug that decreases the availability or action of a neurotransmitter is called an *antagonist*. They bind to receptors and block. For example, risperidone (Risperdal) blocks dopamine at the postsynaptic membrane. Keep these concepts in mind. They will be revisited in later chapters with respect to specific diseases and medications.

In summary, a few neurotransmitters are particularly important for those in the mental health field. The following gives you a general foundation for each one.

- *Acetylcholine.* In the central nervous system, acetylcholine is widely distributed and thought to play a role in memory, learning, behavioral arousal, attention, mood, and rapid eye movement that occurs during sleep. In the peripheral nervous system, acetylcholine is found at synapses where the nerve terminals meet skeletal muscles, causing excitation leading to muscle contractions.
- *Epinephrine or adrenaline.* This neurotransmitter is probably more active in the peripheral nervous system than in the central nervous system. Epinephrine is secreted by the adrenal glands, small endocrine glands above the kidneys. In the peripheral nervous system, epinephrine regulates our fight-or-flight response. Its role is described in more detail in Chapter 7.
- *Norepinephrine.* Primarily, norepinephrine is an excitatory neurotransmitter in the central nervous system. Norepinephrine cell bodies in the brainstem have axons projecting into the limbic system (brain structures involved in emotions) and the frontal lobes. Wakefulness and alertness are the two major functions of norepinephrine. The role of norepinephrine is discussed later in Chapter 7 and Chapter 9.
- *Dopamine.* Another major neurotransmitter, dopamine is involved with behavioral regulation, movement, learning, mood, and attention. Dopamine may have both excitatory and inhibitory effects in the brain. It is believed that overactivity of dopamine or oversensitivity of dopamine receptors is responsible for the major symptoms in schizophrenia. Amphetamines, cocaine, and other drugs of abuse directly activate dopamine receptors. The resulting excitation helps account for the psychotic symptoms commonly seen when these drugs are abused.
- *Serotonin.* Another major neurotransmitter in the central nervous system is serotonin, which involves the inhibition of activity and behavior, and it also is a key neurotransmitter involved in maintaining *homeostasis* in the brain (the brain's equilibrium or "resting" state). Other areas where serotonin plays a significant role include mood regulation, control of appetite, sleep and arousal, and pain regulation. Serotonin and norepinephrine axons project into almost the same areas of the brain and are thought to have opposing actions.

- ***Other neurotransmitters.*** By virtue of its inhibitory nature, GABA makes the brain more stable by decreasing the neural transmission that prevents overexcitation. Benzodiazepines and barbiturates are two good examples that act to increase GABA. (See Chapter 7 for more about GABA.) Glycine is another inhibitory amino acid neurotransmitter that is present mostly in the spinal cord. When glycine receptors are activated, the cell becomes hyperpolarized and less likely to transmit a signal. Strychnine, a toxin that causes convulsions, acts by blocking these glycine receptors, leading to overexcitation and possibly death. Glutamate, another amino acid neurotransmitter, is definitely excitatory. More neurotransmission occurs because glutamate lowers the threshold for neural excitation. Glutamate is often found in Asian food in the form of monosodium glutamate (MSG), which excites the taste buds on the tongue (for further reading see Carlson, 2004).

CHAPTER **3**

Psychopharmacology and Pharmacokinetics

This chapter will address issues related to psychopharmacology and pharmacokinetics, how drugs work and bring about chemical and behavioral changes in the body, and how drugs are dispensed and prescribed. It will provide some basic information that is helpful in understanding the patient.

Topics to be addressed include the following:

- Routes of drug administration
- Drug absorption, distribution, and metabolism
- Other pharmacokinetic principles
- Prescription and pharmacy terms

When we talk about pharmacology and more specifically, psychopharmacology, we need to start with some basic concepts. In Chapter 2 we described *pharmacodynamics*, which may be defined as the study of how drugs affect receptor sites, send signals, and cause some neurochemical changes. On the other hand, *pharmacokinetics* refers to the administration, absorption, distribution, metabolism, and elimination of a drug inside the body.

ROUTES OF DRUG ADMINISTRATION

Medications may be introduced into the body by various methods, including orally (by mouth), subcutaneously (deep tissue injection), intramuscularly or IM (muscle injection), intradermally (dermal injection), intranasally (nasal spray), inhalational (respiratory infusion), sublingually (dissolution under the tongue), transdermally (skin absorption), and intravenously or IV (venous injection). The most common way that a drug is administered is orally. In recent times, a few medications have been delivered orally in the form of a "soltab" or orally dissolving tablet. Many psychiatric drugs are introduced into the body in this way. Examples of medications available as soltabs include olanzepine (Zyprexa Zydis), mirtazapine (Remeron Soltabs), risperidone (Risperdal M-tabs), and clonazepam (Klonopin Wafers).

In more acute settings such as a hospital or clinic, intramuscular injections are commonly used to control behavior. Long-acting intramuscular injections such as haloperidol (Haldol Decanoate), fluphenazine (Prolixin Decanoate), or risperidone (Risperdal Consta) are used for more chronically mentally ill patients.

DRUG ABSORPTION, DISTRIBUTION, AND METABOLISM

Drug Absorption

When a drug is introduced orally, the rate of absorption is determined by the form of the drug. For example, liquids are absorbed faster than capsules or tablets. Over the last few years, many slow- or extended-release forms of medications have become available. They allow for fewer doses per day and cause fewer side effects because of the slower rate of absorption. Oral administration has the slowest rate of absorption when compared to intramuscular, intravenous, and other available forms. Absorption usually occurs in the stomach and duodenum (the first segment of the small intestines). Some medications need to be given with food for better absorption (e.g., ziprasidone); some need to be given without food, which might interfere with absorption. Some gastrointestinal diseases and their treatments may also interfere with drug absorption; for example, antacids interfere with certain antibiotics.

Drug Distribution

After administration and absorption into the venous system, drugs are delivered throughout the body by the circulatory system. The liver is the first organ encountered by orally absorbed drugs. It will break down some of the drug into active metabolites that the body can more readily absorb, as well as nonactive metabolites that the body can expel. This process in the liver is known as *first-pass metabolism*. After leaving the liver, the active metabolites are delivered to their target organs via the bloodstream. The central nervous system is the target for psychotropic drugs. Other factors that affect drug absorption include protein binding, drug half-life, and lipid solubility.

PROTEIN BINDING Some drugs bind tightly to plasma proteins such as albumin in the bloodstream. This *protein-binding* phenomenon determines how much drug is available to act on the brain. Drug protein binding also hinders a drug's metabolism and excretion, which causes it to remain in the circulatory system longer.

DRUG HALF-LIFE The *half-life* of a drug is the average time required to eliminate one-half of the drug's concentration. For example, alprazolam (Xanax) has a half-life of 11 hours. Thus, the concentration of alprazolam will be reduced by about 50% after 11 hours, by 75% after 22 hours, and so on. In general, it takes approximately five half-lives for any drug to be eliminated completely from the body.

LIPID SOLUBILITY The *lipid* or fat *solubility* of a drug determines how easily it crosses a cell membrane, which is important for absorption and effectiveness at its target site. Drugs that are more lipid soluble (lipophilic) cross membranes easily and are more likely to cross over the blood–brain barrier. Some drugs do not cross this barrier and do not exert their effects on the central nervous system.

Drug Metabolism

In ways that can get very complex, drugs are metabolized or broken down primarily in the liver by the *P450* family of *enzymes*. These enzymes are important because of the potential for drug interactions when multiple drugs compete for the same pathways. The liver breaks down the drug into other forms or metabolites that are later excreted in the urine. Geriatric patients have decreased liver enzyme activity that requires drug dosages to be reduced to avoid toxicity. Other medical conditions, such as viral hepatitis or liver cirrhosis, might also decrease a drug's metabolism. A few of the psychiatric medications, such as lithium (Lithobid), are not metabolized by the liver and are excreted unchanged by the kidneys in urine. A patient with kidney dysfunction may not excrete the drug normally, and the concentration may become elevated or toxic.

OTHER PHARMACOKINETIC PRINCIPLES

Therapeutic Index and Dose

The concept of *therapeutic index* is a pharmacokinetic principle that must be addressed. When a certain drug concentration gives a desired response, it is referred to as a *therapeutic dose*. When a drug concentration causes mild or severe side effects, it is referred to as a *toxic dose*. The *therapeutic index* then is the ratio of the *toxic dose* to the *therapeutic dose*. Desirable drugs have a high therapeutic index because the risk of toxicity at therapeutic doses is minimal. On the other hand, drugs that have a low therapeutic index carry more risk because the therapeutic concentration is relatively close to its toxic level. For example, lithium is difficult to use because the toxic level is only slightly higher than the typical therapeutic level (see Chapter 6 for further details).

When determining a drug's therapeutic dose, it might be helpful to consider a dose-response curve (see Figure 3.1). When a drug is introduced into the body, a slow titration upward of the dose usually corresponds to an increasing response. This effect is true up to a certain point, at which the response of the drug levels off despite significant increases in the drug dose. As you might expect, increasing the drug's dose at this point only increases the risk of side effects and toxicity. Although most medications are introduced slowly into the body, some drugs may be initiated at high doses to obtain a certain desired response. We call this a *loading dose* of the medication. After *loading* the patient, further dosage adjustments are seldom needed because we have introduced the therapeutic dose into the body all at once.

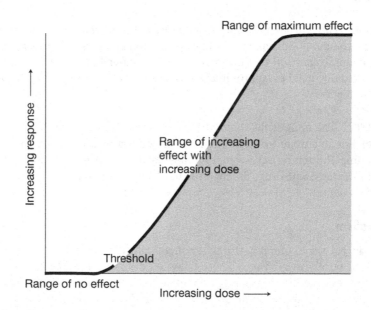

FIGURE 3.1 Dose-Response Curve

Tolerance and Withdrawal

Two important concepts that need to be defined are tolerance and withdrawal. If a patient develops *tolerance* for a drug, he or she needs greater amounts of the drug over time to produce the desired effect. *Withdrawal* from a drug is defined as a set of characteristic symptoms that emerge when a drug is abruptly discontinued after heavy and prolonged use. Depending on the substance, withdrawal symptoms can be medically dangerous and require inpatient treatment. Tolerance and withdrawal are relatively easy to understand when considering alcohol. Tolerance to alcohol develops over time, causing a person to increase the amount consumed to obtain the desired effect. Withdrawal from alcohol develops when an alcoholic suddenly stops drinking, thus throwing his or her body into a state of shock. This withdrawal causes an expected array of symptoms, such as tremors, agitation, insomnia, hallucinations, and even seizures. *Tolerance* and *withdrawal* are terms commonly used when working in the field of chemical dependency or addictions. In the *Diagnostic and Statistical Manual of Mental Disorders,* Fifth Edition (DSM-5), addiction is more specifically defined as *substance abuse and dependence.* Addiction is discussed in more detail in Chapter 13.

Discontinuation Syndrome

A related concept in the field of psychopharmacology is *discontinuation syndrome.* This syndrome is distinct from withdrawal because it is not medically dangerous, although some people claim that they are going through withdrawal. For example, patients who take paroxetine (Paxil) or venlafaxine (Effexor XR) often report that when they miss a dose or stop taking the medication, they feel malaise and other flulike symptoms.

Potentiation and Synergism

A therapist must understand the concepts of potentiation and synergism. *Potentiation* means that one drug may enhance the effect of a second drug. For example, drug X added to drug Y may potentially cause drug Y to be more sedating. One drug that potentiates another drug may increase the sedation effect only twofold or so. *Synergism* refers to the fact that one drug may enhance the effect of a second drug significantly more than expected. For example, drug X added to drug Y may increase the sedation effect of drug Y sixfold. Because of synergism, a patient should not mix alcohol with benzodiazepines.

Placebo Response

A discussion about psychopharmacology and pharmacokinetics would not be complete without mentioning the *placebo response.* During any patient interaction, a complex series of events and communications occurs in addition to any prescribed drug effects. Some patients respond regardless of the specific therapeutic intervention just because of a helper's "therapeutic interaction" with them. Many patients have shown actual chemical changes in their brain when they receive a placebo even when an actual drug is not present. The brain acts "as if" the drug were present even though it is not. When this effect is negative, the term *nocebo* is used. The power of the placebo response should never be underestimated.

PRESCRIPTION AND PHARMACY TERMS

Therapists will encounter numerous Latin abbreviations when reviewing records, dealing with prescriptions, and discussing issues with their prescribing professional (see Table 3.1). Although these abbreviations seem quite foreign at first, they become familiar with use over time.

Table 3.1	Latin Abbreviations	
Abbreviation	**Meaning**	**Latin**
a.c.	before food	ante cibum
b.i.d.	twice a day	bis in die
cap.	capsule	capula
c with bar on top (c)	with	cum
h.	hour	hora
hs	at bedtime	hora somni
p.c.	after food	post cibum
p.o.	by mouth	per os
p.r.n.	as occasion requires	pro re nata
q4h	every 4 hours	quaque 4 hora
q6h	every 6 hours	quaque 6 hora
qd*	every day	quaque 1 die
q.i.d.	four times a day	quater in die
q.o.d.*	every other day	quaque altera die
Rx	prescription	recipere
stat.	immediately	statim
tab.	tablet	tabella
t.i.d.	three times a day	ter in die

* These abbreviations are on the Joint Commission's DO NOT USE LIST as of June 2017. The Joint Commission is a not-for-profit organization that accredits healthcare organizations, with the goal of improving healthcare quality and safety. www.jointcommission.org

It is always good practice to record a patient's medication regimen in his or her chart. This information might be necessary when consulting with other professionals involved in the patient's care. Chapter 4 describes history taking and assessment techniques in further detail.

CHAPTER 4

History Taking and Assessment Techniques

This chapter reminds the clinician that good history taking is essential to a good diagnosis, and a good diagnosis is essential before any referral or recommendation for medication.

Topics to be addressed include the following:

- Obtaining patient history
- Mental status examination
- Patient questionnaires and assessment instruments
- Structuring the initial interview

OBTAINING PATIENT HISTORY

No mental health professional should underestimate the importance of good history taking. It is always important to inquire about a patient's physical and spiritual health before starting any counseling relationship, especially when a patient presents with issues of depression, anxiety, psychoticism, or other highly intrusive behavior. By getting all of the facts surrounding a presenting issue, a therapist is assured that all relevant contributing factors have been considered.

It is critical to take a thorough history from a patient and to use assessment instruments that address the issue the patient presents. Depending on the setting where the history is taken, a few simple questions on the presenting problem, nature of concern, history of the problem, relevant family history, physical findings, and history of treatment might be sufficient. If time allows, however, a more detailed assessment may be in order. The following outline provides a detailed history and assessment of the patient.

Patient's History Format
I. Identifying Information
   Name, age, identified gender, biological gender, race, grade, religion or spiritual beliefs, marital status, occupation, and diagnosis (if applicable)
II. Presenting Problem
   a. Chief complaint
   b. How the person was referred to you
   c. Dates of treatment or assessment including any medications taken
   d. How the person defines the problem
   e. Duration, intensity of concern (history of presenting problem)
   f. Any history of counseling or therapy
III. Personal/Family History
   a. Grandparents, parents, or other relatives, and the quality of the relationships
   b. Spouse, significant other, or lover, and the quality of the relationship
   c. Children, stepchildren, and the quality of the relationships
   d. Siblings and the quality of the relationships
   e. Friends and the quality of the relationships

      f. Religion or other spiritual beliefs

      g. Complete school history (elementary, high school, military, college)

      h. Present career status and beliefs about work

      i. Physical health or chronic illnesses

      j. Sexual history or concerns

      k. Any cultural or environmental issues

IV. Summary of Psychometric Information

      a. Summarize the results of any test instruments used. Be sure to mention the type of test, norms, and all scores collected.

      b. If you are interpreting test results administered by another professional, be sure to state all observations as quotes and compare with your findings.

      c. Accurately summarize reports from other sources such as family and friends. Give reasons for using this source of information.

V. Diagnostic Assessment

      a. Present a developed, logical summary of the status of the patient. This summary should include a mental status exam, the clinician's observations, and conclusions about the patient's level of functioning. Be sure to comment on the patient's intellect and maturity level.

      b. Assess the patient's coping abilities and comment on ego strengths and defense mechanisms.

      c. Give an example of the patient's insight level and his/her strengths and weaknesses.

      d. Make a complete diagnostic statement, including an appropriate DSM-5 diagnosis.

      e. Be sure not to diagnose family members or others who have not been seen or evaluated personally.

VI. Proposed Treatment Goals and Methods

      a. Be sure that all goals and methods relate to the diagnostic assessment.

      b. Define the goals and the objectives leading to them.

      c. Differentiate between short- and long-term goals.

      d. Describe the length and frequency of planned sessions.

      e. Describe the theoretical approach chosen.

      f. Describe any special issues anticipated during treatment—for example, transference, countertransference, financial limitations, or other ethical issues.

      g. List other resources or professionals to contact (psychiatrist, nurse, psychologist, clergy, social services, etc.).

      h. List referrals to make to other professionals or agencies.

      i. Set a time to reevaluate the treatment approach.

      j. Describe the complete prognosis.

VII. Other Information

      a. Describe special circumstances encountered—for example, the sudden death of a loved one.

      b. List releases needed for consults.

MENTAL STATUS EXAMINATION

It is wise to obtain a baseline measure of mental status from all patients. This information not only gives a snapshot of how the patient is doing, but it gives a general sense of the patient in several different realms, including cognitive capacity, intelligence, memory impairment, abstract reasoning, and judgment. If done properly, a good mental status exam (MSE) can help to predict a patient's behavior and provide valuable information for making a diagnosis. A full MSE should include information from the following sources:

Mental Status Information
Attitude and Behavior
• Describe appearance, including hygiene, makeup, and dress.
• Describe mannerisms: lethargic, hyperactive, echopraxia, posture, etc.
• Describe attitude toward self and others.
• Describe affect: sad, flat, labile, etc.

Stream of Mental Activity
• Describe flow of speech: tangential, rapid, spontaneous, blocked, etc.
• Describe language deviations: clang associations or echolalia.

Emotional Reactions
• Describe displays: tearful, anxious, flat. Congruent with stated mood?

Mental Trend and Thought Content
• Describe major themes of conversation: anger, regret, revenge, etc.
• Describe evidence of auditory, visual, gustatory, tactile, olfactory, or visceral hallucinations.
• Describe delusions, ideas of reference, paranoia, or grandiosity.
• Describe somatizations, suicidal or homicidal ideation: Is there a means, intent, or plan?
• Describe history of substance abuse and list current medications and prescriber.

Sensorium, Mental Grasp, and Capacity
Ask questions to determine the following:
• Oriented × 3 (person, place, and time)
• Memory: Immediate (recall of three items after five minutes); recent (events of last evening); remote (name last nine presidents). *Note:* If from another culture or country, ask patient who their last four leaders were, and you can verify the answers later.
• Calculations: Serial 7s and 3s; digits forward and backward
• General intelligence and similarities: Abstract reasoning and proverbs

General Fund of Knowledge
• Ask questions of common knowledge and current events and of items that assess past academic achievements—for example, how many stars and stripes are present in the U.S. flag and why.

Judgment and Insight
• Ask questions to assess the patient's common sense (ego strengths) and ability to live independently—for example, what to do if their home is flooded or what they would do with $10,000.

A typical narrative description for the findings of the mental status exam would be worded in the following fashion, depending on the particular questions asked of the patient and his or her level of cooperation:

Mrs. Jane Doe is a 30-year-old, African American female of average height and weight. Her hygiene and dress were appropriate for the evaluation. She was oriented X3, and while her speech appeared normal, she began to stutter when she became nervous. She denied hallucinations or other psychotic manifestations. Memory appeared intact with good immediate, recent, and remote memory. She appeared to have no educational or learning deficits. The patient appeared to have an above-average level of intelligence. She denied suicidal/homicidal ideation and chemical dependency. Judgment and insight appeared sound and within normal limits.

PATIENT QUESTIONNAIRES AND ASSESSMENT INSTRUMENTS

For therapists, including those who are not psychologists, several patient checklists and questionnaires are available that can be used for patients who present with depression and/or anxiety. These instruments are designed to be easy to use by both the clinician and the patient. While some psychometric knowledge is helpful, most of these self-report format instruments are designed to be administered by mental health professionals with at least a master's degree and some relevant clinical experience. Some assume that the clinician has special training in their use, and some may require the practitioner to be a licensed psychologist. A test's publisher may require professional credentials before selling the instrument. The following list is by no means exhaustive, but it represents some popular tools used in the field today. To learn more about them, type in the name of the test as a keyword on the Internet for publisher and research information.

Assessments for Depression
- The Beck Depression Inventory II: 21 items, easy to score
- The Hamilton Depression Inventory: available in a 17- or 21-item format; better for assessing somatic, less cognitive-related depression
- The Geriatric Depression Inventory: helpful to use with an older population
- The PHQ-9 Patient Health Questionnaire: simple 11-question instrument; available online; helps to determine if the patient is experiencing depression

Assessments for Anxiety
- The Beck Anxiety Inventory: brief, easy to score, and helpful in differentiating between generalized anxiety and panic disorder
- The State-Trait Anxiety Inventory: helpful in determining if the anxiety is one of an emotional reaction "state" versus more of a personality "trait"
- The GAD-7: 7-question instrument; helps clinician to determine if generalized anxiety disorder may be present; also available online

General Assessment of Personality Including Depression, Anxiety, and Other Manifestations
- The Minnesota Multiphasic Personality Inventory (MMPI-2): consists of 567 true/false questions over 10 clinical scales including depression, somatization, anxiety, antisocial tendencies, paranoia, mania, and psychoticism; also available in an adolescent version (MMPI-A)
- The Millon Clinical Multiaxial Inventory-IV (MCMI-IV): a shorter test with 195 items; better for assessing the presence of a personality disorder; maps well on the DSM-5
- The Personality Assessment Inventory (PAI): consists of 344 items; shorter version, called the PAS or Personality Assessment Screener, contains only 22 items and takes less than six minutes to administer

STRUCTURING THE INITIAL INTERVIEW

When a patient presents for counseling services and the therapist is aware that the patient may need medication to treat a serious affective, anxiety, or thought disorder, it is very important to gather as much information as possible. The following are information-gathering suggestions to keep in mind.

1. Document the name of the patient's primary care physician or provider (PCP) and the date of his or her last history and physical. Be sure to include any information on known diseases such as hypertension, diabetes, cancer, stroke, thyroid conditions, and so on. If the patient does not have a PCP, then he or she should be referred to one for a workup as soon as possible. Be sure to ask the physician to assess for thyroid function, glucose tolerance, and electrolyte imbalances. Typical tests would include complete blood count (CBC), thyroid function tests, a basic metabolic panel, and urine toxicology.

2. Take a complete history of any treatment for the presenting problem. This history should include the types of symptoms—that is, depression, panic, anxiety, and so on. Be sure to include all professionals the patient has seen and any medications he or she has taken. Ask the patient if the medications were helpful, effective, or intolerable. What side effects, if any, did the patient experience, and did they lead to noncompliance?

3. Prepare a complete mental status using other assessment instruments as appropriate to confirm initial impressions. It would be appropriate for the therapist to formulate some initial short-term goals for proceeding with this patient.

Good treatment starts with a good history and assessment. Taking a few extra moments with the patient to address the issues mentioned above will assure both the patient and the therapist that no stone was left unturned. Be sure to review the treatment plan with the patient to confirm that he or she is also in agreement. By knowing the patient's history, the therapist can save time later by not reexposing the patient to medication regimes that did not work or that interacted with other medications the patient was taking for a medical condition. Pleading ignorance or claiming not to be a physician is no protection from a malpractice claim. Always remember that you are treating the whole patient.

CHAPTER 5

Treatment of Unipolar Depression

In this chapter, we examine the medications and other treatment considerations for patients with unipolar depression. Depression is the most common presenting concern in all treatment settings. Assessing the nature and type of depression is key to suggesting proper medication.

Topics to be addressed include the following:

- Biological versus environmental depression
- Causes of biological depression
- Counseling and psychotherapy
- Medications for depression
- Herbal and holistic substances
- Light therapy for major depressive disorder (MDD) and seasonal affective disorders (SAD)
- Importance of exercise
- Electroconvulsive therapy (ECT) and other treatments
- Procedural steps for patient treatment
- Case vignettes

BIOLOGICAL VERSUS ENVIRONMENTAL DEPRESSION

Depression is probably the most frequently presented issue in any mental health setting. Researchers have estimated that at least 3% of the population suffers from chronic depression at any one time. More than 17% have had at least one episode in their lifetime, and another 10% reported an episode in the last 12 months (Sutherland, Sutherland, & Hoehns, 2003). It is interesting and sad that despite the recent advances in both psychotherapy and medications for depression, only 30% of those with depression seek treatment for the condition (Rakel, 1999). In addition, less than 20% of those who seek treatment take antidepressants (McIntyre, Muller, Mancini, & Silver, 2003). The lifetime prevalence of major depressive disorder (MDD) in the United States is about 16% in a given year, with about 7% of the population experiencing an episode of MDD, half of which will be moderate in severity. In patients with chronic medical illness, the annual prevalence rate for MDD is up to 25%. Risk factors are multifactorial and include genetic, medical, social, and environmental factors (Bentley, Pagalilauan, & Simpson, 2014). According to Pratt and Brody (2014), recent information indicates that depression is more prevalent among females and people ages 40 to 59. As we might expect, people living below the poverty level were nearly 2.5 times more likely to have depression than those at or above the poverty level. In addition, almost 43% of people with severe depressive symptoms reported serious difficulties in work, home, and social activities. Finally, when looking at those with severe depressive symptoms, only 35% reported having contact with a mental health professional in the past year (Pratt & Brody, 2014). Thus, there is a huge unmet medical need that we must address.

Therapists have many issues to consider when treating depression. First, they must determine the nature of the depression. Some forms of depression are biological or *endogenous*: It is believed they stem from *within* the person. This form of depression is likely to have a biological link or perhaps a family link to others who also have depression. In fact, Rakel (1999) mentions that monozygotic twins have a 65% concordance rate, and dizygotic twins have a 14% rate. According to Lohoff (2010), twin studies suggest a heritability of 40% to 50%, and family studies indicate a twofold to threefold increase in lifetime risk of developing MDD among first-degree relatives. Some forms of depression are more reactive or *exogenous* and are typically caused from forces *outside* of the body. In these cases, stress or grief may be the cause. Therapists often find that both internal and external factors play a role in many patients' depression (Barlow & Durand, 2005).

It is important for the therapist to determine the nature and source of a patient's depression. At times it may be rather clinical or endogenous in nature. Typically, major depression and the depressive phases of bipolar conditions meet these criteria, but therapists are also aware that dysthymia, cyclothymia, and grief reactions have some biological components. Further, the clinician must determine the role of other complicating factors, such as substance use, psychotic features, physical diseases, and medications that may cause depression.

CAUSES OF BIOLOGICAL DEPRESSION

For many patients presenting with depression, the cause can be related to another physical disorder that they may have. The following is a list of diseases and disorders that can cause or exacerbate depression:

Addison's disease	Diabetes mellitus	Multiple sclerosis
Alzheimer's disease	Fibromyalgia	Myocardial infarction
Anemia	Hepatitis	Pancreatitis
Asthma	HIV/AIDS	Parkinson's disease
Brain tumor	Huntington's disease	Porphyria
Cancer	Hyperthyroidism	Postpartum hormonal changes
Cardiovascular conditions	Hypothyroidism	Premenstrual dysphoric disorder
Chronic fatigue syndrome	Influenza	Rheumatoid arthritis
Chronic infections	Lupus	Stroke
Chronic pain syndrome	Malnutrition	Syphilis
Colitis	Menopause	Tuberculosis
Congestive heart failure	Mental retardation	Uremia
Cushing's disease	Metabolic abnormalities	
	Mononucleosis	

In addition to these diseases and disorders, many medications and other substances have been known to cause or worsen a patient's depression. The following is a list of these medications and substances:

- Alcohol
- Antianxiety medications: diazepam, chlordiazepoxide, alprazolam, lorazepam, clonazepam, phenobarbital

- Antihypertensive medications: reserpine, propranolol, methyldopa, guanethidine sulfate, clonidine, hydralazine, metoprolol, prazosin
- Anti-inflammatory medications: indomethacin, butazolidin, rofecoxib (withdrawn from U.S. market in 2004), celecoxib
- Antiparkinsonian medications: levodopa/carbidopa, amantadine
- Cold remedies: antihistamines, others containing alcohol
- Corticosteroids and other hormones: estrogen, progesterone, cortisone acetate, most oral contraceptives, etc.
- Drugs of abuse: marijuana, codeine, morphine, PCP, crystal methamphetamine, psychedelics, opium derivatives, synthetic pain killers
- Sedative–hypnotic medications: zolpidem, zaleplon, triazolam, flurazepam, temazepam, meprobamate

If after careful history and assessment the therapist determines that the patient's depression appears to have little or no physical cause, a treatment plan is proposed to address the concern. While it is a well-known fact that psychotherapy and counseling alone are very effective treatments for depression, psychotherapy and medication together are most efficacious (Segal, Kennedy, Cohen, & CANMAT Depression Work Group, 2000); combining the two increases response rates, with estimates of the increase ranging from 6% to 33% (Hollon et al., 2014). In cases of dysthymia (chronic-mild depression), psychotherapy alone may be attempted. If little response is noticed, an antidepressant may be added. In cases of a grief reaction with sleep disturbances, medications to improve sleep may be used without an antidepressant. Only when the grief is prolonged, severe, and accompanied by suicidal ideation should antidepressants be considered. Suicide assessment is very important to keep in mind, as up to 80% of depressed patients also have suicidal ideation (Sonawalla & Fava, 2001). Those suffering from depression are at 25 times greater risk for suicide than is the general population (American Association of Suicidology, 2014).

The following is a list of treatment options for the patient with moderate to severe depression:

- Counseling and psychotherapy
- Medication, including pharmaceuticals and herbal remedies
- Light therapy for those with seasonally influenced depression
- Exercise
- Electroconvulsive therapy (ECT) and other treatments

COUNSELING AND PSYCHOTHERAPY

Psychotherapists often underestimate the effective nature of therapy. However, psychotherapy as a medical treatment has been found to be more effective than bypass surgery, drug treatments for arthritis, and even aspirin for heart attack (Lipsey & Wilson, 1993). Further, research on the percentage of improved patients at selected sessions has demonstrated that patients typically show the greatest gains in the first 16 to 20 sessions (Howard, Kopta, Krause, & Orlinsky, 1986). While nearly every form or approach of counseling or psychotherapy is helpful, some therapists believe that solution-focused therapy or briefer forms of therapy offer quicker solutions. Still others believe that cognitive-behavioral approaches work better than other forms (Rakel, 1999). To further support this position, a recent randomized controlled trial in Finland showed the effectiveness of three treatment regimens (interpersonal psychotherapy, psychoeducational group therapy, and treatment as usual) with marked improvement over one year

(Saloheimo el al., 2016). Current guidelines from the Anxiety and Depression Association of America (2017) support the use of multiple psychotherapies over waitlists or other minimal contact treatments. Meta-analyses that compare the effectiveness of cognitive-behavioral therapy, interpersonal psychotherapy, and problem-solving therapy indicate no large differences in effectiveness between these treatments.

MEDICATIONS FOR DEPRESSION

For the most part, antidepressants can be divided into five main categories: tricyclic antidepressants (TCAs), monoamine oxidase inhibitors (MAOIs), selective serotonin reuptake inhibitors (SSRIs), serotonin-norepinephrine reuptake inhibitors (SNRIs), and atypicals or "others."

The oldest antidepressants are the TCAs. Tricyclic antidepressants have been around for more than 60 years. They prevent the reuptake of neurotransmitter substance back into the presynaptic cell. Although effective, TCAs are not "clean" medications, and, therefore, they affect many nontarget organs and systems in the body. They have troublesome anticholinergic side effects that include sedation, weight gain, difficulty urinating, dizziness, dry mouth, sexual dysfunction, orthostatic hypotension, and blurred vision. Typically, these medications are not safe for children or the elderly. Due to their toxic cardiovascular nature, TCAs pose a serious risk of overdose for patients with significant suicidal ideation.

As was mentioned in Chapter 2, a patient's depression may be caused by depletions in the neurotransmitters serotonin (5-HT), norepinephrine (NE), dopamine (D), or all three. Table 5.1 lists TCAs with their trade and generic names, typical daily doses, neurotransmitter action, and level of sedation.

Table 5.1	Tricyclic Antidepressants (TCAs)				
Trade Name	Generic Name	Typical Dose (mg/day)	Neurotransmitter 5-HT	Neurotransmitter NE	Level of Sedation
Anafranil	clomipramine	100–250	***	*	Heavy
Ascendin	amoxapine	150–400	*	***	Moderate-heavy
Elavil	amitriptyline	150–300	***	*	Heavy
Ludiomil	maprotiline	150–225	***	0	Moderate
Norpramin	desipramine	150–300	0	***	Light
Pamelor, Aventyl	nortriptyline	75–125	**	***	Moderate-heavy
Sinequan, Adapin, Silenor	doxepin	150–300	**	***	Heavy
Surmontil	trimipramine	100–300	**	**	Moderate
Tofranil	imipramine	150–300	***	**	Light-moderate
Vivactil	protriptyline	15–60	*	***	Light

* Minimal neurotransmission
** Moderate neurotransmission
*** Significant neurotransmission

The second major classification of antidepressants is known as monoamine oxidase inhibitors or MAOIs. These drugs work a bit differently than the others. They inhibit monoamine oxidase (MAO), the enzyme that breaks down neurotransmitters and renders them ineffective. MAOIs exert most of their influence in the presynaptic cell. While the side effects of MAOIs closely resemble those of TCAs, MAOIs are usually well tolerated. Patients taking MAOIs must adhere to strict dietary restrictions, as ingestion of any food containing tyramine may cause a hypertensive crisis. MAOIs have fallen out of use in the United States but are still widely used in Europe. Many prescribers use them as a last-resort drug for patients who do not respond well to other medications (see Table 5.2).

In the early 1980s, another drug was introduced with the trade name Desyrel and the generic name trazodone. This medication primarily affects serotonin but acts more as a 5-HT2 receptor antagonist. Trazodone is less likely to cause sexual side effects but may cause priapism, a condition resulting in a prolonged, painful erection in men. Overall, it has fewer side effects than older TCAs and is less of a suicidal risk, but the typical side effects of sedation and dry mouth remain. Trazodone is often used as a general sedating medication without the risk of addiction to sedative hypnotics for those who have trouble sleeping. Less expensive generic TCAs are available, making this class of medication more affordable for many patients.

In the late 1980s, a new generation of drugs was born. Selective serotonin reuptake inhibitors (SSRIs) block the reuptake of serotonin back into the presynaptic cell. This blocking action allows more serotonin to exert its influence on the postsynaptic cell. Research has found no statistical differences between the various SSRIs with relation to effectiveness, but some research maintains that escitalopram (Lexapro) and sertraline (Zoloft) may be better tolerated, and are, therefore, more likely to be continued than others (Cipriani et al., 2009; Hansen et al., 2008). Table 5.3 lists SSRIs, their trade and generic names, typical daily dose, and level of sedation.

The side effects for SSRIs are considerably less severe than those for older TCAs. Typical side effects include headache, nausea, diarrhea, dry mouth, anorexia, weight gain, restlessness, insomnia, tremor, sweating, yawning, dizziness, inhibited sexual desire, and inhibited orgasm for some (Hansen et al., 2008). As mentioned, SSRIs are "cleaner" and interact with few other medications the patient may be taking. They are considered safer medications for children, seniors, and

Table 5.2   Monoamine Oxidase Inhibitors (MAOIs)

Trade Name	Generic Name	Typical Dose (mg/day)	Neuro-transmitter 5-HT	Neuro-transmitter NE	Neuro-transmitter DA	Level of Sedation
EMSAM	selegiline transdermal system	3 mg/24 hrs–12 mg/24 hrs	**	**	**	None
Marplan	isocarboxazid	10–40	**	**	**	Light
Nardil	phenelzine	30–90	**	**	**	Light
Parnate	tranylcypromine	20–60	**	**	**	Light

* Minimal neurotransmission
** Moderate neurotransmission
*** Significant neurotransmission

Table 5.3	Selective Serotonin Reuptake Inhibitors (SSRIs) Antidepressants		
Trade Name	**Generic Name**	**Typical Dose (mg/day)**	**Level of Sedation**
Celexa	citalopram	10–60	Light
Lexapro	escitalopram	5–20	None
Luvox	fluvoxamine	50–300	Light
Paxil, Paxil CR, Pexeva	paroxetine	20–50/25–50	Moderate-heavy
Prozac, Sarafem	fluoxetine	20–80	None
Prozac Weekly	fluoxetine	90 (weekly)	None
Zoloft	sertraline	50–200	None

patients who may be at risk for a suicide overdose; however, FDA warnings suggest that 4% on drugs versus 2% on placebo of children and adolescents demonstrate an increase in suicidal thinking and behavior (see the FDA website, https://www.fda.gov/drugs/drugsafety/postmarketdrugsafetyinformationforpatientsandproviders/ucm161679.htm). Many clinicians believe that the benefits of SSRIs outweigh their risks because severely depressed children and teenagers without treatment are at serious risk of suicide. Although research has found that SSRIs and medications like them (e.g., venlafaxine) increase the risk of gastrointestinal bleeding, newer research has found that this may be to a lesser degree than once thought due to alcohol abuse among subjects (Opatrny, Delaney, & Suissa, 2008).

If serotonin levels inside the central nervous system become too elevated from using SSRIs or other medications, some patients may experience *serotonin syndrome*. Symptoms may include agitation, confusion, insomnia, flushing, fever, shivering, muscle rigidity, hyperreflexia, incoordination, diarrhea, and hypotension. Many of these symptoms can be life-threatening; therefore, any patient started on medication for the first time should be closely monitored.

In the 1990s, a new class of antidepressants were developed known as serotonin-norepinephrine reuptake inhibitors (SNRIs). Venlafaxine (Effexor/Effexor XR) is usually well tolerated and has been shown to be helpful in general depression, generalized anxiety, and postpartum depression (Cohen, 1997). It has been known to increase blood pressure at higher doses. Desvenlafaxine succinate (Pristiq) is the succinate salt of the isolated major active metabolite of venlafaxine, O-desmethylvenlafaxine. This drug was approved by the FDA in 2008. Its potential advantages over other SNRIs include a narrow dose range, requiring less adjustment and more effectiveness at lower dosing. Since the drug is mainly excreted in urine, it has minimal effect on the CYP450 pathway in the liver, and, therefore, it may be a preference for medically ill patients without renal impairment who may be taking multiple medications (Lourenco & Kennedy, 2009). Duloxetine (Cymbalta), released in 2004, is similar to venlafaxine and desvenlafaxine in that it has a dual mechanism of action. Duloxetine has the advantage of equally stimulating both serotonin and norepinephrine at all doses. Venlafaxine is more serotonergic at lower doses.

The latest SNRI is levomilnacipran (Fetzima) which was approved in 2009. It is unique among other SNRIs in that it predominantly potentiates norepinephrine over serotonin; it has more than a 15-fold higher selectivity for norepinephrine versus serotonin reuptake inhibition compared with duloxetine, desvenlafaxine, or venlafaxine (Asnis & Henderson, 2015). See Table 5.4 for more details.

Table 5.4	Serotonin-Norepinephrine Reuptake Inhibitor Antidepressants (SNRIs)					
Trade Name	Generic Name	Typical Dose (mg/day)	Neuro-transmitter 5-HT	Neuro-transmitter NE	Neuro-transmitter DA	Level of Sedation
Cymbalta	duloxetine	20–60	***	***	0	None
Effexor	venlafaxine	50–300	***	***	*?	None
Effexor XR	venlafaxine XR	75–300	***	***	*?	None
Fetzima	levomilnacipran	40–120	**	****	0	None
Pristiq	desvenlafaxine	50–400	***	***	*?	None

* Minimal neurotransmission
** Moderate neurotransmission
*** Significant neurotransmission
**** Major neurotransmission

Table 5.5	Atypical or Other Antidepressants					
Trade Name	Generic Name	Typical Dose (mg/day)	Neuro-transmitter 5-HT	Neuro-transmitter NE	Neuro-transmitter DA	Level of Sedation
Aplenzin	bupropion hydrobromide	174–522	0	**	**	None
Desyrel, Oleptro	trazodone	50–400	***	0	0	Heavy
Remeron, Remeron Soltab	mirtazapine	15–45	***	***	0	Heavy
Serzone[1]	nefazodone	100–500	***	*	0	Moderate
Trintellix	vortioxetine	5–20	***	0	0	None
Viibryd	vilazodone	20–40	***	0	0	None
Wellbutrin	bupropion	75–450	0	**	**	None
Wellbutrin SR	bupropion SR	100–400	0	**	**	None
Wellbutrin XL	bupropion XL	150–450	0	**	**	None

[1] Serzone is no longer available by prescription; the generic, nefazodone, is available by prescription.
* Minimal neurotransmission
** Moderate neurotransmission
*** Significant neurotransmission

In the last few years, atypical or other antidepressant medications have been introduced. These medications offer many possibilities as noted in Table 5.5. Atypical antidepressants have side effects similar to SSRIs, but they have less possibility of sexual dysfunction. Mirtazapine (Remeron) is helpful in restoring normal sleep patterns. It has also been found to increase appetite, which is an undesirable side effect for overweight, depressed patients. However, because of this side effect, mirtazapine may work wonders in depressed HIV or cancer patients who are having trouble with weight loss. Like mirtazapine, nefazodone (Serzone) may help restore sleep patterns and cause sedation for many. Unfortunately, the medication has an FDA "black-box" warning due to its increased risk of liver failure and must be used only with caution, especially for patients taking other medications that also use the CYP450 3A4 pathway for drug elimination in the liver. Patients who begin nefazodone therapy should have a baseline liver function test and periodic tests for at least the first six months (Stewart, 2002). Bupropion (Wellbutrin) is well tolerated but is rather uplifting and agitating for some. While bupropion has not been associated with sexual dysfunction, it is not appropriate for patients with seizure or eating disorders, as it lowers the seizure threshold and reduces appetite. Vilazodone (Viibryd) was approved in 2011 for MDD and is both a serotonin transport inhibitor and a 5-HT1A receptor partial agonist (Caraci, Leggio, Salomone, & Drago, 2017). It has been referred to as a serotonin partial agonist-reuptake inhibitor (SPARI) (Wang et al., 2016). Finally, Trintellix (vortioxetine) was approved in 2013 for MDD. The mechanism of action of Trintellix is selective blockade of serotonin reuptake (by inhibiting the serotonin transporter [SERT]) and direct modulation of 5-HT receptors activity (such as 5-HT3, 5-HT7, 5-HT1D, and 5-HT1B). Trintellix is considered an SSRI and a serotonin modulator given the other effects as already noted (Sowa-Kucma et al., 2017).

To be comprehensive, lithium must be mentioned as a possible treatment option for unipolar depression, as well as for bipolar depression. This strategy is usually reserved for more difficult and treatment-resistant cases. Lithium will be explored further in Chapter 6.

HERBAL AND HOLISTIC SUBSTANCES

St. John's wort is a plant that is said to have medicinal properties. Research, primarily conducted in Europe, claims that St. John's wort helps to control mild to moderate levels of depression with virtually no side effects (Bloomfield, Nordfors, & McWilliams, 1996). Most practicing clinicians believe that few patients are helped by St. John's wort, and they are now learning that it may interfere with or react to other medications that patients may be taking. For example, St. John's wort potentiates blood thinners such as warfarin (Coumadin) and lessens the effectiveness of other heart medications such as digoxin (Lanoxin). It may also interfere with protease inhibitors taken by HIV/AIDS patients. The active ingredient in St. John's wort is *hypericin*. The Latin name of the plant is *hypericum perforatum*. Patients who are allergic to plant derivatives should not take St. John's wort because they might break out in a rash or become seriously photophobic to it and experience severe burn when exposed to the sun. Patients who take hypericum perforatum should take it in its liquid form, which ensures that they get a true dose. Health food stores sell brands that may contain more inactive plant parts and less hypericum. St. John's wort should not be taken with other antidepressants because it may potentiate their effects and cause serotonin syndrome. Recent information indicates that St. John's wort demonstrates comparable response and remission rates, and a significantly lower discontinuation rate compared to SSRIs, which are first-line drugs recommended for depression in most countries worldwide (Ng, Venkatanarayanan, & Ho, 2017).

Ginkgo biloba is a tree of Chinese origin. An extract from it is said to relieve mild depression and increase memory and concentration. While 60 mg/day of ginkgo biloba is typical for depression and mild memory concerns, as much as 240 mg/day has been used with Alzheimer's patients (Trebatická1 & Duracková, 2015). Since it is said to have blood-thinning properties, ginkgo biloba should be used with caution by those taking blood-thinning medications. In our experience, it has not been as effective as antidepressants in the treatment of moderate to severe depression.

The hormone *dehydroepiandrosterone* or *DHEA* is normally secreted by the adrenal gland and is a precursor to testosterone and estrogen. Typically, adolescents have high levels of this substance, but the levels decrease with age. Some clinicians believe that when DHEA is taken orally (90–450 mg daily), it reduces mild to moderate depression, causes weight loss, increases large muscle mass, and may increase sexual appetite. While these claims have yet to be fully proven, many practicing endocrinologists believe DHEA may increase the risk of certain types of cancer. Side effects are usually mild but may include oily skin, acne, irritability, and even psychosis (Qureshi & Al-Bedah, 2013).

*S-adenosyl-*L-*methionine* (SAM-e) is a substance that is endogenous to the body. It is essential to many biological processes, such as cell methylation. The body converts SAM-e into the amino acid homocysteine, which accumulates and can cause depression, joint problems, and cancer. Homocysteine can be converted back into SAM-e by utilizing vitamins B_6, B_{12}, and folic acid. Research conducted in Italy has shown that depressed patients have much lower levels of SAM-e than nondepressed patients. Patients with poor diet typically make less SAM-e. It is now available as a synthesized substance and has been shown to be as effective at 1600 mg daily as many prescription antidepressants for relieving depression. It is available as a prescription in many European countries. SAM-e may also be helpful in relieving joint pain and for cleansing the liver of other toxins. Researchers believe that SAM-e may increase the synthesis of serotonin and dopamine and aid chemical communication between cells by potentiating the postsynaptic membrane (Martínez-Cengotitabengoa & González-Pinto, 2017).

Animal research has also demonstrated that zinc and magnesium may possess antidepressant properties and may serve as valuable agents in enhancing the activity of conventional antidepressants (Szewczyk et al., 2008). Other substances have been studied, including *Rhodiola rosea*, saffron, lavender, other herbs, omega-3 fatty acids, and Ayurvedic medicines with mixed results (Qureshi & Al-Bedah, 2013).

In addition to the substances mentioned, research into the use of ketamine demonstrates that it may reduce depressive symptoms, and especially reduce suicidal ideation, but the potential for abuse, the potential cardiovascular and respiratory issues, and the cost of administration still warrant further research and investigation to determine if this will prove to be a viable option for treatment (Sanacora et al., 2017). NAC or N-acetylcysteine, an antioxidant that is often used in the treatment of acetaminophen overdose and pulmonary conditions, may prove to be helpful in the treatment of depression, especially bipolar depression at 2,400 mg daily. Side effects are minimal, but results of research suggest it is worth considering along with more conventional medications (Berk et al., 2008; Muskin, Gerbard, & Brown, 2013).

LIGHT THERAPY FOR MAJOR DEPRESSIVE DISORDER (MDD) AND SEASONAL AFFECTIVE DISORDER (SAD)

Antidepressants have been shown to be helpful for patients with MDD and seasonal affective disorder; however, the use of light boxes is also effective. Therapists who treat patients living in colder, darker climates and suffering from seasonal depression might consider suggesting the use of a light box first unless the patient's depression worsens and he or she becomes suicidal. Several commercially produced lamps or boxes are available for $50 to $300. The light source should produce at least 10,000 lux of full-spectrum light. Patients need to be directly exposed to the light for 30 to 60 minutes per day and sit approximately 10 to 12 inches from most light sources. Bulbs sold in hardware stores for use in overhead fixtures and in doorways may be esthetically pleasing, but they offer little in the form of treatment. Most good-quality lamps can be found by searching the Internet under *seasonal affective disorders* or *full-spectrum lamps*. In some cases, a letter from a physician or psychologist is required for the patient to purchase such lamps. In a randomized controlled trial, Lam et al. (2016) demonstrated that bright-light treatment, both as monotherapy and in combination with fluoxetine, was efficacious and well tolerated in the treatment of adults with nonseasonal MDD.

IMPORTANCE OF EXERCISE

Therapists should always encourage depressed patients to exercise. Not only does exercise lead to weight loss and increased levels of motivation, but it also helps to release important endorphins and neuromodulators such as phenylethylamine (PEA). The presence of PEA is associated with increased levels of endorphins and improvement in motivation, energy, and mood. A meta-analysis of the literature by Josefsson, Lindwall, and Archer (2014) showed a significant and large overall effect favoring exercise interventions. Exercise may be recommended for people with mild and moderate depression who are willing, motivated, and physically healthy enough to engage in such a program.

ELECTROCONVULSIVE THERAPY (ECT) AND OTHER TREATMENTS

In some cases, patients with severe depression do not respond to antidepressants. If their depression worsens and includes suicidal ideation, they may be referred for ECT. Electroconvulsive therapy is given when the patient is anesthetized and paralyzed. Electrodes are placed on the scalp, usually on the nonspeech-dominant hemisphere to avoid later damage to verbal memories. Electricity is then administered, resulting in a seizure. No movement is noted because the patient is paralyzed or immobilized. Most patients receive three sessions per week for up to four weeks, or until improvement is noted. While excessive use of ECT may cause brain damage and memory loss, some researchers have noted that naloxone (Narcan), a drug that blocks opioid receptors, may reduce some of the adverse cognitive side effects of ECT (Prudic, Fitzsimons, Nobler, & Sackeim, 1999). Some clinicians, especially those who treat elderly and medically ill patients, believe that the risks associated with ECT are equivalent or even preferable to those associated with many medications used to treat depression (Kelly & Zisselman, 2000).

For patients who may not be good candidates for ECT, new research into the use of repetitive transcranial magnetic stimulation or rTMS to the prefrontal cortex, stimulation of the vagus nerve, and stimulation of other areas of the brain through deep brain stimulation may offer some relief (Klein et al., 1999; Triggs et al., 1999). In addition, a meta-analysis and systematic review of ECT and rTMS by Chen, Zhao, Liu, Fan, and Xie (2017) showed that ECT was the most efficacious treatment for MDD but not well tolerated, whereas rTMS was the best tolerated. Bilateral rTMS appears to have the most favorable balance between efficacy and acceptability.

PROCEDURAL STEPS FOR PATIENT TREATMENT

When a decision is made to use medication to treat a patient's depression, the therapist should follow a *treatment protocol* or procedural steps to decide on the appropriate medications and how to use them.

Step 1   Most prescribing professionals start with the easier medications first. These include the SSRIs such as fluoxetine (Prozac), sertraline (Zoloft), escitalopram (Lexapro), and so on. These medications have fewer side effects and interact with fewer other medications. In many cases, the patient is started on a low dose and titrated up. The patient must end up on a therapeutic dose of the medication to truly determine if the medication is helpful. Research suggests that too many patients are maintained on too small a dose of antidepressants, which are no better than no dose at all (Leon et al., 2003). (This is a common problem when primary care physicians write prescriptions.) If the patient has a satisfactory response and all symptoms appear to remit, the therapist should continue with psychotherapy and not increase the medication. The clinician may need to wait at least four to five weeks to determine the level of response.

Step 2   In some cases the patient has only a partial response to SSRIs, even when the dose is increased to maximum dose. Since SSRIs affect only the neurotransmitter serotonin, the patient's depression may be related to norepinephrine and/or dopamine. In such cases, additional medications aimed at the other neurotrans-mitters might need to be added or substituted. It is not unusual for such patients to be taking an SSRI like fluoxetine or an SNRI like venlafaxine (Effexor) with bupropion (Wellbutrin). Polypharmacy is more complicated and should not be attempted by the patient's primary care physician. In addition, antidepressants can be augmented or boosted by adding a low dose of lithium, or by adding a stimulant such as methylphenidate (Ritalin). Buspirone (Buspar), a nonbenzodi-azepine anxiety medication with antidepressant qualities, and folic acid may also boost the antidepressant response.

Step 3   If the patient appears to have psychotic features in addition to his or her depression, an appropriate neuroleptic or antipsychotic medication might need to be added to the regimen. In rare cases, the patient may also have racing thoughts that interfere with his or her ability to relax. In these cases, neuroleptics may also be added to calm the thoughts and allow the patient to sleep better (Baune, 2008; Nelson, Pikalov, & Ber-man, 2008). Refer to Chapter 8 for further information on these medications.

Step 4   If the therapist and the prescriber have tried several drugs with no response, they should check with the patient to determine if he or she is using alcohol or other substances, taking the medication as directed, not taking the medication at all, and/or taking an unreported dietary supplement. Adherence to the medication regimen is crucial to achieve the desired outcome.

Step 5   The therapist should keep in mind that certain medications are contraindicated for certain types of patients. For patients with poor appetite or eating disorders, do not use bupropion as it may decrease appetite. For overweight patients, use mirtazapine (Remeron) and TCAs with caution, as they have been shown to cause an increase in weight and appetite. Patients with a history of seizure should not take bupropion because it lowers the seizure threshold. Nefazodone (Serzone) must be used with extra caution because it may cause liver failure in some patients. It is important to remember that MAOIs do not mix with other antidepressants and can cause a hypertensive crisis. It is imperative to wait at least two weeks after using an MAOI before starting another antidepressant because of potential drug interactions; the prescriber must wait two weeks after stopping another medication before trying MAOIs. There is one exception: The prescriber should wait five weeks after dis-continuing fluoxetine before MAOIs are used. This is called the "washout period."

Effective therapy includes *patient education*. As mentioned, patients with dysthymia or minor depression typically are not placed on medication unless they are experiencing sleep difficulties, or the depression is seriously affecting their ability to function, which is true for patients who are experiencing serious complications related to grief. For patients who are suffering from major depressive episodes and who are found to be good candidates for pharmacology, the therapist should inform them of the following five facts where appropriate:

1. Antidepressant medications take time to work. Typically a patient waits between one and four weeks before an antidepressant begins to work. Advise the patient to be patient! Some medications, like venlafaxine and desvenlafaxine (Effexor/Pristiq) may begin to work within a couple of days, but this is the exception, not the rule.

2. Inform the patient about the types of side effects to expect from the medication he or she is taking. It is easy to remember the major side effects with antidepressants, as they all start with the letter S. The side effects include sedation, seizure, sexual symptoms, and stomach-related symptoms. In most cases, these side effects are minimal, and most of them disappear within a few days. Try not to spend too much time talking about side effects because the patient may begin to fear the medication and refuse to take it. The following is a list of typical side effects and how best to resolve them.

- *Dry mouth:* Increase water consumption, chew gum, and use hard candy (avoid TCAs).
- *Inability to reach orgasm:* Reduce dose of SSRI; switch to bupropion (Wellbutrin); add low-dose bupropion, mirtazapine (Remeron), buspirone (Buspar), nefazodone (Serzone), or cyproheptadine; also, consider switching to duloxetine (Cymbalta).
- *Forgetfulness:* Add bupropion, ginkgo biloba, or stimulant.
- *Insomnia:* Check for serotonin syndrome; add sedative-hypnotic, trazodone or nefazodone.
- *Sedation:* Avoid TCAs, paroxetine (Paxil), and nefazodone; use fluoxetine (Prozac), venlafaxine, or bupropion.
- *Weight gain:* Avoid TCAs or mirtazapine; consider bupropion or other SSRIs.
- *Stomach upset:* Take with food, avoid SSRIs if GI upset is severe.
- *Headache:* Treat with acetaminophen (Tylenol) or aspirin if severe.
- *Hand tremors:* Reduce dose, add low-dose benzodiazepine.

3. Remind the patient that he or she should never stop the medications abruptly. This may cause the patient to experience a type of withdrawal known as discontinuation syndrome, which is accompanied by severe flulike symptoms. If the patient is concerned about the medications, he or she needs to discuss the problem with the therapist and the prescribing professional. If a decision is made to stop a medication, it should be done gradually and under medical supervision. Watch for an increase in depression or suicidal ideation.

4. Pregnant patients should probably not take antidepressants (or any other medication) if they can help it. The clinician should consider antidepressant only if the patient is severely depressed and cannot function without them. Typically, antidepressants are most dangerous in the first trimester. Teratogenicity data and practice experience have indicated that SSRIs and bupropion are generally safer than other antidepressants. Lithium and antipsychotic medication should be avoided or used only under strict medical supervision. Breastfeeding mothers should consult their physician before they proceed (Howland, 2009). Medical decision making is often complex and seldom free of risks. Obviously, as providers we cannot guarantee that fetal exposure to antidepressants is totally free of risk, yet this is true for any medicine taken in pregnancy. However, to date, perinatal psychiatry has collected enough evidence to suggest that, if the clinical picture warrants it, the use of many antidepressants, especially the SSRIs, is favorable compared to exposing mother and child to untreated depressive illness (Muzik & Hamilton, 2016). Furthermore, breastfeeding mothers should consult their physician before they proceed (Howland, 2009).

5. Typically, antidepressants relieve symptoms of depression and associated anxiety. Many patients today are concerned about taking drugs and resist the therapist's recommendations. When working with a severely depressed patient for whom psychotherapy alone has not helped, the therapist must help the patient to see that medication may be a very effective part of treatment. The therapist may find it helpful to use the analogy of prescribing vitamins for the person who is malnourished. Antidepressants allow the brain and neurotransmitters to work better, leading to improved emotional functioning.

CASE VIGNETTES

Case 1

CLINICAL HISTORY

Justin is a 22-year-old Hispanic male who works full-time in an auto parts warehouse and attends community college part-time in the evening. He recently sought counseling for depression at the urging of his new girlfriend. He claims that he has always had a problem with depression, even as a youngster, but attributed it to the chaotic household he grew up in. His parents divorced when he was very young due in part to his dad's heavy drinking. Justin claims he does not remember his father very much. His mother told him his father moved back to Guatemala when Justin was just three years old. Justin has one older sister, who is a nurse. While she often looks and acts as if she is depressed, she claims she is not, nor has she sought treatment of any kind. Justin's mother, however, has been placed on antidepressants by her PCP at various times.

Justin admits that he used alcohol in his teen years to self-medicate his depression. His alcohol use became problematic in the last two years, and this led to a breakup with his fiancée Marta four months ago. He decided shortly after that to refrain from using alcohol when he met his current girlfriend, Elena, at a work-related event. He has noticed that his depressive symptoms worsened when he didn't have something to "soothe it." He is most bothered by poor sleeping and difficulty concentrating at work. While he is very happy about meeting Elena, his depression has escalated recently, leading to thoughts of suicide on at least two occasions.

POSTCASE DISCUSSION AND DIAGNOSIS

Justin is suffering with Major Depressive Disorder that appears to be rather Chronic and Severe in nature (F33.2). He reports problems with poor sleeping—namely, terminal insomnia. He further presents with concentration concerns, feelings of sadness, and suicidal ideation. There also appears to be positive family history for mood disorders. Although he reports past issues with alcohol, there appears to be no reason for detox at this time. Since gaining sobriety, he has noticed an increase in depressive symptoms, indicating a need to treat depression as a causal factor for his drinking. A complete physical was conducted with his PCP and all blood work and other findings were within normal limits.

PSYCHOPHARMACOLOGICAL TREATMENT

Justin was started on a conservative starting dose of 5 mg daily of Lexapro by his family doctor. He was watched closely by his physician and therapist for any signs of mood changes or an increase in suicidal thinking. Within two weeks he reported an improvement in both mood and outlook. Elena also noticed a big change, but Justin reported that his early morning awakening, although better, has not fully improved. His dose was increased to 10 mg daily. Within a month, he reported that he was able to sleep through the night without awakening. At one visit with his therapist, Justin complained that although he was happy with his overall level of improvement, he had noticed that it was much more difficult to have an orgasm when he was with Elena. Upon consultation with his doctor, a low dose of bupropion was added each day. Three weeks later, Justin reported that he was doing well, with no problems "in the sex department."

Case 2

CLINICAL HISTORY

Helen is a 45-year-old African American female who separated two months ago from her husband of 25 years after he had an extramarital affair. In addition to running the household and managing 18-year-old fraternal twins, she works part-time at a local dry cleaning business. Helen started experiencing increased anxiety, lack of ability to fall asleep, and daytime tiredness over the last three months. The symptoms have progressed over the last four weeks to increasing sadness, inappropriate guilt, poor appetite, and decreased energy levels. Helen is struggling to maintain her usual activities and is starting to feel that "life is not worth living," but she has not had any suicide ideation per se. Helen has no personal or family history of psychiatric illness. She uses alcohol once or twice a month but not to excess. Helen's medical history is significant for lower-extremity neuropathy of unknown origin.

POSTCASE DISCUSSION AND DIAGNOSIS

Helen is suffering with Major Depressive Disorder of Moderate Severity (F32.1) that appears to be triggered by her marital stress and separation. In addition to her other depressive symptoms (noted above), she is experiencing passive suicide ideation but is able to contract for her safety. A complete physical was conducted with her PCP, and all blood work and other findings were within normal limits. Helen agreed to initiate psychotherapy immediately to help manage her distress and figure out whether she wanted to continue the relationship with her husband or not.

PSYCHOPHARMACOLOGICAL TREATMENT

Helen mentioned that she heard about Cymbalta and wondered if it would help her depression and neuropathy. Due to her neuropathy, Helen was treated by her PCP with Cymbalta 30 mg daily for one week, followed by 60 mg daily thereafter. She continued her weekly psychotherapy, which focused on managing her depression, improving her functioning, looking at her self-esteem, and considering her long-term goals. Over the next two weeks, her passive suicide ideation resolved and her mood started to improve. After four weeks of treatment with Cymbalta, the depression symptoms resolved and Helen did not have any significant side effects. She continued her pharmacological and psychotherapeutic treatment over the next six months and was able to move on with her life, relationship, and getting her family back together again.

CHAPTER **6**

Treatment of Bipolar Disorder

This chapter reviews the types and causes of bipolar illness, as well as current information on treatment options for this population. Polypharmacy and family education will also be discussed.

Topics to be addressed include the following:

- Prevalence and types of bipolar illness
- Causes of bipolar disorder
- Counseling and psychotherapy
- Medications for bipolar disorder
- Electroconvulsive therapy (ECT)
- Treatment resistance and protocol
- Patient and family education
- Case vignettes

PREVALENCE AND TYPES OF BIPOLAR ILLNESS

Bipolar illness is a disorder of mood regulation characterized by cycling between extreme highs or *mania* and extreme lows or *depression*. Although effective treatments are available, three out of four patients fail on maintenance treatment within five years (Moller & Nasrallah, 2003). The lifetime prevalence of *bipolar disorder* is approximately 1% of the general population when a strict DSM-5 definition is used (Malhi, Mitchell, & Salim, 2003; Merikangas et al., 2007; Vieta et al., 2018). When the broader term *bipolar spectrum disorders* is used, Grunze, Schlosser, and Walden (2000) report that the lifetime prevalence increases from 3% to 6%. Bipolar disorder usually begins with an index depressive episode about 50% of the time. The average age of onset of the first depressive episode is 18.7 years, and the average age of onset of the first manic episode is 24.5 years. Unfortunately, obtaining the correct bipolar diagnosis is typically delayed until the patient reaches age 33.5 years. Bipolar disorders are the 17th-leading cause of global burden of disease (Vieta et al., 2018).

In contrast to unipolar depression, bipolar disorder is thought to originate endogenously but may be triggered by exogenous or environmental stimuli. Monozygotic twins have a 40% to 45% concordance rate, whereas dizygotic twins or first-degree relatives have only a 5% to 9% chance of inheriting the illness (Barnett & Smoller, 2009; Craddock & Jones, 1999). The mainstay of treatment is, therefore, derived from a biological perspective—that is, medications. Psychosocial stressors may trigger the patient to *cycle* or may cause a more severe cycle. Although some environmental factors influence the disorder, it is commonly known that a genetic predisposition or vulnerability is necessary.

There are many different types of bipolar spectrum disorders. Bipolar Disorder Type I is a well-defined symptom cluster that may present as manic features, depressive features, or mixed mood states. Bipolar Disorder Type II is similar but limited to hypomanic states. In addition, cyclothymia is considered to be the milder form of the classic disease that is characterized by cycles between hypomania and low-level depression. Another useful term to know is *rapid cycling*, which is defined as the occurrence of four or more episodes of mania or depression in a 12-month period. The most common cause of rapid cycling is the uncritical use of antidepressant medications (Grunze et al., 2000).

When compared to unipolar depression, bipolar depression is associated with higher rates of suicide and psychosis. Primarily during the depressive cycle, approximately 15% to 20% of bipolar patients complete suicide (Goodwin, 2002; Vieta et al., 2018). According to Bowden (2001), psychotic symptoms occur in the context of Bipolar Disorder Type I about 50% to 90% of the time. Comorbidity commonly occurs in bipolar patients, with anxiety disorders and substance abuse problems being the most prevalent. Comorbidity is covered more extensively in Chapter 14.

CAUSES OF BIPOLAR DISORDER

When evaluating a bipolar patient, the psychiatric symptoms are only one component of a larger, dynamic, functioning person. While an exact cause of bipolar conditions is not well understood, it is theorized that the cause may be related to neurotransmitter dysregulation or possibly abnormal permeability of the postsynaptic membrane. The clinician needs to exclude medical issues that might cause or contribute to a patient's cycling mood disorder. The following is a list of diseases and disorders that have been associated with or are known to exacerbate mania:

Brain tumors	Metastatic cancer
Carcinoid syndrome	Multiple sclerosis
CNS syphilis	Parkinson's disease
CNS trauma	Pellagra (deficiency of nicotinic acid)
Delirium (multiple etiologies)	Postpartum metabolic changes
Encephalitis (herpes and other viruses)	Renal failure and hemodialysis
Huntington's disease	Stroke
Influenza	Temporal lobe epilepsy
Hyperthyroidism	Vitamin B_{12} deficiency
Metabolic changes (electrolyte abnormalities)	Wilson's disease

Furthermore, many medications and other substances have been known to cause or worsen a patient's mania. These substances are often overlooked when a patient presents to medical providers. The following is a list of these medications and substances:

Antidepressants (pharmaceuticals and herbals)
Antihypertensive medications: captopril, hydralazine
Baclofen

Bromides

Bromocryptine

Cimetidine

Corticosteroids and other hormones: prednisone, testosterone

Cyclosporine

Disulfiram

Drugs of abuse: amphetamines, cocaine, ephedra, hallucinogens, PCP

Isoniazid

Levodopa

Opiates and opioids

Procarbazine

Procyclidine

Psychostimulants: dextroamphetamine, methylphenidate

Yohimbine

COUNSELING AND PSYCHOTHERAPY

After a thorough clinical assessment and medical evaluation, the therapist prepares an appropriate treatment plan for the patient. In addition to pharmacotherapy and possible hospitalization, the patient will most likely need psychotherapy when he or she has stabilized on medications. Remember that mild forms of unipolar depression may be treated with psychotherapy alone. However, pharmacotherapy is the cornerstone of treatment, with psychotherapy playing a lesser role with bipolar mood disorder. Suicide assessment is still an important part of any evaluation. Bipolar patients have a higher risk of suicide because of their erratic and chaotic mood swings and behaviors.

One of the first steps a counselor or psychotherapist should address is basic family education regarding the illness. Most families have little understanding of the symptoms, behavioral management, causes, or treatments needed for the identified patient. Many educational resources are available through organizations such as the National Institute of Mental Health (NIMH), National Alliance on Mental Illness (NAMI), or Depression and Bipolar Support Alliance (formerly National Depressive and Manic Depressive Association). Family therapy should focus on establishing a safe environment, constructive communication, and solving problems together. The patient might benefit from individual psychotherapy by better understanding the illness, accepting the diagnosis, and learning to manage the chronic nature of the disorder. Psychotherapists know that various forms of psychotherapy may be appropriate, including psychodynamic, cognitive-behavioral, or solution focused.

MEDICATIONS FOR BIPOLAR DISORDER

Psychopharmacology for bipolar disorder involves a class of medications known as *mood stabilizers*. The list of mood stabilizers consists of three broad categories: lithium, anticonvulsants, and atypical antipsychotics. The choice of treatment options depends on whether the patient is in the manic, depressed, or mixed phase of the illness. These options will be discussed in more detail in the following sections.

Lithium

Lithium has been the gold standard for treating bipolar disorder since the early 1970s. It is indicated for treatment of acute mania and as maintenance therapy to prevent subsequent cycling. Furthermore, both manic and depressive phases of the bipolar cycle may be treated with lithium. Research by Sondergard, Lopez, Andersen, and Kessing (2008) has demonstrated that lithium may be superior to many other bipolar medications in the prevention of suicide. Although lithium's mechanism of action is still unknown, Schatzberg, Cole, and DeBattista (1997) found that there are multiple biochemical effects, including the following:

- Increases synthesis of serotonin
- Enhances release of serotonin
- Increases rate of synthesis/excretion of norepinephrine in depressed patients
- Decreases rate of synthesis/excretion of norepinephrine in manic patients
- Blocks postsynaptic dopamine receptors' supersensitivity
- Has direct or indirect effect on G proteins that mediates the balance of neurotransmitters
- Inhibits enzymes in the phosphoinositide (PI) second-messenger system that may affect receptor activity of many neurotransmitters

Since lithium acts as a salt in the body, lithium concentration is determined by the patient's body fluid status. Lithium is not metabolized in the liver and is excreted unchanged by the kidneys. Thus, when dehydration occurs, the kidneys may reabsorb more lithium, which might lead to toxicity. Because of the pharmacokinetics of lithium, the therapeutic level is close to the toxic level; thus, this medication has a low *therapeutic index* (refer to Chapter 3 for more explanation).

The most common side effects of lithium include increased thirst, increased urination, rash, tremor, dry mouth, increased appetite with weight gain, nausea, bloating, diarrhea, edema, and thyroid dysfunction. The side effects of the drug may be diminished by using divided doses throughout the day rather than one daily dose. In rare cases, lithium toxicity may cause renal insufficiency or failure. Although this effect sounds terrible, lithium may be used with success when it is monitored appropriately by the prescribing professional.

Lithium is usually started at 300 mg/day and increased to a therapeutic dose of 600 to 1,200 mg/day (see Table 6.1). Laboratory testing is usually done before initiating therapy and subsequently at regular intervals (about every six months) when the patient is stable. Therapeutic levels of lithium are usually in the range of 0.7 to 0.9 mEq/L, and the toxic range is typically 1.5 mEq/L or above.

Signs of lithium toxicity include ataxia, poor coordination, slurred speech, poor attention span, severe tremors, severe nausea/vomiting, lethargy, arrhythmias, hypotension, seizure, coma, and death. Lithium use in pregnancy has been contraindicated because of an association with congenital heart malformation. In the past, the risk was rated as only moderate (Viguera, Cohen, Baldessarini, & Nonacs, 2002). However, more recently published guidelines report a disproportionate-to-low or no risk of teratogenesis with lithium treatment, and the British Association of Psychopharmacology identified the risk of cardiac malformation at 0.05% to 0.1% in the first trimester, correcting previously reported relative risks of teratogenicity (e.g., Ebstein's anomaly) as being 10 to 20 times greater than the risk in general population (Malhi, Gessler, & Outhred, 2017).

Table 6.1	Mood Stabilizers		
Trade Name	**Generic Name**	**Typical Dose (mg/day)**	**Proposed Mechanism of Action**
Abilify, Abilify Discmelt, Abilify MyCite	aripiprazole	15–30	Partial agonism at dopamine type 2 and serotonin type 1A, serotonin type 2A antagonism
Abilify Maintena	aripiprazole	300 mg–400 mg/month	Partial agonism at dopamine type 2 and serotonin type 1A, serotonin type 2A antagonism
Clozaril, Fazaclo	clozapine	300–600	Low dopamine type 2 antagonism, high dopamine type 1 and type 4 antagonism, high serotonin type 2 antagonism
Depakote, Depakote ER, Depakene, Stavzor	valproate or valproic acid	500–2,000	Inhibition of sodium and/or calcium channels, increases GABA, releases glutamate
Fanapt	iloperidone	12–24	Dopamine type 2 and serotonin type 2 antagonism
Gabitril	tiagabine	8–16	Increases GABA
Geodon	ziprasidone	80–160	Dopamine type 2 and serotonin type 2 antagonism
Invega, Invega Sustenna	paliperidone	6–12	Dopamine type 2 and serotonin type 2 antagonism
Klonopin, Klonopin Wafer	clonazepam	2–6	Increases GABA
Lamictal, Lamictal XR, Lamictal ODT, Lamictal CD	lamotrigine	200–400	Inhibition of sodium channels, presynaptic modulation of glutamate release
Latuda	lurasidone	20–120	Dopamine type 2 and serotonin type 2 antagonism
Lithobid, Eskalith CR	lithium carbonate or lithium citrate	600–1,200	Enhances serotonin, increases or decreases norepinephrine, blocks dopamine receptors' supersensitivity, alters second messengers
Neurontin, Gabarone	gabapentin	300–3,600	Enhances GABA
Risperdal, Risperdal M-tab, Risperdal Consta	risperidone	2–6	Dopamine type 2 and serotonin type 2 antagonism
Saphris	asenapine	10–20	Dopamine type 2 and serotonin type 2 antagonism
Seroquel, Seroquel XR	quetiapine	400–600	Dopamine type 2 and serotonin type 2 antagonism
Symbyax	olanzapine/ fluoxetine	3/25–12/50	Inhibition of serotonin reuptake/dopamine type 2 and serotonin type 2 antagonism

Trade Name	Generic Name	Typical Dose (mg/day)	Proposed Mechanism of Action
Tegretol, Tegretol XR, Carbatrol, Equetro	carbamazepine	600–1,200	Inhibition of sodium channels
Trileptal	oxcarbazepine	600–1,200	Inhibition of sodium channels, modulation of calcium channels
Topamax	topiramate	100–500	Increases GABA, blocks glutamate receptors
Verelan PM, Covera-HS, Ispotin SR, Calan SR	verapamil	200–400	Calcium channel blocker
Vraylar	cariprazine	3–6	Partial agonism at dopamine type 2 and serotonin type 1A, serotonin type 2A antagonism
Zonegran	zonisamide	200–400	Inhibition of sodium and/or calcium channels, facilitates dopaminergic and serotonergic neurotransmission
Zyprexa, Zyprexa Zydis, Zyprexa Relprevv	olanzapine	10–30	Dopamine type 2 and serotonin type 2 antagonism

Anticonvulsants

In addition to lithium, there is another class of mood stabilizers known as anticonvulsants or antiseizure medications. Researchers believe that some of the anticonvulsants increase the concentration of GABA, the inhibitory neurotransmitter. By increasing inhibition, electrical activity is diminished and less neurotransmission occurs.

VALPROATE   The best-known medication in the anticonvulsant group is valproic acid or valproate (Depakote). Unlike lithium, valproate may be more useful in patients with rapid cycling, atypical features, or mixed mood states. Valproate has been approved by the U.S. Food and Drug Administration (FDA) for treatment of acute mania and as an adjunctive therapy with other agents. The most common side effects of valproate include nausea, diarrhea, hair loss, rash, weight gain, and tremor. Laboratory testing is required with valproate to evaluate the serum concentration, complete blood count, and liver function tests. Although the therapeutic index is wider when compared to lithium, valproate serum concentrations of 150 mcg/ml or greater lead only to more side effects, without any improved clinical response. Valproate is not used during pregnancy because of the high risk of neural tube defects—for example, spina bifida and anencephaly.

CARBAMAZEPINE   Another anticonvulsant that has widespread use as a mood stabilizer is carbamazepine (Tegretol). Although this medication has been extensively studied, it does not have FDA approval for use as a mood stabilizer. The most common side effects of carbamazepine include rash, fatigue, nausea, dizziness, and sedation. As with lithium and valproate, carbamazepine requires laboratory monitoring because of the possibility of agranulocytosis (decreased white blood cell count) and aplastic anemia (decreased production of all blood cells); however, both of these effects are rare. Drug interactions with carbamazepine may be more problematic, and the prescribing professional should be aware of the pitfalls. As with valproate, the use of carbamazepine in pregnancy carries a high risk of multiple fetal anomalies.

LAMOTRIGINE Lamotrigine (Lamictal) is another anticonvulsant that obtained FDA approval in 2003 for maintenance treatment of bipolar disorder. This medication appears to be superior to the other mood stabilizers for bipolar depression (Chang, Wagner, Garrett, Howe, & Reiss, 2008; Geddes, Calabrese, & Goodwin, 2009). The most important side effect to remember about lamotrigine is the potential for a *toxic rash* (Stevens–Johnson syndrome). Other common side effects include headache, dizziness, and sedation. The risk of this medication in pregnancy is virtually unknown; however, some research suggests that it may be a safer alternative for pregnant women with bipolar illness than lithium or other anticonvulsants (Newport et al., 2008).

GABAPENTIN Gabapentin (Neurontin) is also used in the treatment of bipolar disorder, primarily as an adjunctive treatment. This drug has been used clinically and has some research basis but has not been approved by the FDA for use in bipolar disorder. The most common side effects of gabapentin include sedation, tremors, nausea, dizziness, and weight gain. The use of gabapentin during pregnancy is not recommended.

TOPIRAMATE Topiramate (Topamax) might be another useful alternative, but like gabapentin, it does not have the FDA indication. This drug may have one major advantage over the others: It does not cause weight gain. While not an advantage in terms of efficacy, weight loss is an important factor for patients on so many medications shown to alter blood glucose and increase weight and blood pressure (Roy Chengappa et al., 2007). The most common side effects of topiramate include weight loss, sedation, cognitive dulling, fatigue, headache, and paresthesia (numbness in extremities). The use of topiramate during pregnancy is not recommended.

OXCARBAZEPINE Oxcarbazepine (Trileptal) is a medication similar to carbamazepine but does not carry the risk of agranulocytosis or aplastic anemia. Oxcarbazepine shares the same general side effect profile as carbamazepine but in much milder form, with the exception of hyponatremia, which is more common with oxcarbazepine (Gitlin & Frye, 2012).

OTHER ANTICONVULSANT MEDICATIONS A few other anticonvulsant mood stabilizers worth mentioning include tiagabine (Gabitril) and zonisamide (Zonegran). They are similar to the other medications mentioned that are being researched for use in bipolar disorder. Clonazepam (Klonopin) is another anticonvulsant medication, which happens to be a benzodiazepine. It is used primarily as an adjunctive treatment in patients who do not have a history of chemical dependency.

Atypical Antipsychotic Medications

In addition to lithium and the anticonvulsants, the final category of mood stabilizers is the atypical antipsychotic medications.

OLANZAPINE   The first antipsychotic medication to receive FDA approval for acute mania was olanzapine (Zyprexa). When a patient presents with mania and psychosis, olanzapine is the drug of choice because it functions both as a mood stabilizer and an antipsychotic. Olanzapine has received FDA approval for acute monotherapy treatment, maintenance monotherapy treatment, and combination treatment for bipolar disorder. The medication also comes in an alternative form, Zyprexa Zydis (orally disintegrating tablet), which is used in hospital settings where compliance is called into question. The most common side effects of olanzapine include sedation, weight gain, constipation, dry mouth, dizziness, orthostatic hypotension, and weakness. When a patient takes olanzapine, laboratory monitoring of glucose, lipids, and liver functions is recommended because of the likelihood of the drug causing diabetes, hypercholesterolemia, and liver dysfunction. The use of olanzapine in pregnancy is not recommended.

SYMBYAX   Another medication approved by the FDA, specifically for the depressive phase of bipolar disorder, is known as Symbyax. This medication is a combination of fluoxetine (Prozac) and olanzapine (Zyprexa). More information about the individual medications can be found in Chapter 5 and Chapter 8.

RISPERIDONE.   Another antipsychotic medication that has mood-stabilizing properties is risperidone (Risperdal). It has been approved by the FDA as monotherapy or adjunctive therapy for treatment of acute manic or mixed episodes. As with Zyprexa Zydis, Risperdal can be delivered as the orally disintegrating tablet Risperdal M-tab. The most common side effects include restlessness, insomnia, constipation, and dizziness. Recommendations for laboratory monitoring are basically the same as with olanzapine. Risperidone use during pregnancy carries significant risk and is not recommended. Paliperidone (Invega) is the major metabolite of risperidone. One advantage of this newer formulation is that approximately 59% is eliminated through the kidneys as an unchanged drug. The cytochrome P450 enzyme system, therefore, plays a minimum role in drug elimination (Fowler, Bettinger, & Argo, 2008). Neither paliperidone or the injectable version (Sustenna) are currently FDA approved for the treatment of bipolar illness.

QUETIAPINE   Quetiapine (Seroquel) is an antipsychotic medication that may be useful with acute mania. It is currently approved by the FDA for acute mania, either as monotherapy or adjunctive therapy. Quetiapine's side effects include sedation, dizziness, constipation, and dry mouth. As with the other atypical antipsychotic medications, laboratory monitoring of blood sugar and lipids is recommended when using quetiapine. It is not recommended during pregnancy.

ZIPRASIDONE   Ziprasidone (Geodon) is another option available for acute mania, with or without psychosis. Compared with the other atypical agents, ziprasidone is more likely to cause QT prolongation on EKG, which is associated with a potentially fatal arrhythmia. The most common side effects include somnolence, dizziness, rash, anxiety, and nausea. Laboratory monitoring of glucose, lipids, and liver functions is recommended. Ziprasidone use during pregnancy is not recommended unless the potential benefit to the mother outweighs the potential risk to the fetus.

ARIPIPRAZOLE   Another atypical antipsychotic available is aripiprazole (Abilify). This medication is also clinically effective as a mood stabilizer. In late 2004, the FDA approved Abilify for use in acute manic or mixed episodes. The most common side effects of aripiprazole include headache, nausea, insomnia, and somnolence. Laboratory monitoring is again necessary. As with other newer medications, aripiprazole is not recommended during pregnancy. In addition, Abilify Maintena was approved by the FDA in 2017 for maintenance monotherapy treatment of Bipolar Disorder Type I in adults.

CLOZAPINE   Another atypical antipsychotic medication that is worth noting is clozapine (Clozaril). Although this medication is only approved for treatment-resistant schizophrenia, clozapine has been used for the last decade to manage severe mania in some circumstances. This drug is used only in select cases because it may have very severe side effects, including agranulocytosis and seizures. Clozapine requires weekly monitoring of the white blood cell (WBC) count for the first six months, then every other week while the patient remains on the drug. Other common side effects include weight gain, sedation, headache, orthostatic hypotension, constipation, salivation, tachycardia (increased heart rate), and myocarditis (inflammation of the heart). Clozapine is definitely an effective medication but requires more intense monitoring by the prescribing professional. Interestingly, clozapine is not known to be teratogenic and may be used in pregnancy if the benefits outweigh the risks. Clozapine comes in an orally disintegrating tablet form known as Fazaclo.

ASENAPINE   Asenapine (Saphris) is another FDA-approved atypical antipsychotic for Bipolar Disorder Type I as acute monotherapy treatment of manic or mixed episodes, in adults and pediatric patients 10 to 17 years of age, as adjunctive treatment to lithium or valproate in adults, and as maintenance monotherapy treatment in adults.

CARIPRAZINE   In addition, cariprazine (Vraylar) is FDA approved for acute treatment of manic or mixed episodes associated with Bipolar Disorder Type I in adults. A recent phase 3 study showed positive results for cariprazine use for treatment of bipolar depression, but this has not been approved by the FDA as of this writing.

LURASIDONE   Lurasidone (Latuda) is the also FDA approved for depressive episode associated with bipolar depression in adults and pediatric patients (10 to 17 years) as monotherapy, and it is FDA approved for depressive episode associated with bipolar depression in adults as adjunctive therapy with lithium or valproate.

Typical Antipsychotic Medications

As opposed to *atypical* antipsychotic medications, a multitude of other *typical* antipsychotic medications are used adjunctively with other mood stabilizers. Haloperidol (Haldol), fluphenazine (Prolixin), trifluoperazine (Stelazine), thioridazine (Mellaril), and chlorpromazine (Thorazine) are a few of the best-known agents. These medications are used primarily for acute agitation while the patient is hospitalized. Haloperidol and some of the other medications may be given intramuscularly or by mouth, depending on the acuity of the situation. Although this class may cause major side effects, including extrapyramidal symptoms, typical antipsychotics are used for behavioral management only in the short term (less than one week). More information about these medications may be found in Chapter 8, Treatment of Psychotic Disorders.

Other Medications

In addition to the medications already discussed, some other options are worth mentioning. Verapamil is a calcium channel blocker that is primarily used in the treatment of hypertension, angina, and supraventricular arrhythmias. A small number of open trials suggest that the drug has antimanic properties. One randomized, double-blind, placebo-controlled study did not show any antimanic effect (Bowden, 2001). Other drug classes, including NSAIDs (celecoxib), dopamine agonists (bromocriptine), protein kinase C inhibitors (tamoxifen), and xanthine oxidase inhibitors (allopurinol), have also been studied in acute mania as monotherapy or adjunctive therapy. The sample sizes of those studies were small, and the results were generally inconclusive (Vieta et al., 2018).

Benzodiazepines are useful medications that may be used adjunctively with other mood stabilizers. For example, lorazepam (Ativan) is commonly given to manic patients early in their treatment to decrease agitation, which helps with behavioral management, until the primary mood stabilizer becomes effective. There is little evidence that supports the possible benefits of thyroid hormone, acetylcholinesterase inhibitors, acetyl-L-carnitine, pregnenolone, naltrexone (Revia), or lisdexamfetamine (Vyvanse) for bipolar depression. However, studies with a small sample size have shown efficacy of pramipexole (Mirapex), ketamine (Ketalar), and scopolamine (Transderm Scop) for bipolar depression. Anti-inflammatory agents such as NSAIDs, N-acetylcysteine, omega-3 polyunsaturated fatty acids, and pioglitazone (Actos) might also have antidepressant effects in bipolar depression when used adjunctive to conventional therapy (Vieta et al., 2018).

ELECTROCONVULSIVE THERAPY (ECT)

In some severe manic patients, who are unresponsive to medications, a course of electroconvulsive therapy (ECT) is appropriate. During the depressed phase of the illness with suicidality present, ECT may be an option for a rapid response. As with any treatment option, the benefits of ECT must be weighed against the risks before proceeding. See the discussion in Chapter 5 for more information.

TREATMENT RESISTANCE AND PROTOCOL

Mania Treatment Protocol

As with depression, making decisions on medication for bipolar disorder requires a logical approach, depending on the phase of the bipolar cycle.

Step 1   The first place to start is with FDA-approved medications for treatment of acute mania. For example, lithium or valproate would be first-line agents. If psychotic symptoms are present, olanzapine or another atypical antipsychotic might also be appropriate. The acutely manic patient is typically hospitalized during this phase of treatment. As noted, a therapeutic dose or level of a particular medication is necessary. These medications need 5 to 15 days in a patient's system before a response may be evaluated.

Step 2   If the first drug trial fails or the patient is unable to tolerate the side effects, an alternative is chosen. For example, if the patient started with lithium first, he or she may then be switched to valproate or vice versa.

Step 3   If monotherapy fails, the next step would be a two-drug combination. Lithium plus an anticonvulsant, two anticonvulsants, or either of these combinations with an atypical antipsychotic would be reasonable choices. If the patient fails to respond or only partially responds, a different two-drug combination therapy would be indicated. Most experts recommend continuing the various two-drug combinations until all are exhausted or the patient responds.

Step 4   If the two-drug combinations fail, the next step would be a three-drug combination. The most common formula would include one drug from each of the main categories: lithium, anticonvulsant, and atypical antipsychotic. For the patient who gets to this level of difficulty, ECT or clozapine would also be appropriate options to consider. Remember that benzodiazepines and typical antipsychotics are used as adjunctive therapies throughout each step that is presented here.

Step 5   If the patient is not responding to the treatment plan, the clinician should take a step back and reassess the diagnosis, comorbid medical conditions, compliance issues, and/or substance abuse issues. Clinicians must stay alert to changes in the patient's illness and must reassess the situation at every step along the way.

Depression Treatment Protocol

In addition to the mania protocol, the depressive phase of bipolar disorder requires the prescriber to consider some alternative issues.

Step 1   The primary medication to treat bipolar disorder, regardless of phase, is a mood stabilizer. When a patient is in the depressive phase, the mood stabilizer should be optimized first, usually by increasing the dosage. For example, lithium therapy should be increased to obtain a serum concentration of 0.7 to 0.9 mEq/L.

Step 2   If the first drug trial fails or the patient is unable to tolerate the side effects, an alternative is chosen. For example, if the patient started with lithium or valproate, he or she may then be switched to an atypical antipsychotic like lurasidone.

Step 3   The addition of an antidepressant, such as an SSRI or bupropion, to the mood stabilizer or atypical antipsychotic would be the next choice. Remember that each medication must be given at an adequate dose and for an appropriate amount of time to see if the patient will respond. The prescriber must be cautious when using lamotrigine with valproate because of the significantly elevated risk for the toxic rash.

Step 4   The next choice in this process would include adding an atypical antipsychotic medication or a monoamine oxidase inhibitor (MAOI). Further steps beyond this include using ECT, typical antipsychotics, NSAIDs, hormones, omega-3 fatty acids, N-acetylcysteine, and so on.

Treatment Protocol for Mixed Mood States

Although there may be some similarities with the mania protocol, the treatment of mixed mood states needs to be further explained.

Step 1   Atypical forms of bipolar disorder respond preferentially to anticonvulsants or atypical antipsychotics rather than to lithium. For example, valproate or olanzapine would be first-line treatments. As noted in the other protocols, the prescriber may need to optimize the dose in order to achieve the maximum response.

Step 2   If monotherapy with one medication fails, then monotherapy with the other agent would be appropriate. For example, valproate would be given if olanzapine was unsuccessful or vice versa.

Step 3   As noted in the mania protocol, two-drug combinations would reasonably be followed by three-drug combinations, and so on. The most important factor to consider is keeping a logical approach to this complex behavioral disorder. In other words, keep the treatment plan simple.

PATIENT AND FAMILY EDUCATION

Patient Education

The counselor or psychotherapist must assess the patient's level of understanding of his or her illness and try to fill in the gaps when necessary. The first step in this process is basic patient education about the natural history, symptoms, comorbidities, and various treatments of bipolar disorder. The best way for the patient to learn about his or her own illness is by reading and by talking to others who have the same problems. Support groups give patients an opportunity to learn from others and to help normalize their experiences. Compliance with medications is an enormous problem with bipolar patients because they often miss the euphoric mania. In fact, lithium is known to be less effective the more it is started and stopped for whatever reasons.

Comorbid alcohol or drug abuse is also common with bipolar patients and should be assessed routinely. Controlling excessive alcohol use in bipolar patients may provide a more promising treatment outcome with less novelty seeking, suicidality, aggressivity, and impulsivity. Further, the use of medications like topiramate may reduce alcohol cravings in patients who drink regularly (Frye & Salloum, 2006). It is also not uncommon for a patient to minimize his or her use of "recreational" methamphetamine, which may be complicating the patient's response or lack thereof to the medications. Patients often "forget" to inform the prescriber about drinking one or two martinis before or during dinner, which is likely contributing to the patient's symptomatology. The clinician should keep in mind that these patients have little concept of balance in their life because they live between the extremes.

Family Education

As noted, family education is very important because the patient's life has a context that family members need to understand. Remember that the manic phase of the illness, primarily the euphoria, feels really great to the patient. The clinician can help the family to understand that the patient may not want to lose this feeling. Family members may be helpful in monitoring the patient's compliance with medications and appointments. Any competent clinician would enlist the patient's family to assess symptomatology, consider compliance issues, and be involved in implementing the treatment plan. Moreover, the family is the clinician's eyes and ears while the patient is at home.

The psychotherapist can be helpful by referring family members for their own individual treatment when they are having difficulty coping with the patient's behaviors. Although the most experienced clinician may be overwhelmed at times by the patient's bipolar illness, keep in mind that the family assists the patient on a daily basis to manage the symptoms.

CASE VIGNETTES

Case 1

CLINICAL HISTORY

Trisha is a 28-year-old, unemployed white female. She is no stranger to therapy, having seen counselors for most of her teen and adult years. Her friends would describe her as a "wild woman" who takes no crap from anyone. She has held various part-time jobs for the last few years because she usually gets angry at her boss or coworkers and quits. While she has had a string of boyfriends over the years, she has been seeing one man for the last year or so. He too is unemployed and has both an alcohol and methamphetamine problem. She describes the relationship as "addictive and dysfunctional, yet exciting and hot." Trisha is back in treatment at the urging of her parents, who describe her behavior as erratic and unpredictable. They also claim that she has periods where she "sleeps little and parties lots." There were also several occasions in the last five years when she was so depressed she didn't eat or want to leave the house. Her father also admits to periods of depression, and Trisha's grandfather was diagnosed with manic depression, resulting in numerous hospitalizations in the 1950s and 1960s. Trisha's only brother died in a car accident several years ago. He was drunk at the time, but she claims he had a long history of depression. Recently Trisha was arrested for disorderly conduct at a friend's party. She had not slept for nearly 24 hours and was drunk and combative. When she was first approached by police, she solicited them for sex. They report that she was rather hyperverbal and hyperactive. They later had to investigate a complaint from local storeowners for bad checks she wrote in excess of $7,000.

POSTCASE DISCUSSION AND DIAGNOSIS

Trisha has Bipolar Disorder Type I, Most Recent Episode Manic (F30.13). She appeared to have boundless energy with little need to rest and was engaging in dangerous, promiscuous and irresponsible behavior. She also meets criteria for recent episodes of major depression. According to Trisha and her parents, she uses alcohol only when she is feeling "high on life" or when she is so depressed she can't get out of bed. There is also a positive family history for both unipolar and bipolar depression.

PSYCHOPHARMACOLOGICAL TREATMENT

Upon consultation with a psychiatrist, Trisha was placed on valproate and titrated to a dose of 750 mg daily. In addition, her psychiatrist added quetiapine 300 mg q.h.s. to assist with sleeping and restlessness at night. Trisha's mood has stabilized, and she has been attending therapy twice weekly and group once weekly. She has also been able to return to a part-time job as a waitress and is no longer dating her boyfriend, who was recently arrested for methamphetamine use. She hopes to attend college next year if she is able to save enough money for her own apartment. She has gained much insight into her illness and now helps other young women in a local support group.

Case 2

CLINICAL HISTORY

Royce is a 23-year-old, mixed-race male who is in his third year of veterinary school at the local university. He has never been hospitalized but has been taking Prozac for depression on and off for the last 6 years (inconsistent use). Lately, Royce has been working long hours on his surgery rotation and has not been sleeping many hours. Since he has "enough energy," he decided to attend a party with some cute undergrads that he met at the gym on his way home. Royce stayed out all night drinking alcohol but was able to show up at work the next day and function appropriately. After several days of erratic behavior, Royce decided that he needed a Nissan GTR and proceeded to buy it on credit. During this time, he was speaking with his family who noted that Royce was speaking quite rapidly and was difficult to interrupt. On his way to work, Royce was driving erratically at 60 mph in a 30-mph zone. When the police pulled him over, he was extremely animated and told police that he was Jesus Christ.

POSTCASE DISCUSSION AND DIAGNOSIS

Royce was involuntary hospitalized with acute mania where the psychiatrist diagnosed him with Bipolar Disorder, Manic, Severe with Psychotic Features (F30.2). He was quite grandiose, trying to convince the hospital staff that he had arisen from the dead 2000 years ago and showing the scars on his hands as evidence. When gathering more information as he stabilized, the psychiatrist obtained a family history that was negative for mood, psychotic, or anxiety disorders. His urine drug screen was also negative.

PSYCHOPHARMACOLOGICAL TREATMENT

Prozac was immediately discontinued, and he was prescribed aripiprazole (Abilify) 10 mg daily in the morning. Lorazepam (Ativan) 2 mg every 4 hours was also prescribed as needed for agitation to maintain control of his behavior. After a few days, aripiprazole was increased to 20 mg daily and his mania started to subside with return of more normal sleep patterns. After the first week in the hospital, Royce decided to stay in the hospital for additional treatment on a voluntary basis. He was discharged home with a normal mood after two weeks and returned to his veterinary school classes.

CHAPTER 7

Treatment of Anxiety Disorders

This chapter explores the symptoms associated with anxiety conditions, the general concept of anxiety, and its role in behavior. A biological explanation for panic states is explored, along with the various treatment options and cautions.

Topics to be addressed include the following:

- Symptoms and causes of anxiety disorders
- Panic disorder with or without agoraphobia
- Generalized anxiety disorder
- Posttraumatic stress disorder
- Obsessive-compulsive disorder
- Social anxiety disorder
- Adjustment disorders and other phobic conditions
- Treatment reminders and cautions
- Case Vignettes

SYMPTOMS AND CAUSES OF ANXIETY DISORDERS

Second only to depression and alcohol abuse, anxiety disorders are commonly presented in both mental health and medical–surgical settings. A well-known fact is that anxious patients overuse medical services and often expect their primary care providers to address their issues (Bandelow et al., 2012; Lindesay, 1991). The pathophysiology of most anxiety disorders is rather complex and most likely linked to abnormal regulation of neurotransmitters such as serotonin, GABA, and glutamate. In addition, a strong comorbidity exists among anxiety disorders, and although they often have similar symptoms, the manifestation or presentation might be different. Since the symptoms of most anxiety disorders are similar, the pharmacological treatment is the same (Bourin & Lambert, 2002).

Anxiety disorders typically include the following symptoms in various forms and intensity: trembling, general nervousness or tension, shortness of breath, diarrhea, hot flashes, feelings of depersonalization, worry, agitation, initial insomnia, poor concentration, tingling, sweating, rapid heartbeat (tachycardia), frequent urination, and dizziness. In assessing these symptoms, the therapist needs to determine the intensity, duration, and quality of these symptoms. This information helps the therapist make the proper diagnosis and treatment.

Anxiety symptoms may result from many other physical conditions, so it is important to rule out any of the following conditions:

Adrenal tumor	Chronic sinus conditions
Alcoholism or other substance abuse	Cushing's disease
Angina	Delirium
Cardiac arrhythmia or other cardio-vascular problem	Hypoglycemia
	Hyperthyroidism

Mitral valve prolapse

Parathyroid disease

Post-concussion syndrome

Premenstrual syndrome (PMS)

Seizure disorders

It is also important to remember that many substances or drugs may cause or exacerbate anxiety. These include amphetamines and other stimulants, diet medications and other appetite suppressants, certain asthma medications, decongestants, cocaine, caffeine, and steroids. Withdrawal from antidepressants, anxiolytics, and other substances of abuse may cause anxiety also.

Once a medical or substance etiology has been ruled out, the therapist needs to determine the type and nature of the anxiety and a likely diagnosis. Anxiety disorders are now categorized as follows:

Panic disorder or PD (with or without agoraphobia)

Agoraphobia with or without panic disorder

Generalized anxiety disorder (GAD)

Posttraumatic stress disorder (PTSD)

Obsessive-compulsive disorder (OCD)

Social anxiety disorder

Adjustment disorder with anxious mood

Simple phobias

Treatment and choice of medication depend on the type and severity of the anxiety disorder. Research has consistently demonstrated that anxiety disorders respond well to psychotherapy and that relaxation, cognitive therapy, and cognitive-behavioral therapy work best (Bourin and Lambert, 2002; Cukor, Spitalnick, Difede, Rizzo, & Rothbaum, 2009; Freire et al., 2017; Gorman, 2002). Further, Gorman (2002) and Freire et al. (2017) maintain that the combination of therapy and medication offers the best prognosis for resistance to relapse of symptoms. Not surprising to many, the continued use of benzodiazepines with or without an antidepressant reduced relapse rates of anxiety, but may create some issues with dependence (Freire et al., 2017). Today, many calming agents, such as serotonin-based antidepressants, atypical antipsychotics, and certain benzodiazepines, are used in place of the older sedative hypnotics that have greater risks for dependence or overdose (Advokat, Comaty, & Julien, 2014). With this in mind, we address each of these disorders with the most efficacious approach based on research and our experience.

PANIC DISORDER WITH OR WITHOUT AGORAPHOBIA

Many patients present to a therapist with complaints of anxiety and believe that they have panic disorder. Patients often confuse periods of uncomfortable anxiety, which many professionals call "anxiety attacks," with actual panic attacks. However, for those patients who experience four or more intense attacks, panic disorder is a seriously debilitating condition. Although some who have panic disorder also experience avoidance behaviors such as agoraphobia, this is not always the case. The DSM-5 suggests that when agoraphobia is present, patients receive a diagnosis of Agoraphobia With Panic Disorder (F40.01), and a diagnosis of Panic Disorder (F41.0) when it is not.

What is happening in the panic-disordered patient? The patient experiences anxiety when the brain perceives a threat. As part of the fight-or-flight response, the limbic system goes on red alert. The body responds to a series of physiological reactions: the limbic system sends signals to the hypothalamus and the locus ceruleus; they in turn send signals to the pituitary, the thyroid, and the adrenal cortex. As a result, various hormones such as cortisol and adrenaline are produced, readying the body for attack, but with panic disorder it is a false alarm with no actual threat. Panic disorder often runs in families, and the cause appears to be biological in nature. A dysregulation of the limbic system, serotonin depletion, excessive glutamate, and insufficient amounts of GABA may all be to blame. Panic can be induced in patients with panic disorder by injecting them with either lactic acid (a by-product of muscular activity) or cholecystokinin (CCK), a peptide produced by cells in the duodenum and in the brain. When large amounts of cortisol and adrenaline are produced, the patient is in a constant or chronic state of arousal. The effects of stress on the body cause these hormones to suppress immune functions and increase blood pressure. These chronic conditions have been linked to other medical illnesses, cardiac problems, and cancer.

On the surface of about 40% of nerve cells in the brain, including the locus ceruleus, are tiny gateways or receptor sites called *chloride ion channels*. Chloride ions, which have a negative charge, are found in the fluid surrounding each cell. The ion channel can be activated or opened when stimulated by the naturally occurring neurotransmitter GABA. As the channel opens, the chloride ions are drawn in. When the cell is infused with negative ions, the cell hyperpolarizes or relaxes. This causes a calming effect of the locus ceruleus. Benzodiazepines also bind at the chloride ion channels, causing a calming effect. This effect is also true for alcohol. (See Figure 7.1.)

The treatment for panic disorder involves three stages: (1) stop the panic, (2) regulate the limbic system with drugs that increase serotonin, and (3) provide appropriate psychotherapy to educate the patient and reduce anticipatory anxiety or self-defeating behaviors.

Stage 1   In this stage, the therapist sees that the patient is experiencing intense anxiety and needs immediate relief. Many patients with panic disorder use or abuse alcohol, which binds with the chloride ion channel to control symptoms. Unfortunately, as tolerance develops, more alcohol is required, resulting in addiction for many patients.

Benzodiazepines are the drugs of choice for quick relief of panic symptoms. Alprazolam (Xanax), lorazepam (Ativan), and oxazepam (Serax) offer the fastest relief because of their short half-lives (see Table 7.1). For many patients with panic disorder, the treatment ends here.

Primary care physicians often provide benzodiazepines to patients with panic disorder and forget to follow up with them. These patients assume that since they are no longer panicking, they must be okay. Although the patients are no longer in a state of anxiety or having panic attacks, the use of benzodiazepines for panic disorder has only relieved the symptoms and the cause remains. Since most of the pharmacologic treatment of anxiety happens at the primary care level, effective protocols are now available to primary care to ensure that effective methods are being used (Bandelow et al., 2012).

Stage 2   In this stage the professional initiates antidepressant therapy. Once panic has been controlled with benzodiazepines, the use of various antidepressants increases serotonin and helps regulate the limbic system. While some of the older tricyclics, such as imipramine, nortriptyline, and amitriptyline, are used, the newer SSRIs and SPARIs offer better relief with fewer side effects. MAOIs do work as well, but dietary restrictions result in poor compliance for panic patients (see Chapter 5).

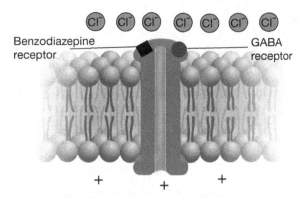

Benzodiazepine receptor

GABA receptor

Phase 1: Choride ion channel closed (patient anxious)

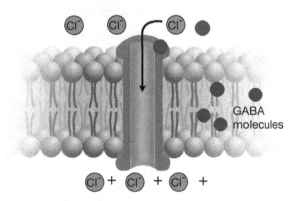

GABA molecules

Phase 2: GABA binds to receptors: Channel begins to open

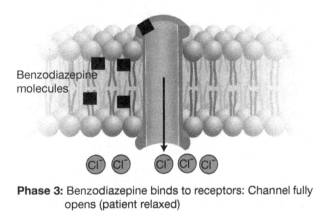

Benzodiazepine molecules

Phase 3: Benzodiazepine binds to receptors: Channel fully opens (patient relaxed)

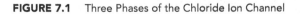

FIGURE 7.1   Three Phases of the Chloride Ion Channel

Table 7.1	Various Medications Used in Anxiety Disorders			
Trade Name	**Generic Name**	**Typical Dose mg/day**	**Medication Class**	**Uses**
Ambien, Ambien CR, Edluar, Zolpimist	zolpidem	5–10	Sedative-hypnotic	Sleep aid
Ativan	lorazepam	1–6	Benzodiazepine	PD, seizure, anxiety NOS
Buspar	buspirone	5–40	Nonbenzodiazepine	GAD, depression, anxiety NOS
Catapres	clonidine	0.1–0.3	Central alpha agonist	Hypertension, social anxiety disorder
Centrax	prazepam	20–60	Benzodiazepine	PD, anxiety NOS
Dalmane	flurazepam	15–30	Sedative-hypnotic	Sleep aid
Doral	quazepam	7.5–15	Sedative-hypnotic	Sleep aid
Halcion	triazolam	0.25–0.50	Sedative-hypnotic	Sleep aid
Inderal	propranolol	20–80	Nonselective beta blocker	Hypertension, social anxiety disorder
Klonopin	clonazepam	0.5–4	Benzodiazepine	PD, seizure, sleep aid, mood stabilizer
Librium	chlordiazepoxide	15–100	Benzodiazepine	Anxiety NOS, muscle relaxation
Lunesta	eszopiclone	1–3	Sedative-hypnotic	Sleep aid
Prosom	estazolam	2–4	Sedative-hypnotic	Sleep aid
Restoril	temazepam	15–30	Sedative-hypnotic	Sleep aid
Rozerem	ramelteon	8	GABA agonist	Sleep aid
Serax	oxazepam	30–120	Benzodiazepine	Anxiety NOS
Sonata	zaleplon	5–10	Sedative-hypnotic	Sleep aid
Tranxene	clorazepate	15–60	Benzodiazepine	Anxiety NOS
Valium	diazepam	5–40	Benzodiazepine	Seizure, anxiety NOS, muscle relaxation
Visken	pindolol	10–60	Nonselective beta blocker	Hypertension, akathisia, sexual dysfunction
Xanax	alprazolam	0.25–4	Benzodiazepine	PD, anxiety NOS

GAD = Generalized panic disorder; PD = Panic disorder; NOS = Not otherwise specified (NOS)

There has been some concern in recent years that the use of benzodiazepines, or benzos, may increase the occurrence of cognitive decline or dementia, especially in the elderly, but current research appears to show no definitive connection (Gray et al., 2016).

Stage 3 In this stage the therapist provides cognitive-behavioral treatment for patients with panic disorder. These patients must learn to manage their anxiety without developing avoidance behaviors that are caused by experiencing panic attacks in places such as shopping malls. This *anticipatory anxiety* is actually more debilitating than the panic itself. For patients with panic disorder and agoraphobia, or agoraphobia alone without panic disorder, the use of in vivo or real-life techniques is helpful. Encouraging patients to take walks outside of the home with the therapist and/or other treatment staff reduces isolation and discourages additional phobias from developing (Sinacola, 1998). For many patients with panic disorder, fears tend to compound the longer they go untreated. It is best to address fears early in therapy. As expected, many patients are reluctant at first and may complain of increased levels of arousal until new relaxation and other therapeutic methods are understood and practiced.

With panic disorder it is very important for the therapist to address all three stages. Once the therapist determines that a patient truly has the condition, benzodiazepines should be started. While the use of benzodiazepines alone or with an antidepressant varies among prescribers, many claim publicly to be conservative in prescribing them, but they are rather loose in monitoring patients on them (Starcevic, 2012). The therapist should inquire about any history of substance abuse because these patients often enjoy the "high" they get from benzodiazepines and may abuse them. Clinicians need to be cautious of patients who take benzos with opioid medications or with alcohol. This may result in an unintended overdose (Sun et al., 2017). It is worth noting here that the longer-acting benzodiazepines, such as clonazepam (Klonopin), are less likely to be abused than alprazolam (Xanax) or lorazepam (Ativan). The prescriber must include an appropriate antidepressant along with the benzodiazepine. The benzodiazepine first controls the panic, and within one or two weeks the antidepressant begins to work. Then the benzodiazepine should be gradually withdrawn. For some, the use of benzodiazepines may need to be extended a bit longer to reduce the possibility of panic returning, and it is crucial not to withdraw the benzodiazepine too quickly, as the panic may return (Freire et al., 2017). Typically, withdrawing the benzodiazepines over two or three weeks is effective unless the patient has been taking the medication for a long time and the dose is high. In such cases, it is wise to taper more slowly, tapering by 0.25 mg each week until the medication is discontinued (Nardi et al., 2010). For some patients who find themselves dependent on benzodiazepines after successful treatment with serotonergic antidepressants, the use of flumazenil (Anexate) may help in reducing benzodiazepine usage (Hood, Norman, Hince, Melichar, & Hulse, 2014). Further studies also suggest that co-occurring use of antidepressants and benzodiazepines may in fact create the possibility of benzo dependence if the use of benzos is not reduced when prescribed along with antidepressants (Bushnell, Stürmer, Gaynes, Pate, & Miller, 2017).

The antidepressant should maintain patients if they are not abusing alcohol or other drugs, as these reduce the effectiveness of the medication. Psychotherapy may be attempted at any time during this process once the patient is calm enough to focus and concentrate in the session.

GENERALIZED ANXIETY DISORDER

Many practicing clinicians believe that generalized anxiety disorder (GAD) is a behavioral condition and should not be treated with medication. Further, some researchers believe that GAD is more closely related to depression than to anxiety, and for this reason, medications used to treat major depression are typically effective for treating various forms of anxiety (Sheehan, 1999; Sowa-Kucma et al., 2017). Sheehan also found that people with GAD utilized medical services more than those without the diagnosis.

Most patients with GAD respond well to a combination of medication and psychotherapy (Sheehan, 2002). Cognitive therapy is helpful as a form of psychoeducation that allows patients to see patterns in their perceptions of issues and the behaviors or actions that follow. While benzodiazepines have been used to treat GAD in the past, this use is not the best approach because it does not teach patients to manage their condition.

Typically, the best medications for GAD include venlafaxine/desvenlafaxine (Effexor/ Pristiq); buspirone (Buspar); and most of the SSRIs, such as fluoxetine (Prozac), paroxetine (Paxil), and escitalopram (Lexapro). It also includes the newer SPARI medications of vortioxetine (Trintellix) and vilazodone (Viibryd). These newer medications are thought to have fewer sexual and cognitive side effects than other SSRIs, and they typically do perform better than placebo, but they were not found to be superior to other medications (Sowa-Kucma et al., 2017). However, some studies found no statistical difference between vortioxetine and placebo in the treatment of GAD specifically (Rothschild, Mahableshwarkar, Jacobsen, Yan, & Sheehan, 2012). Some research performed by Pae et al. (2015), however, suggests that Trintellix may be more helpful than traditional medications when a patient with generalized anxiety disorder has more severe and debilitating symptoms. When patients also present with pain symptoms, research has demonstrated the efficacy of using venlafaxine (Effexor) and duloxetine (Cymbalta) even pregabalin (Lyrica) to control both the anxiety and pain brought on by chronic tension (Bandelow et al., 2012; Beesdo et al., 2009; Khan & Macaluso, 2009). Buspirone is a nonbenzodiazepine antianxiety drug with properties more similar to an antidepressant. As mentioned in Chapter 5, buspirone may alleviate depression for the anxious patient with co-occurring mood concerns. Unlike benzodiazepines, buspirone and the other antidepressants may take three to four weeks before they take effect. Patients need to be informed of this fact, and they must be patient. Patients also need to be told that these medications should be taken as directed and not only as needed. If the patient is concerned about sedation, fluoxetine (Prozac), venlafaxine (Effexor), sertraline (Zoloft), citalopram (Celexa), and escitalopram (Lexapro) may be better choices. If the patient has serious trouble relaxing, buspirone or paroxetine may be better because they have a more relaxing and calming effect.

For many patients with GAD, initial insomnia is a problem. Sleep aids may be helpful for the short term, but many of them, such as the drugs zolpidem (Ambien), eszopiclone (Lunesta), zaleplon (Sonata), and the newer drug suvorexant (Belsomra), may be habit forming in the long term. Suvorexant works a little differently than the others as it is an orexin receptor antagonist. It is probably better to begin the antidepressant therapy and wait a week or two to see if sleep improves as serotonin levels increase. If the patient is persistent, the clinician could recommend a low dose of a sedative-hypnotic. For example, 5 to 10 mg of zolpidem at bedtime for only one week reduces the likelihood of dependence. If the patient is concerned about taking prescription sleep aids, the clinician could recommend over-the-counter diphenhydramine (Benadryl) at 25 to 50 mg before bedtime. For patients with severe agitation and racing thoughts at bedtime, gabapentin (Neurontin) may enhance sleep. Research has also demonstrated that adding an atypical antipsychotic such as quetiapine may not only enhance the effectiveness of SSRIs but may also reduce racing thoughts at bedtime (Baune, 2008; see Chapter 5, Chapter 6, and Table 7.1).

POSTTRAUMATIC STRESS DISORDER

Historically, benzodiazepines and neuroleptics have been used to treat patients with posttraumatic stress disorder (PTSD), especially patients who demonstrate psychotic behaviors (Albucher & Liberzon, 2002). Today, considering reported overall efficacy and side-effect profiles, clinicians have found much success with SSRIs and SPARIs. In some cases, mood stabilizers, such as lamotrigine (Lamictal), and atypical neuroleptics, such as risperidone, quetiapine, aripiprazole, or olanzapine, might be needed if the patient becomes agitated, combative, or psychotic (Berger et al., 2009). While sertraline and paroxetine are the only FDA-approved antidepressant drugs for PTSD, Veterans Administration (VA) practice guidelines also suggest fluoxetine and venlafaxine (Berlin, 2017). Berlin further suggests in her research that newer medications, such as steroids, MDMA, and ketamine, have shown promise, but further research is needed to address issues related to risk and efficacy over time.

Research has examined the role of various medications in the prevention of PTSD symptoms by interfering with how memories are chemically stored in the brain. Medications such as propranolol appear to interfere with how emotional memories are stored and may prove to be an effective prophylactic for those recently traumatized or as an adjunct to current medications (Chamberlain, Muller, Blackwell, Robbins, & Sahakian, 2006; Henry, Fishman, & Youngner, 2007; Nugent et al., 2010). Propranolol may also help with hypervigilance (Berlin, 2017). Recent research suggests that both medication and exposure therapy offer the best probability of success in treatment (Bandelow et al., 2012; Berlin, 2017). Some question the ethics of altering memory or experience, or using exposure, but agree that for severe cases, the benefits outweigh the risks (Bell, 2008; Rothbaum et al., 2012). Prazosin, an adrenergic-inhibiting agent, may also be a promising medication when trauma-related nightmares and sleep disturbances are prominent symptoms (Berger et al., 2009; Berlin, 2017; Reardon & Factor, 2008).

Psychotherapy is a very important part of the treatment for PTSD. Patients may need to slowly expose themselves to the event or events that contributed to the condition. Various behavioral therapies, imagery rescripting, and rehearsal have been found to be effective (Cukor et al., 2009). Like bipolar patients, PTSD patients typically abuse substances in an attempt to dull the pain and anxiety. Detoxification may be needed first to ensure successful use of psychotropic medications. Although any antidepressant would be helpful, SSRIs, such as paroxetine and sertraline, have been approved for such use.

OBSESSIVE-COMPULSIVE DISORDER

Obsessive-compulsive disorder (OCD) is more of a worldwide health problem than once thought. According to the World Health Organization and other researchers, approximately 2% to 3% of the general population suffers from OCD, with typical onset in patients in their twenties (Jenike, 2001). Psychotherapy alone has not been shown to be very effective; behavioral and cognitive-behavioral treatments along with medication offer the best possibilities.

The cause of OCD remains unknown, but a familial link might exist, since patients with OCD typically have a close relative who has OCD or OCD co-occurring with a tic disorder. The most likely cause of OCD is dysfunction in one or more of several segregated corticostriatal pathways.

According to Jenike (2001), OCD seems to involve subtle structural abnormalities in the caudate nucleus, as well as functional dysregulation of neural circuits of the orbital frontal cortex, cingulate cortex, and caudate nucleus. Some researchers believe that childhood infections may contribute to the development of OCD (Insel, 1992). In any case, serotonergic systems have been implicated.

The treatment of choice for OCD involves the use of SSRIs and SPARIs (Bandelow et al., 2012). The tricyclic clomipramine (Anafranil) has been used, but sedation and anticholinergic side effects are troublesome and have been shown to lead to problems with compliance (Choi, 2009). SSRIs affect serotonin levels and typically relieve symptoms. It is important to remember that the doses used for depression and other anxiety disorders might not be high enough for the OCD patient. Therefore, a dose of 60 to 80 mg of fluoxetine (Prozac) or 200 to 300 mg of fluvoxamine (Luvox) may be needed for OCD relief. Escitalopram (Lexapro) may be a bit more effective due to its lower side-effect profile and demonstrated effectiveness when compared to similar SSRIs (Montgomery & Moller, 2009; see Chapter 5 and Table 7.1).

In some cases the obsessions are severely intrusive, and the patient may complain of racing thoughts and insomnia. Low-dose, atypical neuroleptics, such as risperidone (Risperdal), could be added along with a sleep aid if needed. While most atypicals are helpful as adjuncts to SSRIs in reducing symptoms in patients with severe OCD, quetiapine may not be as effective in reducing OCD symptoms as the others; however, it may still be helpful in reducing agitation and racing thoughts before bedtime (Kordon et al., 2008). Further, newer medications may offer reductions in severe OCD and depression without the troublesome side effects of severe weight gain, sedation, or akathisia (Thase et al., 2015).

In cases of severe treatment-resistant OCD in children and teens, memantine (Namenda), an N-methyl-D-aspartate (NMDA) receptor agonist, may be an effective augmenting agent when added to a standard SSRI regimen (Hezel, Beattie, & Stewart, 2009).

SOCIAL ANXIETY DISORDER

Social anxiety disorder or social phobia is a common presenting issue in private practices and public clinics. In such cases the therapist needs to determine that the patient has never had a history of panic disorder. Many professionals believe that social anxiety should be treated with psychotherapy alone and that medications should not be used; however, several medications have been found to be useful (Davidson, 2003). Many patients with social anxiety have found that alcohol relieves their symptoms, but they demonstrate obvious alcohol dysfunction in social situations. This dysfunction may lead to social or occupational problems or, worse, alcohol dependence. Typically, primary care physicians offer benzodiazepines to socially phobic patients. Although these drugs may lessen patients' fears a bit, they do not afford patients an opportunity to understand their fears and subsequent behaviors.

SSRIs and MAOIs offer the best results for social anxiety patients. Tricyclics, benzodiazepines, and buspirone (Buspar) offer little benefit in the long run. In some cases, when the patient reports only situational anxiety—for example, when he or she has to speak publicly—the use of beta blockers such as propranolol (Inderal) or clonidine (Catapres, an alpha agonist), might prove helpful. In these cases the patient may take the medication an hour before the speech and notice less sweating, heart palpitations, and general anxiety without the need to take medication on an ongoing basis.

Psychotherapy, especially behaviorally based treatments, helps the patient to see the connection between environments and the fears they produce. Cognitive rehearsal and role-playing may assist the patient to achieve a more lasting recovery.

ADJUSTMENT DISORDERS AND OTHER PHOBIC CONDITIONS

When a patient presents with anxiety and sleep disturbance related to a stressful event, the clinician must rule out PTSD, GAD, or another long-standing anxiety disorder. If the patient appears to have no history of an anxiety disorder and he or she seems to be aware of the stressor that might be responsible, counseling and psychotherapy are recommended. In most cases the symptoms remit within six months. A sleep aid could be used for a short time if the patient complains of ongoing problems with insomnia. If the patient appears to have significant anxiety, a low-dose SSRI or SPARI could be used for four to six months. If the patient is agitated and cannot relax enough to work or concentrate, sedating antidepressants, such as paroxetine (Paxil), trazodone (Desyrel), or amitriptyline (Elavil), could be used. If there are concerns related to a recent loss, such as the death of a loved one, referral to a grief counselor or other professional experienced in loss may be appropriate.

For patients who present with simple phobias, such as fear of cats, spiders, or elevators, a therapist competent in behavioral techniques might be the answer. Typically, various exposure techniques are preferred rather than medication for phobias.

OTHER ANXIETY-RELATED IMPULSE ISSUES

Several other disorders on the anxiety spectrum would have been considered more of an impulse issue in previous editions of the DSM. The anxiety-based impulse disorders are characterized by the failure to resist an impulse, drive, or temptation to perform some act that is harmful to the patient or potentially to others. In most cases, the patient senses increasing tension or arousal prior to the act and experiences pleasure, gratification, or relief during or following the act. These disorders are now addressed in the DSM-5 as OCD-related disorders. These include conditions such as trichotillomania, excoriation or skin picking, as well as issues such as hoarding and other disorders not currently addressed in the DSM that are under further study, such as excessive buying or shopping. In addition, disorders and conditions such as excessive gambling have also been addressed with pharmacotherapy, especially serotonergic medications as the neurotransmitter serotonin has been implicated.

Trichotillomania has been successfully treated with serotonergic medications such as fluoxetine (Prozac) or escitalopram (Lexapro), as well as TCAs such as clomipramine. There is further clinical evidence that mood stabilizers such as valproate (Depakote) may also be helpful, especially in children (Milanlioglu & Kilic, 2011). Kleptomania, like trichotillomania, typically responds to SSRIs as well, especially escitalopram (Lexapro), the mood stabilizer topiramate (Topamax), and naltrexone (Schreiber, Odlaug, & Grant, 2011). (See more on this in Chapter 14.) Chronic skin picking has been clinically reduced with the use of SSRIs as well, especially citalopram (Celexa) and fluoxetine (Prozac). The use of the antioxidant NAC or N-acetyl-cysteine has been found to be helpful, but mood stabilizers were not found to be especially effective (Schreiber et al., 2011).

In gambling disorders, lithium was shown to be far more efficacious than placebo in reducing gambling behaviors. The opioid antagonist naltrexone (Revia) was found to reduce these behaviors; however, the drug nalmefene (Revex) demonstrated overall reduction in gambling behaviors compared to placebo. N-acetyl-cysteine (NAC) may also reduce gambling urges in patients. Similar results were found incidentally in one study using NAC with trichotillomania. Compulsive buying was found to respond to citalopram (Celexa). It is interesting to note that Prozac and Lexapro did not show efficacy in reducing buying in studies where they were the primary medications (Coccaro, Lee, & McCloskey, 2014; Leung & Cottler, 2008; Myrseth & Pallesen, 2010; Schreiber et al., 2011).

TREATMENT REMINDERS AND CAUTIONS

For all patients with anxiety disorders, the therapist should advise them to eliminate or reduce the consumption of caffeine and caffeine-based energy drinks. In fact, patients may wish to evaluate their general diet and watch for excessive amounts of sugar or stimulants such as sodas, candy, and cigarettes.

For most anxiety disorders, the four "Bs" are used. These include *benzodiazepines* such as diazepam (Valium), alprazolam (Xanax), lorazepam (Ativan), and clonazepam (Klonopin); *barbiturates* such as pentobarbital (Nembutal) and secobarbital (Seconal), which may potentiate GABA but are very sedating and habit forming; *buspirone* (Buspar) for GAD; and *beta blockers* for specific forms of social anxiety.

Side effects for anxiety medications vary according to the type used. Benzodiazepines are usually well tolerated, and the side effects are minimal, but the symptoms of benzodiazepine intoxication include slurred speech, severe sedation, dizziness, cognitive slowing, gait abnormalities, and an exaggerated sense of "high." Since some patients enjoy this feeling, therapists must watch for tolerance and abuse. Benzodiazepines should be given cautiously to seniors because an excess may lead to falls and broken bones. Failure to assess the patient for a more serious depressive disorder or a psychotic disorder can result in a worsening of the condition when treated with benzodiazepines alone. The therapist should warn the patient that sudden withdrawal from benzodiazepines may cause an increase in anxiety and insomnia. Benzodiazepines should never be taken with alcohol or other opioids, which will potentiate their effects and could lead to overdose (Sun et al., 2017). Discontinuing the medication should be done gradually, under medical supervision, and only after the patient has discussed other options with the therapist and the prescribing professional (see Hood et al., 2014; Nardi et al., 2010).

The side effects for buspirone are usually mild and similar to those for antidepressants. They include drowsiness, dry mouth, nausea, headache, dizziness, and insomnia. As with the benzodiazepines, the patient must watch for dizziness, especially if operating heavy machinery.

Sleep aids should be used judiciously—that is, only when necessary and only for one to two weeks maximum if taken daily. In some cases, patients may take sleep aids for long periods if they use them only for intermittent insomnia. Side effects are minimal but include, of course, drowsiness, amnesia, dizziness, falling, lethargy, disorientation, cognitive slowing, and possible depression.

In conclusion, since clinicians prescribing medication for anxiety disorders must make a quick and accurate assessment of the condition, they need to have confidence that patients will comply with treatment. Clinicians should obtain information about the duration and intensity of the condition, as well as a history of substance abuse and previous treatment attempts.

CASE VIGNETTES

Case 1

CLINICAL HISTORY

Beth is a 23-year-old Asian American graduate student. She is currently in treatment with a psychologist for anxiety. She claims that her cognitive therapy has helped her control her worry and anxiety, but she has noticed that her symptoms have worsened this year with all of the pressures of school. In addition to worry, her mind races at night when she tries to sleep, and she claims it may often take her two to three hours to finally fall asleep. She describes herself as a "type A" person who is rather "anal" about doing well. She worries nonstop about grades but also worries nonstop about her health, money, her parents' health, and world affairs. She is very insightful about her condition and agrees the worry is excessive and unwanted. She admits that there is really no basis for the worry, as she has a full scholarship, she and her parents are in good health, and she currently has a 3.9 GPA. She claims that she has always been rather tense, but it didn't get to the point that she sought treatment until her senior year in college. She was worried about getting accepted to grad school and "obsessed" over getting straight A's. She sought the help of a psychologist at the university counseling service, was placed on Paxil, and began therapy. For the most part, her symptoms disappeared, but she remembers feeling tired during the day.

POSTCASE DISCUSSION AND DIAGNOSIS

Beth appears to have a rather classic case of Generalized Anxiety Disorder (F41.1). Her worry is rather chronic, baseless, and interferes with sleep and concentration. After additional history, it appears that both her mother and sister have had problems with anxiety, and her sister currently takes Celexa to address the issue. Beth denies that she has ever had a panic attack and states that she feels comfortable in most social situations. She has refrained from dating because she fears that a boyfriend would distract her from her studies. She hopes to be accepted into a Ph.D. program when she completes the M.A.

PSYCHOPHARMACOLOGICAL TREATMENT

In addition to psychotherapy, Beth was placed on Pristiq 50 mg every morning. While paroxetine was helpful in the past, she did not like the sedation during the day. Since she also complains of muscle tension in her neck, Pristiq and medicines like it help to reduce pain symptoms. In a follow-up session with her psychiatrist two weeks after starting the medication, she reported sleeping better and stated that her level of worry was drastically reduced. She still obsesses over grades but expects to get into the doctoral program with her current GPA.

Case 2

CLINICAL HISTORY

Robert is a 24-year-old Hispanic male who recently took a job as a cable installer with a major communications company. He had a series of low-paying jobs until he completed the training and started this job two months ago. He always considered himself a little "anal" about his work and often worries that he is doing a good job. Recently, at a meeting with his supervisor and five other installers, his supervisor reminded them that someone would be going out to their jobs after they were finished and inspecting them to make sure they were done properly. This news made Robert very anxious, and soon he was having trouble sleeping at night and obsessing over the quality of his work. He would check and recheck his work several times, often returning to various homes after he had left the job. He also started to return to his truck several times while on a job because he feared he had left the truck unlocked. This caused several of his customers to ask him why he was doing this. This behavior was causing him to fall behind on his schedule, thus upsetting his next customer. He started to notice that he was having difficulty falling asleep at night as he would lie awake and wonder about a particular job and whether he had remembered to install it correctly. He also began to notice that he would drive back to many jobs because he thought he had left his tools there, only to find them later in the truck.

POSTCASE DISCUSSION AND DIAGNOSIS

Robert most likely has Obsessive Compulsive Disorder (F42). He appears plagued by a constant need to check and recheck his work to alleviate his level of anxiety. It even interferes with his ability to relax and sleep at night and causes severe initial insomnia. Robert's mother has severe GAD, and his sister was diagnosed with OCD two years ago. Robert feels these behaviors are ruining his life and driving him crazy, but he can't seem to stop them on his own.

PSYCHOPHARMACOLOGICAL TREATMENT

In addition to seeing a psychotherapist who specializes in treating patients with OCD, Robert was seen by a psychiatrist who prescribed the antidepressant/anti-obsessional Prozac (fluoxetine) with a starting dose of 20 mg each morning. Within a week he started to notice a reduction in the obsessive thoughts, and his dose was increased to 40 mg. He was also given 5 mg of zolpidem (Ambien) to help with sleep, but he complained that, even though it made him sleepy, he would still lie awake and think about work. He was then switched from the zolpidem to a low dose of 25 mg quetiapine before bed, and this allowed him to fall asleep within minutes. Within two months, Robert was symptom free but still attending therapy sessions with his therapist as he was learning other ways to reduce his anxiety and manage his thoughts.

CHAPTER **8**

Treatment of Psychotic Disorders

In this chapter we explore the various schizophrenia spectrum disorders, their prevalence, causes, and treatment. The role of both typical and atypical antipsychotics is explored, with advantages and disadvantages presented.

Topics to be addressed include the following:

- Schizophrenia spectrum disorders
- Causes of psychotic disorders
- Medication for psychotic behaviors
- Treatment protocol
- Other significant issues to consider
- Case vignettes

SCHIZOPHRENIA SPECTRUM DISORDERS

Schizophrenia and the other psychotic disorders affect more than 1% of the world's population and cost society a tremendous amount of financial and medical resources (Kahn et al., 2015; Sadock, Sadock, & Ruiz, 2015). These authors also report that there are various schizophrenia spectrum disorders, including schizoid personality disorder, schizotypal personality disorder, schizoaffective disorder, delusional disorder, and psychotic disorder not otherwise specified (NOS), which are reported to be less prevalent but still significant. Although hard data are scarce, Baethge (2002) reports the prevalence of schizoaffective disorder to be about 0.5%, one-half the prevalence of schizophrenia. Patients with schizophrenia need treatment in the earlier stages; this will help prevent relapse because of the higher morbidity and mortality associated with the earlier phases (Tandon & Jibson, 2003). In fact, Lambert, Conus, Lambert, and McGorry (2003) report that during the untreated phase and first-year treatment period, 10% to 15% of first-episode psychotic patients attempt suicide. People with schizophrenia have, on average, a shorter life than the rest of the population; suicide is the main contributor early in the course of the illness, whereas cardiovascular disease is the main contributor later in the illness (Kahn et al., 2015). Overall, the disorder is associated with an increased risk of mortality due to lifestyle and chronic illness associated with the disorder (Seeman, 2007).

Schizophrenia

Schizophrenia is first and foremost a brain disease with numerous abnormalities in structure, function, and neurochemistry. In regard to brain structure, the most common finding is an enlargement of the lateral ventricles, followed by a decreased volume of gray and white matter. The medial temporal structures, including the hippocampus and amygdala, have been noted to be smaller in size when compared to normal brains. When looking at brain function, the clinician notes a relative decrease in cerebral blood flow and metabolism in the frontal lobes.

Studies of the most common neurochemical abnormalities in patients with schizophrenia have focused on the dopamine hypothesis, in which *too much* dopamine is causing the psychotic symptoms (Di Forti, Lappin, & Murray, 2007). This is referred to as a *hyperdopaminergic* hypothesis. As you may know, the conventional or typical antipsychotics (i.e., haloperidol or chlorpromazine) reduce the symptoms of schizophrenia by blocking postsynaptic dopamine D_2 receptors. The newer atypical antipsychotics (i.e., risperidone or olanzapine) have potent serotonergic 5-HT_2 and dopaminergic D_2 antagonism. Other neurotransmitter systems that may be involved in schizophrenia include glutamate, glycine, acetylcholine, serotonin, norepinephrine, phosphodiesterase (PDE) 10 inhibitors, cannabinoid, GABA, neurokinin, N-acetyl cysteine, and other neuromodulators such as substance P and neurotensin (Keshavan, Lawler, Nasrallah, & Tandon, 2017; Matsumoto et al., 2017). These neuromodulators are localized with other neurochemicals and may influence their action. As noted in Chapter 2, their influence could facilitate, inhibit, or alter the patterns of firing (Buchanan et al., 2007).

As you may recall, schizophrenia and other schizophrenia spectrum disorders occur more commonly in families of patients with schizophrenia. Most researchers agree that monozygotic twins have a 40% to 50% concordance rate for schizophrenia, whereas dizygotic twins have only about a 10% concordance rate. This latter rate is consistent for the rate of occurrence of schizophrenia in other first-degree relatives (Matsumoto et al., 2017; Pinel, 2009). In fact, genetic penetrance of schizophrenia can be more than 70% in affected pedigrees. As we advance research, the implementation of whole genome sequencing on a large scale (e.g., millions) and applying advanced machine learning techniques may allow us to predict disease risk. Considering advances in computational genomics, genetics-based diagnoses for psychiatric disease may come of age within the next generation.

In addition to the genetic theories of schizophrenia, immune and viral hypotheses also have been put forward. In fact, some researchers believe that schizophrenia is more common in urban areas and in lower socioeconomic groups. This *social-drift* phenomenon refers to the fact that vulnerable patients have a tendency to lose their social and occupational status and *drift* toward pockets of poverty and inner-city areas. The prevalence of schizophrenia may have a rising north-to-south gradient in the Northern Hemisphere, whereas it may have a rising south-to-north gradient in the Southern Hemisphere. The illness may be endemic in a few areas, such as colder climates with patients born in the winter months (Kendell & Adams, 1991).

When considering the viral hypotheses, researchers suggest that a retrovirus could insert itself in the genome and alter the patient's genetic code; this altered code could be passed down through generations. Other mechanisms that might result in schizophrenia include a viral infection in early life that creates a vulnerability toward the disease, a viral infection leading to secondary scar tissue formation, a virus triggering an autoimmune response, and so on. Some studies have reported that pregnant women exposed to the influenza virus during their second trimester are more likely to give birth to a child who is at increased risk for schizophrenia. The theory is that a viral infection may interfere with normal brain development during the active migration of neuronal cells (Kneeland & Fatemia, 2013).

Some researchers used to think that poor parenting could cause schizophrenia. In the 1950s, Sullivan (1953) focused on patients' disturbance that affected their capacity to relate to others, and this capacity is thought to reflect dysfunction in the mother–infant dyad. In the *stress–diathesis model*, various internal or external stressors can convert vulnerability for schizophrenia into symptoms.

Another concept worthy of mention is that of *expressed emotion* (EE). Several family factors, including criticism, emotionally overinvolved attitudes and behaviors, and negative-affective style, may precipitate the illness or aggravate its course. Schizophrenic patients living with families with high EE have a higher rate of relapse than those living in families with low EE. The chaotic and stressful family interactions might not be the cause of the dysfunction in schizophrenia; rather, the cause might be the complex collection of problems the patient brings to the family setting (Amaresha & Venkatasubramanian, 2012).

Symptoms in Schizophrenia

There are four different types of symptoms seen in schizophrenia and other psychotic illnesses: positive, negative, cognitive, and mood. Although there is a classic presentation, each patient has a unique relative contribution from each of the four categories.

POSITIVE SYMPTOMS   Positive symptoms involve a break from reality in the areas of perception, behavior, thought content, and thought processes. Hallucinations, delusions, loose associations, and grossly disorganized behavior are examples of positive symptoms. These symptoms may require acute psychiatric hospitalizations.

NEGATIVE SYMPTOMS   Unlike positive symptoms, negative symptoms represent something that is deficient and may include apathy, blunted affect, amotivation, anhedonia, poverty of speech, poverty of thought content, asociality, ambivalence, poor hygiene, and so on. Although these symptoms cause the majority of functional disability associated with schizophrenia, negative symptoms rarely lead to hospitalization.

COGNITIVE SYMPTOMS   Symptoms of the third type are the cognitive symptoms. Schizophrenia is characterized by a broad impairment in cognition and neuropsychological functions, which correlate with functional impairment. Topolov and Getova (2016) have noted that patients suffering from psychosis have widespread, multifaceted impairments in many areas, including executive function, attention, perceptual/motor processing, vigilance, verbal learning and memory, verbal and spatial working memory, and semantic memory.

MOOD   Symptoms of the fourth type are mood symptoms. Some patients exhibit depression, agitation, anxiety, insomnia, irritability, and mood lability.

When a patient is diagnosed with a psychotic illness, it is important to evaluate him or her properly for confounding factors such as substance abuse, medical illness, other psychiatric disorders, developmental disorders, and so on. The psychotic disorders include schizophrenia, schizophreniform disorder, schizoaffective disorder, delusional disorder, brief psychotic disorder, schizotypal (personality) disorder, psychotic disorder due to another medical condition, substance/medication-induced psychotic disorder, and unspecified schizophrenia spectrum and other psychotic disorder. In addition to the psychotic disorders, other diagnoses may have secondary psychotic symptoms. For example, psychotic depression, postpartum depression, and bipolar disorder might possibly present with psychosis, depending on the level of severity. Later in this chapter, we will discuss treatment issues, which are similar among the various diagnoses.

CAUSES OF PSYCHOTIC DISORDERS

As with other psychiatric diagnoses, the etiology of a psychotic illness may be related to a physical rather than a functional disorder. The following is a list of common diseases that may cause or exacerbate psychosis:

Addison's disease (adrenal insufficiency)	Hypothyroidism (myxedema)
Brain tumors	Metabolic abnormalities
CNS infections	Multiple sclerosis
Cushing's disease (hyperadrenalism)	Porphyria
Delirium	Postoperative states
Dementia (Alzheimer's, Parkinson's, etc.)	Pregnancy/postpartum hormonal changes
Encephalitis (herpes, AIDS, neurosyphilis, etc.)	Stroke
Systemic lupus erythematosus	Traumatic brain injury
Epilepsy	Uremia
Huntington's disease	Vitamin deficiency (B_{12}, folate, or zinc)
Hyperthyroidism (thyrotoxicosis)	Wilson's disease

In addition to the medical diagnoses, many medications and other substances may cause or exacerbate psychosis. The following is a list of these psychoactive substances:

Alcohol (intoxication or withdrawal)

Anticholinergic medications (benztropine, trihexyphenidyl, etc.)

Antihistamines (diphenhydramine)

Anti-Parkinson's medications (bromocriptine, amantadine, levodopa)

Appetite suppressants (phentermine)

Barbiturates (intoxication or withdrawal)

Benzodiazepines (intoxication or withdrawal)

Beta-blockers (propranolol, metoprolol, atenolol)

Corticosteroids and other hormones (prednisone, methylprednisolone androgens)

Digoxin

Drugs of abuse (marijuana, amphetamines, PCP, psychedelics, cocaine, heroin/morphine, ephedra and other herbal stimulants)

Environmental toxins (volatile hydrocarbons, organophosphates, and heavy metals)

Narcotic medications (morphine, hydrocodone, etc.)

Psychostimulant medications (dextroamphetamine, methylphenidate)

Tricyclic antidepressants (TCAs)

MEDICATIONS FOR PSYCHOTIC BEHAVIORS

Although a wide range of treatment options is available for treating psychotic behaviors, expert consensus guidelines recommend starting with the atypical antipsychotics. According to Kane, Leucht, Carpenter, and Docherty (2003), risperidone (Risperdal) is the treatment of choice for a first-episode psychotic patient with positive symptoms, negative symptoms, or a combination of both. Aripiprazole (Abilify), olanzapine (Zyprexa), ziprasidone (Geodon), and quetiapine (Seroquel) are additional choices but are secondary to risperidone. Other treatment guidelines include the Schizophrenia Patient Outcomes Research Team (PORT) updated treatment recommendations (Kreyenbuhl, Buchanan, Dickerson, & Dixon, 2010), which have a similar approach. Paliperidone (Invega), the major metabolite of risperidone, has been shown to be as effective as risperidone, but it has the same dose-related extrapyramidal symptoms (EPS). Its primary elimination through the kidneys may make it a drug of choice for patients demonstrating liver abnormalities (Marino & Caballero, 2008). You should note that all these are newer atypical antipsychotic medications, not the older typical (i.e., conventional) antipsychotics. Clozapine (Clozaril) was rated an excellent choice for second-line treatment after adequate trials of at least two of the atypical agents. See Table 8.1 for more information.

Table 8.1   Atypical Antipsychotic Medications

Trade Name	Generic Name	Typical Dose (mg/day)	Sedation	Autonomic Effects	EPS
Abilify, Abilify Discmelt, Abilify MyCite	aripiprazole	10–30	*	*	*
Abilify Maintena	aripiprazole	300 mg–400 mg/month	*	*	*
Aristada	aripiprazole lauroxil	441 mg–1064 mg/month	*	*	*
Clozaril, Fazaclo, Versacloz	clozapine	400–600	***	***	None
Fanapt	iloperidone	12–24	*	**	*
Geodon	ziprasidone	80–160	*	**	*
Invega	paliperidone	3–12	*	**	*
Invega Sustenna	paliperidone	78 mg–156 mg/month	*	**	*
Invega Trinza	paliperidone	273 mg–819 mg/3-months	*	**	*
Latuda	lurasidone	40–160	**	**	**
Nuplazid	pimavanserin	34	*	*	*
Rexulti	brexpiprazole	1–4	*	*	*
Risperdal Consta	risperidone	25–50 mg/2-weeks	*	*	*
Risperdal, Risperdal Mtab	risperidone	3–6	*	**	*

(continued)

Table 8.1	(continued)				
Trade Name	Generic Name	Typical Dose (mg/day)	Sedation	Autonomic Effects	EPS
Saphris	asenapine	5–20	*	*	*
Seroquel, Seroquel XR	quetiapine	300–600	***	***	*
Symbyax	olanzapine/ fluoxetine	3/25–12/50	**	**	*
Vraylar	cariprazine	1.5–6	*	*	**
Zyprexa Relprevv	olanzapine	150 mg/2 wk–405 mg/ 4 wk	**	**	*
Zyprexa, Zyprexa Zydis	olanzapine	10–20	**	**	*

* Minimal, ** Moderate, *** Significant

For multiepisode, psychotic patients, risperidone was again the treatment of choice regardless of predominating symptomatology. In addition to the other choices noted previously, Risperdal Consta, the only long-acting atypical antipsychotic, is considered an excellent second-line choice. Other less desirable choices include a long-acting, intramuscular, conventional neuroleptic (such as Haldol or Prolixin Decanoate); an oral, high-potency neuroleptic, for example, haloperidol (Haldol); fluphenazine (Prolixin); trifluoperazine (Stelazine); or thiothixene (Navane). The oral, lower potency, conventional antipsychotic agents, such as chlorpromazine (Thorazine) and thioridazine (Mellaril), were less desirable to the experts when the literature was reviewed (Kane et al., 2003; see Table 8.2). Although acute treatment of agitation is not the focus here, three atypical antipsychotics that have an intramuscular formulation should be mentioned. The injectables ziprasidone (Geodon IM), olanzapine (Zyprexa IM), and aripiprazole (Abilify IM) are available for use in emergency departments and acute psychiatric hospitals. Long-acting injectable medications are typically well tolerated, but in some patients the injection site swells, forming lumpy, painful nodules. Current research suggests that the deltoid muscle may prove to be an alternative location for such injections (Saxena et al., 2008). Over the last decade, atypical long-acting injectable medications are growing in importance to address issues of nonadherence and ease of dosing. Risperdal Consta, Invega Sustenna, Invega Trinza, Zyprexa Relprevv, Abilify Maintena, and Aristada are all reasonable options that all clinicians should consider (Citrome, 2017a).

Atypical Antipsychotic Medications

The atypical antipsychotics have little or no EPS (dystonia, Parkinsonism, akathisia, and tardive dyskinesia). Also, a broader spectrum of efficacy is thought to be associated with the newer agents. Benefits of the atypical antipsychotic agents versus the typical agents include the following:

- Minimal EPS
- Efficacy for positive symptoms (at least as effective as conventional agents)
- Improved efficacy for negative symptoms
- Improved cognition
- Improved mood

Table 8.2	Typical or Conventional Antipsychotic Medications				
Trade Name	**Generic Name**	**Typical Dose (mg/day)**	**Sedation**	**Autonomic Effects**	**EPS**
Haldol	haloperidol	2–20	*	*	***
Haldol Decanoate	haloperidol decanoate	100–300 mg/ month	*	*	**
Loxitane	loxapine	20–100	**	*	**
Mellaril	thioridazine	200–600	***	***	**
Moban	molindone	20–100	**	*	**
Navane	thiothixene	5–30	*	*	***
Orap	pimozide	1–10	*	*	***
Prolixin	fluphenazine	2–20	*	*	***
Prolixin Decanoate	fluphenazine decanoate	25–50 mg/2 wks	*	*	**
Serentil	mesoridazine	50–400	***	***	*
Stelazine	trifluoperazine	5–30	*	*	***
Thorazine	chlorpromazine	200–600	***	***	**
Trilafon	perphenazine	8–64	**	*	**

* Minimal, ** Moderate, *** Significant

Although the atypical agents have similar efficacy, the side effect profiles have been found to be quite different. Tandon and Jibson (2003) report risperidone (Risperdal) shows a clear dose-related increase in EPS and prolactin level, especially at doses greater than 6 mg daily. Prolactin is a hormone secreted by the pituitary gland that increases when dopamine is blocked or suppressed. Increased prolactin concentrations may lead to breast enlargement, galactorrhea (excessive production of breast milk), irregular menses, and so on. Patients who receive increasing doses of olanzapine (Zyprexa) likely exhibit akathisia, Parkinsonism, modest prolactin elevation, and weight gain. One study concluded that using aripiprazole as adjunctive therapy with olanzapine may mitigate weight gain and adverse effects on lipid metabolism (Henderson et al., 2009). Asenapine (Saphris), although most similar to clozapine, is less likely to cause weight gain and prolactin elevation, but its effects on QTc prolongation are comparable to quetiapine (Bishara & Taylor, 2009).

The use of ziprasidone (Geodon) shows a trend toward an increasing level of anticholinergic effects at higher doses (Daniel et al., 1999), but it may be less likely to elevate prolactin levels or cause weight gain (Rosa et al., 2008).

Quetiapine (Seroquel), although still likely to cause weight gain, may be an alternative for patients who must switch medications due to serious weight gain and cholesterol levels; however, overall efficacy may be compromised (Deberdt et al., 2008). Quetiapine has been found helpful as a sedating agent, but because it has developed a reputation as a drug of abuse, some have reconsidered using it with those who have a history of substance abuse. Street names like "quell" and "Suzie Q" have been associated with quetiapine, but research establishing a clear addictive relationship is still inconclusive (Sansone & Sansone, 2010).

Lurasidone (Latuda) is one of the new antipsychotics that is associated with minimal effects on body weight and low risk for alterations in glucose, lipids, or EKG parameters. However, there is a potential for drug–drug interactions as it is a strong inhibitor or inducer of certain liver enzymes such as CYP3A4 (Citrome, 2016).

Brexpiprazole (Rexulti) and cariprazine (Vraylar) are both similar to aripiprazole in that they are partial dopamine agonists with fewer side effects generally, although brexpiprazole may cause more weight gain/increased appetite, and cariprazine may be associated with more EPS (Frankel & Schwartz, 2017).

Clozapine (Clozaril) results in the most weight gain and sedation of all the agents. Keep in mind that clozapine requires weekly blood monitoring and more intense supervision (see Chapter 6).

In addition, Abilify MyCite, approved in late 2017 by the FDA, is a drug-device combination product made of aripiprazole tablets embedded with an Ingestible Event Marker (IEM) sensor intended to track drug ingestion. Per Kopelowicz et al. (2017)*, this digital medicine system allows objective measurement of adherence and potentially improves rates of adherence in patients with schizophrenia. The Abilify MyCite System is composed of four components:

- Aripiprazole tablet embedded with an IEM sensor (Abilify MyCite)
- MyCite Patch (wearable sensor) that detects the signal from the IEM sensor after ingestion and transmits data to a smartphone
- MyCite App, a smartphone application (app) that is used with a compatible smartphone to display information for the patient
- Web-based portal for healthcare professionals and caregivers.

Finally, pimavanserin (Nuplazid) is a new atypical antipsychotic for the treatment of hallucinations and delusions associated with Parkinson's disease psychosis. The mechanism of action is thought to be a combination of inverse agonist and antagonist activity at the serotonin 2A receptors (5-HT2A) and, to a lesser extent, at the 5-HT2C receptors. During clinical trials, pimavanserin showed no appreciable binding affinity for dopamine (including D_2), histamine, muscarinic, or adrenergic receptors (Cruz, 2017).

Typical Antipsychotic Medications

The typical neuroleptics have similar efficacy with respect to positive symptoms, but they may worsen negative symptoms because of their side-effect profiles. Extrapyramidal symptoms have a tremendous negative impact on treatment. *Acute dystonic reactions* are uncomfortable, frightening, and lead to poor compliance. Bradykinesia, cogwheel rigidity, and stiffness, which are *parkinsonian* side effects, contribute to the negative symptoms of the illness (i.e., reduced facial expression, affective responses, gestures, and vocal intonation) with which the patient is already struggling. *Akathisia* is a common subacute side effect related to these medications and may be experienced as restlessness, anxiety, agitation, or insomnia. *Tardive dyskinesia* is the major chronic extrapyramidal symptom that should be avoided if at all possible. The typical agents also have a negative impact on cognition, which further impairs the patient's ability to think and function independently. EPS is commonly treated with anti-Parkinson's or anticholinergic

---

* For full disclosure, it is noted that one of this text's authors, Timothy Peters-Strickland, is an author of this article.

Table 8.3	Antiparkinsonian and Anticholinergic Medications		
Trade Name	**Generic Name**	**Typical Dose (mg/day)**	**Chemical Class**
Artane	trihexyphenidyl	5–15	anticholinergic
Ativan	lorazepam	1–3	benzodiazepine
Austedo	deutetrabenazine	12–48	vesicular monoamine transporter 2 (VMAT2) inhibitor
Benadryl	diphenhydramine	25–50	antihistamine
Cogentin	benztropine	2–6	anticholinergic
Inderal, Inderal LA	propranolol	40–80	nonselective beta blocker
Ingrezza	valbenazine	40–80	vesicular monoamine transporter 2 (VMAT2) inhibitor
Klonopin	clonazepam	1–3	benzodiazepine
Symmetrel	amantadine	100–300	dopamine agonist
Valium	diazepam	5–10	benzodiazepine
Xenazine	tetrabenazine	12.5–50	vesicular monoamine transporter 2 (VMAT2) inhibitor

medications that may also interfere with cognition (see Table 8.3). All of these side effects contribute to discontinuing therapy and long-term compliance issues.

Adverse Effects of Typical and Atypical Antipsychotics

Adverse drug reactions may be seen with any prescribed or over-the-counter medication. As noted in Table 8.2, typical antipsychotics vary with their ability to cause side effects including sedation, autonomic effects, and EPS. Autonomic side effects refer to the adverse effect of medications on the autonomic nervous system and include dizziness, hypotension, and flushing.

The typical or conventional antipsychotics are known for their EPS effects, which include acute dystonia, parkinsonism, akathisia, and tardive dyskinesia. An acute dystonic reaction may occur immediately following a dose of medication and involves intermittent and/or sustained spasms of the muscles of the trunk, head, and neck. Dystonias usually occur within hours to days of the medication and typically are very frightening to the patient.

Parkinsonism, the second form of EPS, may include rigidity, bradykinesia, shuffling gait, and tremor. Patients who take dopamine receptor blockers may look like they have idiopathic Parkinson's disease. This side effect usually occurs within days to weeks of starting the antipsychotic medications.

The most common extrapyramidal side effect is akathisia, which translates to "inability to sit still." Akathisia usually presents itself clinically as feelings of inner restlessness, inability to keep the legs still, constant shifting of weight from one foot to the other, walking in place, frequent shifting of body positions in a chair, and so on. Like parkinsonism side effects, akathisia typically occurs after days to weeks of treatment. Acute dystonia, parkinsonism, and akathisia occur early in treatment with the typical antipsychotics and remit soon after the drug is discontinued.

The last type of EPS is tardive dyskinesia (TD). It is an involuntary movement disorder that may occur after the patient has been on the medication for months to years. Patients with TD may have abnormal movements including lip smacking, sucking or puckering, facial grimacing, blinking, tremors, trunk movements, and so on. Approximately 10% to 20% of patients who are treated with dopamine receptor antagonists for more than a year are at risk for developing tardive dyskinesia. Certain populations, such as elderly females and patients with mood disorders, are at greater risk. Drugs like lithium may offer some protection from TD; however, experts caution against adding lithium unless a mood stabilizer is clearly needed (Van Harten, Hoek, Matroos, & Van Os, 2008). In 2017, both deutetrabenazine (Austedo) and valbenazine (Ingrezza) are now approved treatments for TD and showed significant decreases in abnormal movements across studies (Meyer, 2016).

TREATMENT PROTOCOL

The following general steps simplify the treatment information, which may be a bit overwhelming and confusing.

Step 1   Most prescribing professionals start with risperidone/paliperidone (Risperdal/ Invega) or a similar atypical agent for the patient's psychotic illness.

Step 2   If the patient is unable to tolerate risperidone because of side effects or does not respond, the next logical choices would be olanzapine (Zyprexa), quetiapine (Seroquel), ziprasidone (Geodon), aripiprazole (Abilify), iloperidone (Fanapt), asenapine (Saphris), lurasidone (Latuda), brexpiprazole (Rexulti), or cariprazine (Vraylar). Preferably, the clinician should try two or more of the atypical agents before moving on to the next steps.

Step 3   This step varies and depends on the art of medicine. Some clinicians would recommend a trial of clozapine (Clozaril), and others would use a typical antipsychotic medication like haloperidol (Haldol) or thiothixene (Navane).

Step 4   Another option the clinician could try is to add a third agent in the atypical antipsychotic class. Remember that the typical LAIs (e.g., Haldol Decanoate or Prolixin Decanoate) and atypical LAIs (e.g., Risperdal Consta, Invega Sustenna, Invega Trinza, Zyprexa Relprevv, Abilify Maintena, or Aristada) are also available for patients who have compliance issues.

OTHER SIGNIFICANT ISSUES TO CONSIDER

In addition to choosing the most appropriate medication, other issues must be considered. An *adequate dose* of the antipsychotic, which is approximately the dose recommended in the package labeling, must be prescribed. For example, the optimal dose of risperidone is 4–6 mg daily, whereas the dose for olanzapine is 15–30 mg daily. Each drug has a different dose because of different potencies, but they are all equally efficacious at therapeutic doses. For chronic patients, the dose may be higher than for first-episode patients.

Information on *therapeutic drug monitoring* with the antipsychotics is limited. Clozapine is the only agent for which researchers have considered the plasma level most clinically useful.

Some experts believe that plasma levels of other neuroleptics can be useful to aid in dosage adjustment, especially when there is an inadequate response or problematic side effects.

Research indicates a relationship between certain patient characteristics and necessary dose adjustments. First, smoking can reduce the plasma levels of some antipsychotic drugs (van der Weide, Steijns, & van Weelden, 2003). A mounting body of evidence suggests that the effects of genetic polymorphisms involve cytochrome P450 liver enzymes and the metabolism of psychotropic drugs. Ethnicity, sex, age, and other medical conditions may be factors in determining the best dose for the patient. For example, geriatric patients and Asian patients who tend to be more sensitive to antipsychotic medications require lower dosages because of their slower metabolic processes in the liver.

Since the patient's response to these medications is delayed, an *adequate treatment trial* is important. Expert consensus guidelines recommend waiting a minimum of three weeks and a maximum of six weeks before making a major change in the treatment regimen (Kane et al., 2003). Some prescribers wait longer than six weeks if the patient is showing a partial response, especially during the second or subsequent trials.

When switching from one atypical agent to another, most prescribers recommend cross-titration as opposed to overlap and taper. *Cross-titration* refers to tapering the dose of the first agent while gradually increasing the dose of the second antipsychotic. In contrast, *overlap* and *taper* refer to continuing the same dose of the first drug while gradually increasing the second drug to a therapeutic level and then tapering the first.

As with the antidepressants, the antipsychotic medications may also be augmented if the patient has a partial response. A combination of an atypical antipsychotic and a mood stabilizer has been used clinically despite the lack of empirical evidence in the literature. Some prescribers use combinations of two atypical antipsychotic agents or one atypical agent and one conventional antipsychotic. Again, there is a lack of data to support these practices. The various combinations of medications usually lead to an increased number of side effects, as well as excessive cost. Symbyax is an example of a combination drug that consists of fluoxetine (Prozac) and olanzapine (Zyprexa) in varying doses. This may be useful in patients with schizophrenia and depression or the depressive phase of bipolar disorder.

Clozapine (Clozaril) is indicated for treatment-refractory schizophrenia. Most clinicians define *treatment refractory* as failing to respond to one or more conventional antipsychotics and two atypical antipsychotics. In addition, approximately 30% to 50% of treatment-refractory patients respond to clozapine. In some instances, electroconvulsive therapy (ECT) may be considered after other options have been exhausted. Remember that the primary goals of treatment are rapid and complete control of acute psychotic symptoms, avoidance of functional deterioration, and prevention of relapse.

CASE VIGNETTES

Case 1

CLINICAL HISTORY

Christopher is a 20-year-old college junior who has just returned from the summer break. He lives in a fraternity on campus that just held its welcome-back beer bash. When the party was over, his two roommates noticed that he was acting strange. At first, they just thought he was drunk and ignored his behavior, but around 3:00 a.m. he started to become paranoid and combative with others in the house. There were reports from observers that he was convinced that his frat brothers were "in a conspiracy with aliens to steal intelligence secrets from the university." It escalated to the point that he barricaded himself in his room and campus security was called. He was taken to a secure psychiatric facility. After examination, it was determined that he was not under the influence of drugs and actually had very little alcohol in his system. He was kept in the facility for 72 hours for further evaluation.

POSTCASE DISCUSSION AND DIAGNOSIS

Christopher's father provided history to the social worker at the facility. As it turns out, Christopher's mother was diagnosed with schizoaffective disorder several years before Christopher's birth and was placed on medication after a stay in the hospital. His older brother was once diagnosed as schizotypal when he was a student in college; he now works as a video game engineer. His maternal grandmother also was diagnosed with a "psychiatric illness" and was hospitalized at various times in her life. There is no psychiatric illness on the father's side of the family. After an examination by the attending psychiatrist, the diagnosis was first-episode Schizophrenia (F20.9).

PSYCHOPHARMACOLOGICAL TREATMENT

Christopher was rather agitated when he arrived at the facility and was given a Zyprexa injection. When he was calmer and had an opportunity to adjust to the unit, he was interviewed by several of the treatment staff. This included a social worker, a psychologist, and the attending psychiatrist. His paranoid ideations continued, and he refused to sit in the dayroom as he was convinced that the TV monitor was beaming messages to the very aliens trying to steal intelligence information. He told staff he could hear their voices even when the monitor was turned off. When staff attempted to work with him and get him to interact with others, he became aggressive and stayed in his room. He was placed on 3 mg daily of risperidone. Over a period of three days, he became less combative and the hallucinations diminished substantially. The dose was increased to 6 mg per day, and Christopher was monitored closely by the staff. His progress continued, and he was discharged two weeks later with a referral for outpatient treatment and medication management.

Case 2

CLINICAL HISTORY

Fiona is a 29-year-old woman who works in a medical factory making medical equipment. She lives with her husband and in-laws. Over the last week, she has been more isolative, saying strange things to her husband, and not sleeping due to unidentified fearfulness. The only stressor that her husband can identify is that they started talking about having children. Fiona refuses to do her ADLs, eats very little, and appears intermittently in a trancelike state. The family was becoming more and more concerned and attempted to get Fiona to see their family doctor, but she was refusing. Finally, police were called due to worsening regressed behavior and Fiona was brought to the local emergency department (ED) for evaluation. The ED physician examined her and reported after labs and neuroimaging that she was medically stable. Although the patient reported no history of psychiatric illness, she did report that her maternal grandmother was in a state hospital for most of her life. The physician recommended psychiatric hospitalization for new onset of a psychotic illness.

POSTCASE DISCUSSION AND DIAGNOSIS

Fiona was admitted to an acute psychiatric unit where she was evaluated by the psychiatrist. After evaluation, observation, and gathering collateral information, the psychiatrist discovered that Fiona had been hospitalized seven years ago at which time she was diagnosed with "probable bipolar disorder or schizophrenia." Although she had been relatively well since then, the psychiatrist believed she has a diagnosis of Schizophrenia (F20.9) given her current presentation. When hospitalized previously, she had taken Abilify 15 mg daily with good response; however, she stopped after a few months as she felt back to normal.

PSYCHOPHARMACOLOGICAL TREATMENT

Fiona was restarted on Abilify 10 mg daily for the first week, which was then increased to 15 mg daily, which was her previous therapeutic dose. After 10 days in the hospital, her psychotic symptoms started to subside and she started acting more like herself per husband. The psychiatrist discussed further treatment options, including a long-acting injectable form of Abilify (e.g., Abilify Maintena). After discussion with the patient and family, Fiona chose the monthly injection rather than having to take pills daily. On the day of discharge, she was given her first injection into her deltoid muscle of Abilify Maintena 400 mg and given a 14-day prescription of Abilify 10 mg daily consistent with the prescribing information. Fiona was set up to see an individual therapist for support and ongoing family counseling as needed. She returned to work within the following week and settled back into life with her family.

CHAPTER 9

Treatment of ADHD and Disorders of Attention

This chapter explores the nature and causes of ADHD and other disorders of attention. Special consideration is given to diagnosis and matching the right behavioral and pharmacological treatment to the needs of patients and their families.

Topics to be addressed include the following:

- Etiology of ADHD
- Diagnostic assessment of attention disorders
- Psychological and pharmacological treatment
- Case vignettes

Attention-deficit disorders are the most common disorders presenting in childhood. Researchers estimate that approximately 3% to 7% of all school-age children have attention-deficit disorders (Kratochvil, Vaughan, Harrington, & Burke, 2003; Polanczyk et al., 2007; Spencer, Biederman, Wilens, & Faraone, 2002). Attention-deficit/hyperactivity disorder (ADHD) is diagnosed two or three times more often in boys than in girls, and it is commonly comorbid with other mental health concerns such as conduct/antisocial personality, substance abuse, anxiety disorders, and mood disorders including pediatric mania (Nevels, Dehone, Alexander, & Gontkovsky, 2010; Solberg et al., 2018; Strange, 2008). Further, it is estimated that as much as 70% of these youth will demonstrate attention-deficit disorder (ADD) or ADHD symptoms into their adult years (Aviram, Rhum, & Levin, 2001; McCann & Roy-Byrne, 2000). The symptoms for adults with these disorders are almost identical to the symptoms seen in children, but adults tend to display less hyperactivity and more internalized restlessness.

Treatment of ADHD can be complicated because many children who meet diagnostic criteria for the disorder may also have comorbid oppositional and conduct disorders (Wilson & Levin, 2001). Wilson and Levin also estimated that approximately 50% of youth treated for substance abuse meet diagnostic criteria for ADHD. Some clinicians are concerned that treating ADHD with stimulants may increase the risk for substance abuse, including possibly abusing the stimulant, but research suggests that treating ADHD early may in fact reduce this risk (Aviram et al., 2001; Wilson & Levin, 2001). Animal studies have indicated that stimulants such as methylphenidate are far less likely to be abused than are other stimulants such as cocaine (Kollins, 2003, 2008). Kollins also found that an ADHD patient is less likely than those without the diagnosis to abuse methylphenidate and other therapeutic stimulants. Moreover, Kollins (2008) found that comorbidity of other psychiatric disorders—especially bipolar disorder, antisocial personality disorder, and eating disorders—were particularly predictive of polydrug and nonmedical stimulant use. Long-acting preparations may be more beneficial because of their higher potential for increased compliance and lower potential for abuse (Bright, 2008; Nair & Moss, 2009). Bright further maintains that mixed amphetamine salts are more likely to be abused than methylphenidate (40% vs. 15%, respectively). Nair and Moss further state that, despite concern about diversion of the drug, recent data suggest that there may be benefits in preventing substance abuse disorders in patients with adult ADHD.

ETIOLOGY OF ADHD

Molecular genetics and neuroimaging studies confirm that disorders of attention like ADHD are heterogeneous neurobiological disorders, mainly of the dopaminergic and noradrenergic pathways (Adler & Chua, 2002). These researchers further found as much as a 50% concordance rate with other first-degree relatives. Subsequent studies have demonstrated frontal lobe dysfunction in the pathophysiology of ADHD and a dysregulation of the neurotransmitters dopamine and norepinephrine in the frontal lobes, the basal ganglia, the amygdala, and possibly the reticular formation (Zimmerman, 2003). More recently, functional MRI scans have shown consistent irregular neurotransmitter activity in the frontal striatal networks and, most important, in the anterior cingulate gyrus (Makris et al., 2010; Weiss & Murray, 2003). These areas of the brain also act like filters, assisting the patient in screening out irrelevant information. In particular, the anterior cingulate acts as a decision-making discrimination system, acting as a "conflict monitor" when making choices (Van Veen & Carter, 2002). Drugs used in the treatment of attention disorders stimulate these brain centers, allowing them to work faster and more efficiently. This stimulation assists the patient with both attention and retention of information.

DIAGNOSTIC ASSESSMENT OF ATTENTION DISORDERS

Attention disorder symptoms for adults and children are essentially the same; however, adults may exhibit less hyperactivity and report more restlessness and agitation. As stated in the DSM-5 diagnostic criteria, considering a childhood history of ADD or ADHD is necessary for the adult diagnosis. A strong family history is usually found. Another important item to remember is the DSM-5 criterion that requires the patient to demonstrate symptoms and behaviors in more than one setting. Various testing and evaluation instruments can assist in making the diagnosis. Common tools used by professionals include: Conners' Rating Scales—Revised (CRS-R), Conners' Adult ADHD Rating Scales (CAARS), Conners' Continuous Performance Test - 3rd Edition (CPT-3), the Attention Deficit/Hyperactivity Disorder Test, the ADHD Problem Checklist, and the Test of Variables of Attention (TOVA) . Once again, to determine if the patient truly has this disorder, the clinician should review all of the DSM criteria and rule out other conditions such as a mood disorder, learning disability, or physical condition (e.g., thyroid abnormality) that could contribute to these symptoms.

PSYCHOLOGICAL AND PHARMACOLOGICAL TREATMENT

Only a few controlled studies have considered the efficacy of psychological treatments for ADHD. Most available studies have emphasized the need for social-skills training, time-management techniques, vocational and career appraisal, and life coaching in addition to addressing poor self-esteem and other stereotypes experienced by these patients (Bemporad, 2001; Weiss & Murray, 2003). Further, studies examining behavioral techniques, such as metacognitive therapy (MCT), and more structured techniques find that such approaches are significantly more effective than traditional unstructured talk therapy for ADHD (Philipsen et al., 2007; Safren et al., 2010; Solanto et al., 2010). These authors and others stress the need for daily coping strategies, including meal planning, conflict resolution, and parenting skills. Good patient education is also necessary to help patients and their families understand the condition and to formulate realistic expectations (Barkley, 2002).

The best treatment approach for attention disorders involves both a psychological and pharmacological approach (Emilsson et al., 2011; Meijer, Faber, van den Ban, & Tobi, 2009).

The use of stimulants and other antidepressants that potentiate levels of dopamine and norepinephrine show the greatest promise. In fact, the pharmacologic treatment of ADHD remains one of the most promising of any disorder in the DSM-5, with a response rate of 70% to 90% in most cases (Strange, 2008). Table 9.1 lists the psychostimulants used in the treatment of ADHD. These are the same stimulants mentioned in Chapter 5 for augmentation of antidepressants. These medications tend to be dose dependent—that is, higher doses typically correspond to better response rates. Typical side effects include hypertension, insomnia, headaches, weight loss, and growth retardation in children. Growth retardation varies from patient to patient and may be mitigated by brief drug holidays, or if pronounced, a treatment interruption (Findling, Childress, Krishnan, & McGough, 2008). In some cases, research on growth suppression is lacking, with insufficient follow-up on patients' final heights (Goldman, 2010). Insomnia is usually controlled by using stimulants with shorter half-lives that wear off before bedtime but may sometimes be treated with the addition of nonstimulant ADHD medications such as guanfacine (Intuniv) (Adler, Reingold, Morrill, & Wilens, 2006; Spencer, Greenbaum, Ginsberg, & Murphy, 2009).

As clinicians know, the potential for abuse with stimulants is high, so they may need to determine the risk of using these substances with patients who have a history of abuse. Also patients who are taking MAOIs; lithium; neuroleptics such as haloperidol (Haldol) and chlorpromazine (Thorazine); certain antidepressants such as amitriptyline (Elavil), nortriptyline (Pamelor), and imipramine (Tofranil); and certain analgesics should refrain from using stimulants unless they are monitored closely.

If the patient is a child who needs to be able to focus during school, after school, and for evening homework, the clinician should consider the longer acting stimulants, such as Adderall XR (a brand of amphetamine salts), Adzenys XR-ODT (a variety of amphetamine with a higher ratio of dextroamphetamine to levoamphetamine), or Concerta (a brand of methylphenidate). If the child has problems with sleeping, the clinician should consider stimulants with shorter half-lives, such as standard dextroamphetamine (Dexedrine) or methylphenidate (Ritalin), or the addition of nonstimulant medications such as guanfacine (Intuniv) that may counteract the insomnia. The longer acting stimulants such as Metadate ER and Ritalin SR (i.e., types of methylphenidate) have a polymer, multiparticulate bead system that allows for breakdown and delivery over several hours. Concerta is a bit more ambitious. It has an outer capsule that delivers an immediate dose and an inner core that is released over 12 hours by gastrointestinal pressure through a laser-drilled hole in the membrane. Once empty, the capsule is passed in the stool. Methylphenidate is also available in a transdermal patch (Daytrana). A transdermal patch eliminates the need for multiple dosing throughout the day and may be helpful for children who show an exaggerated gag reflex when taking oral medications.

Lisdexamfetamine (Vyvanse) is a prodrug psychostimulant of dextroamphetamine available in doses of 30, 50, and 70 mg. The use of a prodrug may greatly reduce the potential for abuse because it depends on first-pass hepatic metabolism. The current formulation is designed to be activated in the liver, and, therefore, any alteration of the original form has decreased pharmacological activity. While research on the long-term use of stimulants is lacking in adults, lisdexamfetamine appears generally well tolerated and effective for long-term use in children with ADHD (Findling et al., 2008). Further, it does not appear to be a significant contributor to insomnia in adults with ADHD (Adler, Goodman, Weisler, Hamdani, & Roth, 2009).

Any patient with ADHD should see a physician for a complete physical. Patients with glaucoma, hypertension, and tic disorders should be evaluated and counseled by their primary care physician before starting stimulants.

Table 9.1	Psychostimulant Medications		
Trade Name	**Generic Name**	**Child/Adult Typical Dose (mg/day)**	**Level of Insomnia**
Adderall,	amphetamine/mixed salts	5–30/5–60	**
Adderall-XR[3]		12.5–30/12.5–50	***
Mydayis[3]			***
Cylert	pemoline	37.5–112.5	**
Dexedrine	dextroamphetamine	5–10/5–60	*
Dextrostat			*
Dexedrine Spansules			**
Desoxyn	methamphetamine	5–25/5–30	*
Evekeo	amphetamine sulfate	2.5–40/5–40	*
Adzenys XR-ODT		3.1–18.8/12.5–18.8	**
Dyanavel XR Oral Susp		2.5–5	**
Focalin[1]	dexmethylphenidate	5–30/5–40	*
Focalin XR[2]		5–40	***
Ritalin[1]	methylphenidate	10–30/10–40	*
Ritalin-SR		10–60	**
Methylin-ER		10–60	**
Metadate-ER[2]		10–60	**
Aptensio XR		10–60	**
Quillivant XR		10–60	**
QuilliChew ER		10–60	**
Cotempla XR-ODT		8.6–51.8	**
Daytrana Transdermal		12.5–37.5 cm^2	***
Concerta[3]		18–54	***
Vyvanse	lisdexamfetamine	30–70	***

[1] Effective for 2–6 hours
[2] Effective for 6–8 hours
[3] Once per day dosing
* Minimal neurotransmission; **Moderate neurotransmission; ***Significant neurotransmission; **** Major neurotransmission

In addition to the psychostimulants, antidepressants and alpha-adrenergic agonists are used in the treatment of ADHD (see Table 9.2). The response from antidepressants and alpha-2 agonists is usually not as robust as stimulants, however. Alpha-2 agonists such as clonidine (Catapres) and guanfacine (Tenex and Intuniv) may enhance prefrontal cortical regulation of attention and impulse control. With optimal prefrontal cortical regulation, the locus ceruleus fires to relevant, but not irrelevant, information, thus improving overall attention (Strange, 2008).

Table 9.2	Antidepressants and Alpha-Adrenergic Agonists Used in the Treatment of ADHD	
Trade Name	**Generic Name**	**Typical Dose (mg/day)**
Catapres, Kapvay	clonidine	0.2–0.9
Effexor	venlafaxine	50–300
Effexor XR		75–300
Intuniv	guanfacine extended release	1–4
Norpramin	desipramine	150–300
Pamelor	nortriptyline	75–125
Strattera	atomoxetine	40–100
Tenex	guanfacine	1–9
Wellbutrin	bupropion	75–450
Wellbutrin SR	bupropion	100–400
Wellbutrin XL	bupropion	150–450

Since the use of alpha-2 agonists may lower blood pressure, regular monitoring and cardiac evaluation are advised. These medications may be a good alternative for patients who cannot tolerate stimulants or the problems with insomnia they may cause. As mentioned in Chapter 5, antidepressants must be prescribed cautiously for children and adolescents because of the FDA warning about an increase in suicidal thinking and behaviors. For more complete information on medication side effects, see Chapter 5 or the Appendix.

Many experts who treat patients with ADHD have found that a combination of psychotherapy, stimulants, and antidepressants offers a complete and direct treatment approach to the condition. Stimulants work for most patients, and in some cases antidepressants offer symptom relief. Atomoxetine (Strattera) is a stimulating antidepressant that increases levels of norepinephrine. It has been shown to be effective in both children and adults, it may be slightly more effective in younger children (6–7 years) than in older children (8–12 years), but younger children may report greater rates of GI upset and somnolence (Kratochvil, Milton, Vaughan, & Greenhill, 2008). Antidepressants with stimulating qualities often are prescribed alone for the condition. Bupropion (Wellbutrin) is most often the antidepressant of choice because it does not interfere with most stimulants and offers enriched levels of dopamine and norepinephrine. Some research may suggest that males and females may respond to bupropion differently. Males appear to respond to bupropion regardless of ADHD type. Females with combined type, but not inattentive type, responded better than those with other ADHD types (Wilens et al., 2005). Though not FDA approved, tricyclics such as desipramine have been shown to be efficacious, but side effects and cardiotoxicity may preclude their use with some patients.

Medications are typically given by titrating doses upward until complete symptomatic relief is obtained. It is not uncommon for parents to request drug holidays for children in the nonschool, summer months. This practice often helps allow growing periods for the child since many stimulants can stunt growth.

Many parents today are concerned about placing their child on drugs, especially stimulants. They will often cite newspaper articles and pieces from popular magazines suggesting that behavioral therapy alone is sufficient. Some parents believe that diet alone will improve their child's symptoms. Although sugary snacks certainly do not help children with ADHD, the connection between sweets and behavior is not conclusive. In most cases, children and adults with moderate-to-severe cases of ADHD do not respond adequately to dietary changes, behavioral interventions, and environmental changes alone. The clinician should educate the parents and the patient about the benefits of medications. The proof will be apparent in the child's behavior and academic performance. Nothing else, aside from counseling, is better for raising self-esteem and ensuring a healthy sense of independence.

CASE VIGNETTES

Case 1

CLINICAL HISTORY

Jacob is an eight-year-old African American boy who lives with his mother and younger sister. His parents are separated, and he sees his father on twice-per-month visits. While Jacob has always been a very active child who loves sports and anything related to video games and wrestling, even his father has noticed that his behavior has gotten a bit out of control. He has noticed that Jacob can be a bit hard to discipline and doesn't seem to listen when he is spoken to directly. In consultation with his teacher and principal, and after speaking with the school counselor, who has spoken with Jacob about several of his detentions after class, it was determined to refer him to the school psychologist for learning disabilities evaluation.

Jacob is essentially a happy child, but he often disrupts his second-grade class with excessive talking and walking around the room, although he returns to his seat when asked. He also often interrupts the teacher to ask to use the restroom or sharpen his pencil. He also blurts out answers and won't let others answer questions without interrupting them. The teacher has also noticed that he can't seem to wait his turn in both board games and in games on the playground. She is concerned about his grades, and he appears to be having trouble with retention of information from one subject to another. Reading comprehension is especially difficult for him.

Various evaluation questionnaires were given to Jacob, his teacher, the principal of his school, and his parents. It is clear that these behaviors are problematic in several settings. In fact, Jacob failed a spelling quiz because he forgot to study for it. He also forgot to take home a permission slip for a field trip to the zoo and was not allowed to go. He frequently loses books, backpacks, and sporting equipment. His coach said he might not be able to stay on the team if he forgets to attend another practice after school.

POSTCASE DISCUSSION AND DIAGNOSIS

After examining the questionnaires completed by Jacob, his parents, his teacher, and his principal, Jacob was referred to the school psychologist for a battery of tests. The results confirm that Jacob appears to have significant evidence for Attention-Deficit/Hyperactivity Disorder, Predominantly Hyperactive Type (F90.1). Jacob's father also had this condition when he was younger, but he did not continue to have symptoms into his adult years. There is no history of other mental illness or substance use in his family, and his sister appears to be without a learning difficulty.

PSYCHOPHARMACOLOGICAL TREATMENT

Jacob was evaluated by his pediatrician. After reading the psychologist's report, the pediatrician agreed with the diagnosis and placed Jacob on 18 mg of Concerta each morning. Within a few weeks, Jacob's grades improved and he was better able to attend to school tasks and homework. He was tolerating the medication well, but there were reports of some insomnia. He was switched to methylphenidate 15 mg every morning and again at 3:00 p.m. This dose appeared to work well without excessive stimulation at bedtime.

Case 2

CLINICAL HISTORY

Sam is a 35-year-old white male who lives with his girlfriend of 10 years. His family lives out of state, and he reports limited contact with them or friends. Sam reports that throughout his childhood school was "easy when [he] wanted to do it" but that he struggled to self-motivate when uninterested in a topic. Sam reports generally earning good grades in school, although he indicates that his assignments were generally "turned in at the last minute." After high school, Sam attended trade school to become a photographer, and he reports previous employment as a photo editor and freelance photographer. Since leaving college, however, Sam reports difficulty maintaining meaningful employment, describing fears that he will "get bored and not return to work" and leading him to "disappoint everyone."

Sam reports that in social settings he often likes to "be the center of attention" and that others often describe his behavior as "loud" and that he "doesn't understand why." During therapy, Sam evidences a similar level of increased volume and tangential speech, often changing topics midsentence when a newer topic becomes more interesting to him. Sam states that prior therapists attempted to treat him for bipolar disorder but that mood stabilizers and antidepressants had minimal therapeutic impact.

Presently, Sam remains unemployed, citing his fears over following through with any work-related tasks. Evaluations of Sam confirm that he struggles staying on task in nearly all settings, often forgetting key tasks until after their respective due dates.

Sam also reports a history of regular marijuana use, as well as occasional recreational use of cocaine "once or twice a year." Sam reports that both drugs lead to temporary improvement of his ability to focus on tasks but that the improvements quickly subside.

POSTCASE DISCUSSION AND DIAGNOSIS

After initial evaluation, Sam was referred to a psychiatrist for further testing. Testing confirmed that Sam's symptoms were likely caused by an underlying, previously undiagnosed Attention-Deficit/Hyperactivity Disorder, Combined Type (F90.2) and not Bipolar Disorder or any other related mood disorder. Sam reports no family history of any psychiatric diagnoses or substance abuse but admits that his mother evidences similar difficulties with staying focused.

PSYCHOPHARMACOLOGICAL TREATMENT

Sam was evaluated by his psychiatrist and placed on 15 mg of dextroamphetamine (Adderall) twice per day (b.i.d.). Within a few days, Sam reported increased ability to focus on individual tasks, as well as a significantly decreased desire for nonmedical drugs such as cocaine or marijuana. Despite otherwise tolerating the medication, Sam complained of severe insomnia, often remaining awake until 1:00 a.m. Sam's Adderall dosage was subsequently decreased to 10 mg b.i.d. However, Sam complained that the medication was no longer effective at this lowered dose. Similarly, attempts to reduce dosage to 15 mg once per day resulted in reduced concentration after about 3:00 p.m. each afternoon. Ultimately, Sam was placed back on 10 mg Adderall b.i.d. with the addition of 2 mg Intuniv (guanfacine) in the evening for its sedating properties. This modified dosing schedule appeared to work well, improving his ADHD symptoms with few significant side effects and reduced insomnia.

CHAPTER | 10

Treatment of Cognitive Disorders

This chapter presents a discussion of the various forms and causes of dementia and how best to treat them and reduce the negative aspects caused by these conditions. The advantages and disadvantages of various medications for cognitive decline are explored and discussed.

Topics to be addressed include the following:

- Forms of dementia
- Alzheimer's disease
- Medical and behavioral evaluation
- Medications for cognitive disorders
- Other approaches to cognitive enhancement
- Other significant issues to consider
- Case vignettes

The cognitive disorders consist of delirium and dementia, although this chapter focuses mainly on dementia. Delirium is an acute confusional state that is basically a medical emergency; the patient needs acute medical treatment to find the etiology of the confusion and treat it accordingly. For the most part, delirium would not be part of a patient's clinical presentation to outpatient treatment setting. On the other hand, dementia is becoming more of an issue as the population ages. Alzheimer's disease (AD), the most common type of dementia, affects more than 15 million people worldwide; the United States has about 4 million people with the disease (Grossberg, 2003). According to the National Institute of Aging, the cost associated with caring for a dementia patient is more than $250,000 per person over their lifetime, which is 57% more than for other illnesses (www.nia.nih.gov/Alzheimers). It is estimated that as much as 20% of the general population over the age of 60 will be affected with mild cognitive impairment (MCI) (Marcos et al., 2015). This research also suggests that conversion rates from MCI to Alzheimer's disease is greater for those with less education and that the rates increase sharply with age. Marcos et al. also estimate that in 4.5 years as many as 15% of patients with DSM-5–diagnosed MCI will develop more serious dementia. Grossberg (2003) further reports that about 1 in 45 Americans will eventually be diagnosed with AD. It is also estimated that 34 million persons worldwide will suffer with some form of dementia by 2025 (Toda, Kaneko, & Kogen, 2010).

FORMS OF DEMENTIA

Dementia has many different forms that include memory disturbance as their central feature. The three most common forms are Alzheimer's disease, dementia with Lewy bodies, and vascular dementia.

Alzheimer's disease accounts for approximately 55% to 60% of all irreversible dementias. To date, no single factor causing AD has been identified (Toda et al., 2010). It will be discussed as the prototype for our purposes although other less common diagnoses may be treated in a similar fashion. In addition to memory problems, Alzheimer's disease is characterized by either aphasia, apraxia, and/or agnosia. Toda et al. (2010) further state that neuropathologically AD is identified by amyloid plaque, neurofibrillary tangles, and synaptic loss. A loss of acetylcholine, a critical neurotransmitter, is also noted. Currently, an autopsy is the only definitive way to diagnose AD, but various cognitive psychological tests and scans are typically used. Maybe one day there will be a blood test to determine if one has Alzheimer's. Some possibilities are currently in testing because using diagnostic tools such as PET and SPECT scans is terribly expensive, and testing of cerebral spinal fluid is very invasive (Paraskevaidi et al., 2017).

Dementia with Lewy bodies (DLB) is the second most common type of dementia, accounting for about 20% to 25% of cases; it is characterized by memory dysfunction with visual hallucinations, Parkinsonism, and/or fluctuating alertness levels. DLB and another cause of dementia, Parkinson's disease, probably have similar neuropathology. Vascular dementia is the third most common type, but it accounts for less than 20% of all cases. Classically, vascular dementia was thought to be the second most common type, ahead of DLB, and it was then known as multi-infarct dementia (MID). The less common forms of dementia include the following: frontotemporal dementia (i.e., Pick's disease), corticobasal degeneration, progressive supranuclear palsy, Creutzfeldt-Jakob disease, neurosyphillis, normal-pressure hydrocephalus, and HIV-associated dementia (Boeve, Silber, & Ferman, 2002).

Overall, these disorders are a significant public health concern because of their economic burden. According to the Alzheimer's Association (2013), the cost of Alzheimer's disease alone is over $605 billion worldwide, or about 1% of the entire world's gross domestic product. These figures are expected to triple in the coming years due to aging baby boomers. It is estimated that 5.5 million Americans are living in 2017 with Alzheimer's, and it is expected to reach 7.1 million by 2025 (Larson et al., 2013). Of the total costs of care, direct patient care accounts for 31%, lost productivity due to illness or premature mortality accounts for 20%, and unpaid caregiver cost accounts for the remaining 49%. As the number of patients and the cost to society increases, we will all be facing this issue at some point, either professionally or personally (Grossberg, 2003; Toda et al., 2010).

ALZHEIMER'S DISEASE

Alzheimer's disease is characterized by gradual onset and is marked by progressive decline in cognition; motor function declines in the later stages. Research indicates that several neurotransmission pathways may be involved, including *cholinergic, glutamatergic, serotonergic,* and *dopaminergic.* Currently, loss of cholinergic neurons appears to be the most important abnormality. In the mid-1970s, researchers discovered a deficit in brain presynaptic cholinergic systems in post mortem brain tissue in patients with AD (Davies & Maloney, 1976). This discovery has led to a major finding: Acetylcholinesterase inhibitors, which increase intrasynaptic acetylcholine levels, produce moderate symptomatic improvement in AD.

Inflammatory processes may also play a role in the disease progression. Beta-amyloid (amyloid-β) plaques are the most widely studied neuropathological change in AD. These plaques do not affect the whole nervous system uniformly but, rather, only certain vulnerable cortical and subcortical areas; the sensory and motor regions of the brain tend to remain unaffected. Chronic neuroinflammation may be responsible for the degeneration of cholinergic neurons via a chain of inflammatory processes initiated by beta-amyloid (Rhein et al., 2009).

Sometimes a faulty gene may cause the problem, as in the familial form of AD. On the other hand, the more common form of the disease is known as sporadic AD. The genes that contribute to AD appear in all cells, but their expression varies in different areas of the brain and in different individuals. Obviously, the neuroanatomy and neurochemistry are very complex and beyond the scope of this chapter.

MEDICAL AND BEHAVIORAL EVALUATION OF COGNITIVE DISORDERS

As part of the medical evaluation of cognitive disorders, an inventory of currently prescribed and over-the-counter medications must be reviewed and analyzed as potential causes. Behavioral toxicity associated with pharmacotherapy is the most common etiology of reversible delirium. Appropriate laboratory evaluation, including serum electrolytes, blood urea nitrogen (BUN) levels, serum B_{12} level, and thyroid-function tests, should be done. Vitamin B_{12} deficiency and hypothyroidism may present as reversible causes of a cognitive disorder if detected in the earlier stages. A diagnostic neuroimaging procedure (CT or MRI of the brain) is commonly used to rule out tumors, subdural hematomas, and normal-pressure hydrocephalus. The clinician should obtain a past psychiatric history from the patient or family because patients with major mental illness can also develop dementia in later life (e.g., schizophrenia complicated by AD).

The medical aspects of cognitive disorders are certainly important. In addition, the clinician also needs to look at behavioral factors that precipitate or contribute to some of the dysfunction. Patients with dementia who have poor short-term memory and disorientation may appear quite compensated as long as they remain in a familiar environment that does not require new learning. Furthermore, when these patients are moved to a hospital, nursing home, or other unfamiliar setting, they may become disoriented and disorganized, leading to physical aggression and acting out. Once the patient adapts to the new environment, behavioral problems may resolve spontaneously over a month or so. If aphasia is part of the dementia, patients have difficulty expressing themselves. This difficulty may present as grabbing or aggressive behaviors when a patient is in pain or needs to go to the restroom. Patients who are apraxic may be unable to carry out their routine activities of daily living, which leads to agitation and/or low frustration tolerance. In addition, family and staff visits are not always welcomed by the patient. If any particular behavior patterns arise, hospital or nursing home staff may need to observe interactions and determine the triggers of these behavioral problems (Goldberg, 2002).

MEDICATIONS FOR COGNITIVE DISORDERS

Only a few approved medications are available for treatment of Alzheimer's disease (see Table 10.1). These drugs improve cognitive function only modestly; however, they are best conceptualized as drugs that "stabilize" cognition, activities of daily living, and behavioral function. Basically, the cholinesterase inhibitors slow the clinical deterioration in AD, but they do not cure it. In the early 1990s, tacrine (Cognex) was the first cholinesterase inhibitor demonstrated to be effective in the treatment of AD. Unfortunately, liver toxicity has significantly limited its use in treatment.

Second-generation cholinesterase inhibitors, such as donepezil (Aricept), have been shown to be as effective as tacrine without the hepatic toxicity. Donepezil has shown positive effects on cognition and overall functioning in AD patients with mild-to-moderate disease (Rogers & Friedhoff, 1996). Although a 23 mg dose is now available, no significant improvements were noted with the higher dose, but patients did experience an increase in side effects (Advokat, Comaty, & Julien, 2014). This medication is easy to use because it is given once daily and has three therapeutic doses: 5 mg, 10 mg, and 23 mg. A patch is also currently being considered for FDA approval. As with all the cholinesterase inhibitors, the most common side effects are gastrointestinal symptoms, including nausea, vomiting, and diarrhea. Donepezil also appears to extend its benefit into more advanced stages of AD than initially thought. Some research maintains that donepezil may also be better tolerated than other AD medications due to a lower risk for GI upset

Table 10.1	Medications for Cognitive Disorders		
Trade Name	**Generic Name**	**Typical Dose (mg/day)**	**Chemical Class**
Aricept	donepezil	5–10–23	cholinesterase inhibitor
Cognex	tacrine	40–160	cholinesterase inhibitor
Exelon	rivastigmine	6–12	cholinesterase inhibitor
Exelon Patch	rivastigmine transdermal system	4.6–9.5 mg/24 hrs	cholinesterase inhibitor
Namenda	memantine	10–20	NMDA receptor antagonist
Namenda XR	memantine	7–14–21–28	NMDA receptor antagonist
Namzaric	memantine/ donepezil	7/10; 14/10; 21/10; 28/10	combination of both medications
Reminyl	galantamine	16–24	cholinesterase inhibitor

when compared to rivastigmine and galantamine (Lockhart, Mitchell, & Kelly, 2009). Feldman et al., (2001) demonstrated significant benefits using cholinesterase inhibitors in moderate to severe AD with continued good tolerability as far as side effects are concerned.

Rivastigmine (Exelon) is another medication used in treatment of AD. In addition to inhibiting acetylcholinesterase, rivastigmine inhibits butyrylcholinesterase. The clinical significance of this latter effect remains to be determined, but butyrylcholinesterase appears to regulate brain acetylcholine levels in animal studies (Blazer, Steffens, & Busse, 2004). Gastrointestinal effects of rivastigmine occur in up to 40% of patients, which is more than with donepezil. Some evidence suggests that rivastigmine may be effective with behavioral problems that are particularly prominent in dementia with Lewy bodies and in patients experiencing a more aggressive course of dementia—in particular, patients with hallucinations (Cummings et al., 2010). The transdermal rivastigmine patch (Exelon Patch), approved in 2007, provides the option of a continuous medication delivery method that is less likely to cause the GI upset associated with oral medications because of fluctuating drug plasma levels (Darreh-Shori & Jelic, 2010; Wentrup, Oertel, & Dodel, 2008).

The final cholinesterase inhibitor is galantamine (Reminyl), which also modulates the nicotinic acetylcholine receptor responsiveness at an allosteric binding site (Blazer et al., 2004). Because a prominent nicotinic cholinergic deficit exists in AD, this additional benefit may be clinically useful. The dosage titration with galantamine is more cumbersome; the maximum dose is 24 mg/day. The side-effect profile looks similar to donepezil if galantamine is slowly increased to a therapeutic dose.

Another class of medications being used are the N-methyl-D-aspartate (NMDA) receptor antagonists. According to the glutamate excitotoxicity hypothesis, beta-amyloid indirectly stimulates the production of excessive glutamate; glutamate in turn overstimulates the NMDA receptors. This process results in neuronal death because of the chronic excitation. To reduce the negative effect of glutamate, experts theorize that intervening as early as possible in the process of AD would help the patient most. Glutamate is thought to play a more prominent role in the early stages of AD rather than the late stages. The medication memantine (Namenda) was approved in late 2003 for use in AD. The most common side effects of memantine include agitation, urinary incontinence, urinary tract infection, and insomnia. Tariot, Farlow, Grossberg, Graham, and McDonald (2004) have reported that memantine, when used in combination with cholinesterase inhibitors, may be useful in patients with more moderate to severe AD. In fact, the use of cholinesterase inhibitors may delay nursing home admissions in cognitively impaired patients, but it may not be helpful in reducing agitation in AD patients (Fox et al., 2012). This effect was significantly enhanced with the addition of memantine (Lopez et al., 2009) and the newer medication Namzaric combines the two (memantine and donepezil) into one medication.

OTHER APPROACHES TO COGNITIVE ENHANCEMENT

Vitamin E and other antioxidants have been used to slow the progression of aging and dementia (Sano et al., 1997). Vitamin E may slow the deterioration associated with AD but not necessarily in the cognitive domain. Some studies found that antioxidants were more effective than placebo in delaying deterioration to functional endpoints such as nursing home placement or substantial loss of ability to perform activities of daily living. The dose of vitamin E recommended in the studies was 1,000 IU given twice daily.

Another medication to consider is selegiline (Eldepryl), which is a selective inhibitor of monoamine oxidase. This medication is used most commonly in Parkinson's disease but may also be used for depression given that it is an MAOI. The doses of selegiline used in the studies were 10 to 40 mg daily. As with vitamin E, treatment with selegiline slows functional deterioration but has little effect on cognitive decline.

Extracts of the leaf of the ginkgo biloba tree have been used in traditional Chinese medications and may have antioxidant, anti-inflammatory, and stimulant properties. A standardized extract of ginkgo biloba has been studied; the results show a small but statistically significant effect on cognitive functioning (Le Bars et al., 1997), but newer studies do not appear to show much effect on memory (Vellas et al., 2012). The improvement was approximately one-half of the effect seen with the cholinesterase inhibitors. Currently, ginkgo biloba is being studied further to evaluate its effectiveness and usefulness.

Studies in postmenopausal women suggest that estrogen replacement therapy decreases the risk of AD for this population. Evidence is still conflicted as to whether conjugated estrogens or more naturally occurring forms are neuroprotective. Keep in mind that treatment with estrogens may also increase the risk of heart disease and breast cancer (Jaturapaptporn et al., 2012; Warren, 2004).

Research suggests that nonsteroidal anti-inflammatory drugs (NSAIDs) might decrease the risk of AD in some patients. By decreasing the inflammation caused by the plaques containing beta-amyloid, the neurons incur less damage and cell death; however, there appears to be little benefit to patients already suffering from AD symptoms (Wentrup et al., 2008). Unfortunately, the potent anti-inflammatory steroid prednisone failed to show any positive effect on cognition or disease progression (Aisen, 2002; Jaturapaptporn et al., 2012). Trials using naproxen (Naprosyn) and rofecoxib (Vioxx) also have been negative. Rofecoxib has been withdrawn from worldwide markets because of the increased risk of heart attack and stroke. Some clinicians have suggested that certain types of NSAIDs and aspirin may decrease beta-amyloid production and that other types do not. At this time, the use of NSAIDs and aspirin does not seem promising in the treatment of AD; however, they may be helpful in prevention.

Agents that lower cholesterol may be useful in preventing AD. Lipid-lowering agents, such as various statin drugs, are associated with a decrease in central nervous system amyloid deposition in animal models (Advokat et al., 2014; Sano, 2003). Atorvastatin (Lipitor), simvastatin (Zocor), and pravastatin (Pravachol) are common examples of statins. Clinical trials are currently underway to evaluate their usefulness in the treatment of AD.

Several investigational medications and nutraceuticals currently are being studied to determine their effectiveness with this population. AD, as has been mentioned, is characterized by deposition of amyloid-β (Aβ) plaques and neurofibrillary tangles in the brain, accompanied by synaptic dysfunction and neurodegeneration. Antibody-based immunotherapy substances, such as aducanumab, appear to work against Aβ to trigger its clearance or mitigate its neurotoxicity (Sevigny et al., 2016). These authors report the generation of aducanumab, a human monoclonal antibody, that selectively targets aggregated Aβ. In a transgenic mouse model of AD, aducanumab is shown to enter the brain, bind parenchymal Aβ, and reduce soluble and insoluble Aβ in a dose-dependent manner. Further studies are planned to determine its effectiveness. Recent research using a tau protein inhibitor, leuco-methylthioninium bis hydromethanesulfanate (LMTM), appears to show that the drug helps improve cognitive functions and activities in daily living for AD patients when it is used as a monotherapy (Gauthier et al., 2016). Ongoing research that is looking at such substances as oleocanthal (a chemical found in certain olive oils), latrepirdine (a Russian antihistamine), zinc, various antioxidants, continine (derived from tobacco), orcein (a red dye compound), fish oils, and cinnamaldehyde (a cinnamon compound) may be helpful to both treat and prevent the development of the disease (Advokat et al., 2014).

OTHER SIGNIFICANT ISSUES TO CONSIDER

Behavioral complications of dementia include physical agitation, verbal aggression, physical aggression, depression, and psychosis. Research suggests that as many as 50% of all AD patients may present with aggressive and agitated symptoms (Advokat et al., 2014; Amann et al., 2009; Larson et al., 2013). An organized way to approach patients with behavioral problems is to define some *target symptoms*, which will dictate the treatment protocol. For example, an atypical antipsychotic agent would be considered a starting point for an AD patient presenting with agitation, aggression, or psychotic symptoms. Risperidone (Risperdal) has been effective in this situation, with dosages up to 2 mg with minimal side effects. However, the use of atypical antipsychotic medications in the elderly has been associated with an increase in cerebrovascular events (stroke and transient ischemic attacks) and even death. Their use should be considered only when behavioral redirection has not worked and when their benefits outweigh their risks (Herrmann & Gauthier, 2008). Low doses of some of the newer medications, such as lurasidone (Latuda) or brexpiprazole (Rexulti), could also be considered. Typical antipsychotic medications, such as haloperidol (Haldol) or chlorpromazine (Thorazine), should be avoided if possible because they present a high risk of tardive dyskinesia (TD) in the elderly (see Chapter 8 for more information on TD).

Another option for a patient with agitation would be mood stabilizers. Carbamazepine (Tegretol) or oxcarbazepine (Trileptal), as well as valproate (Depakote), have been used in low-to-moderate doses with an overall decrease in agitation; however, pharmacokinetic interactions with secondary enzyme induction limit the use of this drug. Lamotrigine (Lamictal), gabapentin (Neurontin), or topiramate (Topamax) may be safer choices (Amann et al., 2009).

If an AD patient primarily has depressive and anxiety symptoms, an SSRI would be an excellent choice. Some research suggests that dual inhibition of cholinesterase and serotonin reuptake would greatly improve the effect of AD medications and perhaps mitigate the dose-related side effects of most AD medications (Toda et al., 2010). Some research also suggests that

SSRIs may delay conversion from mild cognitive impairment to Alzheimer's by as much as three years. It is believed that drugs like Citalopram may reduce the formation of amyloid plaque (Bartels et al., 2017). Although the use of citalopram has reduced agitation in AD patients, its use in patients with full-blown Alzheimer's may actually worsen symptoms and lead to an increase in anorexia, diarrhea, and falls (Porsteinsson, 2014).

The information regarding antidepressant medications discussed in previous chapters will be applicable here. *Note that caution should be used in medicating elderly patients given the high prevalence of polypharmacy and multiple medical diagnoses.*

While several studies suggest that physical exercise does not improve cognitive outcomes for dementia patients, it does improve physical functioning of elderly patients and may delay nursing home placement (Sabia et al., 2017).

Except for Alzheimer's disease, the data on the treatment of other dementia syndromes are sparse. Vascular dementia, for example, rarely occurs in isolation. More commonly, a combination of two neuropathological processes may occur together, referred to as a *mixed dementia*. These types of dementias may respond to the treatment options suggested for Alzheimer's disease alone.

CASE VIGNETTES

Case 1

CLINICAL HISTORY

Eleanor is a 77-year-old white female resident of a skilled nursing facility. Recently her daughter requested an evaluation from the staff psychologist because she noticed that her mother's Alzheimer's symptoms appeared to be getting worse. Eleanor was admitted to the facility six months ago with moderately severe cognitive and physical decline and had to be placed in a skilled facility since she could no longer manage herself at home. Her daughter is a single mother of four teens and works too many hours to care for her mother in her home. She had attempted to care for her until Eleanor left the stove on, resulting in a minor kitchen fire. Eleanor has no history of mental illness, but she began to show signs of cognitive decline in her late fifties. The symptoms became much more pronounced after her husband's death five years ago.

Recently her daughter and other members of the nursing staff noticed that Eleanor has become rather restless and combative. When she gets confused over her surroundings, she wanders through the halls attempting to open fire doors. When nurses attempt to redirect her back to her room, she swears at them and even struck one of them in the face. Her PCP authorized the use of restraints one day after she managed to wander out the front door and was found standing in the middle of the street trying to take a dog away from a woman who was walking it. She yelled at the woman, telling her that she needed the dog to protect her from people who were stealing her clothing in the nursing home.

POSTCASE DISCUSSION AND DIAGNOSIS

Eleanor has Dementia of the Alzheimer's Type with Behavioral Disturbance (F02.81). Her condition has worsened in the last few months. She seldom recognizes her daughter when she visits and now has become rather combative with staff. She often becomes both extremely confused and inconsolable when she is agitated. Staff members have reported that it is difficult to feed her because she often gets angry and throws food on the floor. She will no longer bathe without constant redirection from staff, and they are willing only to assist with sponge baths because she is too much to handle in the shower room.

PSYCHOPHARMACOLOGICAL TREATMENT

Upon evaluation and consultation with the geriatric psychologist and the facility social worker, Eleanor's physician adjusted the medication regimen. In addition to the 10 mg per day of Aricept and 10 mg per day of Namenda that she was already taking, 2 mg of risperidone was added. After one week with partial improvement of symptoms, trazodone 50 mg q.h.s. was added for continued sleep difficulties. Within a week, staff reported that Eleanor was much less agitated and combative. She had no further paranoid delusions, and restraints were no longer needed. Her daughter noticed no changes in her cognitive abilities, and Eleanor was much more pleasant to visit with and would occasionally walk with her in the garden without the need for staff present.

Case 2

CLINICAL HISTORY

Walter is a 74-year-old African American male who is being cared for by his wife and a part-time care assistant at their home. He was diagnosed with AD about four years ago. While he is managed well in the home, both his wife and the caregiver have noticed an increase in cognitive decline, especially in memory and confusion. While Walter is usually able to be left alone for several minutes as he often watches TV or listens to music, lately he has been getting up and walking outside unattended. He recently was found on the street nearly two blocks from their home in a confused state after his wife and the caregiver went to the kitchen to prepare lunch. Both Walter and his wife would like for him to remain in the home as long as possible.

POSTCASE DISCUSSION AND DIAGNOSIS

Walter appears to have Major neurocognitive disorder due to Alzheimer's Disease Without Behavioral Disturbance (F02.80). The condition appears to have gotten worse in the last two months, and although he is not combative or psychotic, he is often frightened by his environment when he travels out of the home or when strangers come to the house.

PSYCHOPHARMACOLOGICAL TREATMENT

The caregiver and his physician agreed that Walter should be allowed to remain in the home as long as he is able. The newer medication Namzaric, which is a combination drug of memantine and donepezil, has been shown to increase cognitive function and delay the necessity for admission to a care facility. Walter was started at the dose of 7/10 mg per day, and this was increased over several weeks to the full dose of 28/10 mg. Other than some mild nausea, Walter was tolerating the medication well and showing fewer signs of confusion and memory loss. He did begin to complain of mild depression, so a low 5 mg dose of escitalopram was added in the morning dose, which appeared to help.

CHAPTER 11

Treatment of Sleep Disorders

This chapter thoroughly explores sleep disturbances, primary sleep disorders, and parasomnias. Various treatment issues and options are presented and discussed.

Topics to be addressed include the following:

- Stages of sleep
- Sleep disorders and conditions
- Behavioral techniques for treating sleep disorders
- Pharmacology for sleep disorders
- Holistic treatments
- Case vignettes

Sleep disturbances are a frequently cited problem by mental health patients. Many of these patients also have comorbid physical conditions that interfere with the quality of their sleep, and many also have other mood or personality disorders that can cause secondary sleep disturbances. Some patients experience sleep disturbances related to substance use or abuse. Research has established that those with sleep disorders are at increased risk for developing hypertension and suffering cardiovascular morbidity and mortality (Richert & Baran, 2003). The most common sleep complaints made by mental health patients involve initial insomnia (difficulty falling asleep) or intermittent awakening throughout the night (middle insomnia). Some patients may fall asleep normally but awaken very early in the morning, with difficulty falling back to sleep (terminal insomnia). A national survey of more than a thousand adults studied by researchers found that 43% reported middle-of-the-night awakening; of those, 26% could not return to sleep and 34% complained of daytime fatigue. A similar study found that as many as 56% had difficulty with initial insomnia, and 67% experienced intermittent awakening (Scharf, 2001). Insomnia is a rather common disorder and can affect nearly everyone at various times of their lives, and it becomes chronic for about 10% of the population (Hardeland, 2009).

STAGES OF SLEEP

There are five distinct stages of sleep. Stages 1 and 2, the theta stages, are rather light stages of sleep. If patients' names were called out during these stages, they would probably awaken without feeling groggy. People spend about 50% of sleep time in stages 1 and 2.

Stages 3 and 4 are the delta stages of sleep, which are characterized by slow brain-wave patterns and very deep, restorative sleep. Here, shaking the patient is necessary to awaken him or her, and the patient would be groggy. People spend about 20% of their sleep time in these stages.

Stage 5 is the rapid eye movement or REM stage. It occupies about 25% of sleep and is characterized by both theta- and delta-type activities that resemble the wave patterns seen while awake. Most dreams occur during this stage. If patients are sleep deprived, they demonstrate additional time spent in stages 3, 4, and REM during their next sleep period, which is called the *rebound phenomenon* (Carlson, 2004). Serotonin is necessary to maintain adequate sleep, especially in stages 1–4 (Monti & Jantos, 2014). Norepinephrine is necessary for REM sleep; so, not surprisingly, depressed patients with lower levels of serotonin and norepinephrine experience problems with the quality of their sleep.

When discussing sleep concerns with a patient, the clinician needs to determine if the patient has a primary sleep disturbance—that is, a sleep disorder that is not caused by a medical, psychiatric, or substance abuse–related issue. In such cases, the clinician must collect adequate history information to ensure that no other complicating conditions or factors exist. The clinician should inquire about such issues as daytime sleepiness, memory/concentration concerns, depression, an increase in accidents, and impaired job functioning. Referral to a neurologist or sleep specialist may be in order to determine the cause.

SLEEP DISORDERS AND CONDITIONS

Patients who present with co-occurring mental illness and sleep disturbances report either initial and/or terminal insomnia. Initial insomnia is usually indicative of an anxiety disorder such as generalized anxiety disorder (GAD) or an adjustment disorder with anxious mood. These patients have great difficulty falling asleep, but once they are asleep, they usually stay asleep throughout the night. Some patients present with middle insomnia (intermittent awakening); they fall asleep but wake up periodically during the night. In addition, some have "early morning awakening" or terminal insomnia. These patients can usually fall asleep easily, but they awaken around 3:00 or 4:00 a.m. and cannot get back to sleep. Most of these patients are likely to have a disorder with an affective component, such as major depression, schizoaffective disorder, Persistent Depressive Disorder, or an adjustment disorder with depressed or mixed features. It is important to note that the relationship between sleep and mood can also be reciprocal: Lack of sleep can exacerbate the same mood symptoms that often lead to the insomnia (Kalmbach, Arnedt, Swanson, Rapier, & Ciesla, 2017).

Sometimes a patient presents what appears to be a sleep-related disorder in addition to the types of poor sleeping patterns that are observed in the depressed or anxious patient. A primary care physician or neurologist should evaluate the patient for the presence of other dyssomnias or primary sleep disorders. The following list describes a few that may affect the patient:

1. *Obstructive Sleep Apnea (OSA).* This condition is troublesome for many patients. A milder form is called *upper airway resistance syndrome.* These conditions are much more common in overweight, middle-aged men or in patients with certain types of oropharyngeal and facial anatomies. The patient is unable to keep the airway open during sleep, and the airway narrows or collapses, leading to gasping or awakening throughout the night. The most common treatment for OSA is the continuous positive airway pressure (CPAP) machine. This device splints the airway open and prevents airway narrowing during sleep. More recently, the FDA has approved the use of modafinil (Provigil) in some patients as an effective pharmacological intervention as well (Arnold, Feifel, Earl, Yang, & Adler, 2012). Surgery is an option for some, but it is rather drastic and effective in only about 50% of cases (Richert & Baran, 2003). Various mouth appliances have been designed to reposition the mandible, tongue, or both when sleeping. They have mixed, less promising results and are usually attempted only by those with mild OSA.

2. *Sleep Bruxism.* Sleep-related teeth grinding is a parasomnia much more common among children, but it can be seen in adults during times of stress. In many cases, psychotherapy and/or anxiety-reducing medications may improve this condition. A dentist may be consulted,

and a mouth guard could be used to reduce the possibility of tooth damage or chronic headaches. In more severe cases, Onabotulinum toxin-A (aka Botox) injections can also be utilized (Ondo et al., 2018).

3. *Sleepwalking and Night Terrors.* These conditions are also typically seen in about 10% of children. Since patients usually outgrow these conditions, the use of medications such as benzodiazepines is not recommended for children or those patients with a history of substance dependence.

4. *Narcolepsy.* This condition consists of uncontrolled attacks of short-duration, restful sleep. The attacks are usually triggered by strong emotions, such as laughter or anger. Since this condition may cause excessive daytime sleepiness, patients should receive counseling to assist with the stigma of the disorder and the perception that they are lazy or unmotivated. Short naps during the day, as well as consistent sleep/wake times, are suggested.

Narcolepsy is typically treated with various psychostimulants, such as methylphenidate (Ritalin) and pemoline (Cylert). However, pemoline is rarely used due to hepatic concerns. Modafinil (Provigil) and the newer armodafinil (Nuvigil) are also used. Historically, stimulants have been used to reduce daytime sleepiness and sleep attacks, along with antidepressants to increase sleep quality. Modafinil and armodafinil are not considered stimulants per se, and research on modafinil suggests it may be less effective for narcoleptic patients, especially if they have been successfully treated with stimulants in the past (Brooks & Kushida, 2002). Armodafinil, also used for narcolepsy, was found to be especially helpful for shift workers who need to remain alert during the night but are seeking a medication that will not affect their daytime sleeping patterns (Czeisler, Walsh, Wesnes, Arora, & Roth, 2009). The clinician needs to watch for signs of tolerance or dependency with all stimulants used in the treatment of narcolepsy.

Gamma-hydroxybutyrate (GHB) or sodium oxybate is also known by the trade name Xyrem. The FDA approved Xyrem in 2002 for excessive daytime sleepiness and cataplexy in patients with narcolepsy. It is a CNS depressant that received the street name *date-rape drug* along with flunitrazepam (Rohypnol) because both are abused as party drugs and are often slipped into an alcoholic beverage in the hope that someone taking the drug would be mentally impaired and willing to participate in sexual relations. Many patients often have impaired memory upon awakening. When taken for sleep disorders including narcolepsy, GHB increases the quality of both REM and non-REM sleep cycles, especially slow-wave (stages 3 and 4) sleep (Antelmi et al., 2017). Side effects of GHB include excessive grogginess and mental confusion before the drug wears off.

5. *Restless Leg Syndrome (RLS) and Periodic Leg Movement Disorder (PLMD).* These conditions often occur together, but they are distinct entities. RLS usually occurs in the evening and throughout the night. Patients complain of feeling restless or jittery and may not be able to relax. They often report that this feeling starts deep within their legs, and they often move or tap their feet to gain relief. PLMD, which was previously known as nocturnal myoclonus, can cause sleep fragmentation and daytime sleepiness. With this disorder, the legs often jerk every few seconds, and this movement can increase in intensity to a point where sleep is seriously disturbed. Some researchers have also pointed out that RLS can be caused or exacerbated by various drugs, including several common antidepressants, so it is vitally important for evaluating physicians to inquire about medications taken for mood conditions (Hoque & Chesson, 2010).

Treatment for both disorders involves either the use of benzodiazepines such as clonazepam (Klonopin) or the use of dopaminergic agents such as levodopa/carbidopa (Sinemet) or pramipexole (Mirapex). Ropinirole (Requip) is another alternative used in the treatment of RLS.

Pregabalin (Lyrica) has not received FDA approval yet but is used off label for limb movement concerns. In severe cases, opioids may be considered. Research has shown that some patients with PLMD have iron, vitamin B_{12}, and folate deficiencies, so complete blood counts with differential should be ordered and evaluated (Richert & Baran, 2003).

In all cases of serious sleep disturbances, the clinician should order a complete sleep study or nocturnal polysomnogram (NPSG). This study is conducted at night in a sleep laboratory under the supervision of a neurologist or a sleep specialist. It involves recording multiple neurophysiologic and respiratory parameters during a patient's typical sleep period (often at night). Data are recorded from several places on the body including the following:

electroencephalogram (EEG) or brain-wave activity

electrocardiogram (EKG) and pulse

facial muscle movement

leg muscle movement

respiratory effort (chest and abdominal wall excursion)

oxygen saturation and carbon dioxide output

With the NPSG information, the clinician can more easily pinpoint the causes of various sleep disturbances and institute the appropriate treatment plan. For patients unable to participate in a sleep study in the lab, doctors can now perform many of these tests remotely with home-based equipment.

Before prescribing professionals consider medication, they should also determine if the sleep problem is chronic or brief in nature. Having occasional sleepless nights might be due to transient stress, poor sleeping environments, or lifestyle incompatibilities. Patients should be instructed in ways to improve their environments and make necessary lifestyle changes to reduce the frequency and intensity of these episodes. Most professionals would probably agree that occasional sleeplessness could be addressed with counseling or therapy sessions. If the patient is concerned about taking a prescription sleep medication, the clinician can suggest over-the-counter sleep aids such as Nidol, Sominex, Tylenol PM, or even Benadryl (brand of diphenhydramine).

BEHAVIORAL TECHNIQUES FOR TREATING SLEEP DISORDERS

Behavioral approaches such as relaxation training and biofeedback may be helpful in teaching patients ways to manage their sleep disturbances. These techniques typically take longer to learn and do not offer immediate relief, although they have been shown to have lasting effects that patients can employ long after medications have been discontinued (Doghramji, 2003). Many professionals use these behavioral techniques along with various medications for both immediate and lasting relief. Research suggests that patients may not be aware that options such as cognitive-behavioral therapy and relaxation training are effective and may work well alone or in conjunction with medications (Neubauer, 2009). All patients with sleep disturbances should consider the following sleep-hygiene (chronotherapy) tips:

1. Avoid exposure to bright light, especially blue light, in the evening hours (Tosini, Ferguson, & Tsubota, 2016). Modern electronic devices now often feature a "Night" mode that reduces the amount of blue light emitted from their displays.

2. Reduce or eliminate the use of nicotine, alcohol, caffeine, or other stimulating substances, except those suggested by a healthcare provider.

3. Try to maintain a regular sleep–wake cycle—that is, sleep and rise at the same time each day.

4. Avoid napping during the day unless advised to do so.

5. Use the bed only for sleeping and sex, not for thinking, working, reading, or watching TV.

6. Try to relax and unwind an hour before going to bed.

7. Try not to go to bed hungry; a light snack is permissible an hour before bed.

8. If you cannot sleep, don't lie there staring at the clock. Get up, read, watch TV, or engage in a nonstimulating activity in another room until you are tired.

9. Moderate exercise during the day, or light exercise, such as walking an hour or so before bed, often helps you to feel tired and sleep better.

10. A warm bath before bed helps to relax sore muscles and induce sleep.

11. Make a list two hours before bed of all activities you need to accomplish the next day. This prevents dwelling on them while you are trying to relax and sleep.

12. Counseling or psychotherapy helps to identify issues and to reduce stress associated with sleep disturbances. Professionals can assist patients with coping skills and relaxation training.

13. Adjust temperature and noise and light levels in the room before you retire.

PHARMACOLOGY FOR SLEEP DISORDERS

Sedative-hypnotics are indicated in the treatment of most sleep disturbances. If the sleep disturbance is intermittent or temporary, these agents can be used safely in the short run without much concern for tolerance and dependence. If the patient appears to have a chronic problem, however, a careful examination must be made by the professional to evaluate the efficacy of using these medications in the long term, especially with patients who have a history of substance abuse or affective disorders. Except where indicated, patients should not use these medications, especially the benzodiazepines, for more than two to three weeks. Adequate evaluation and diagnosis should indicate the best course of action, which may include a sleep study, physical examination, and psychotherapy if helpful.

Benzodiazepines such as alprazolam (Xanax), triazolam (Halcion), lorazepam (Ativan), or diazepam (Valium) should be used sparingly and only by patients without a history of substance abuse. These medications have been known to increase the risk of cognitive impairment and of slip/fall accidents in the elderly. Newer medications have emerged in recent years that are safer overall and offer the prescriber alternatives. See Table 11.1 for a list of medications used in the treatment of sleep disturbances.

In determining the best type of medication to use, half-life and onset of action are key points to consider. Sedating antidepressants such as mirtazapine (Remeron), nefazodone (Serzone), or trazodone (Desyrel) may be helpful, especially when the patient has an affective disorder (see Chapter 5). These medications should be used primarily before bedtime to avoid daytime sleepiness. Trazodone Contramid (an formulation), an extended-release version of trazodone, has been found to improve the quality of sleep for both depressed and nondepressed patients. It allows for the ease of once per day dosing but may increase daytime dizziness and sleepiness (Sheehan et al., 2009). The older tricyclic antidepressants can also be used, but most of these medications increase anticholinergic side effects such as weight gain, daytime drowsiness, dizziness, and orthostatic hypotension.

Table 11.1	Medications Used in Treating Sleep Disturbances		
Trade Name	**Generic Name**	**Typical Dose (mg/day)**	**Onset of Action**
Nonbenzodiazepines			
Ambien, Edluar, Zolpimist	zolpidem	5–10	Rapid
Ambien CR			
Intermezzo			
Lunesta	eszopiclone	2–3	Rapid
Sonata	zaleplon	10–20	Rapid
Benzodiazepines			
Dalmane	flurazepam	15–30	Rapid
Doral	quazepam	7.5–15	Rapid
Halcion	triazolam	0.125–0.25	Rapid
Prosom	estazolam	2–4	Rapid
Restoril	temazepam	15–30	Intermediate
Eugeroics			
Nuvigil	armodafinil	150–250	Intermediate
Provigil	modafinil	200–400	Intermediate
Other			
Belsomra	suvorexant	5–20	Rapid
Benadryl	diphenhydramine	25–50	Intermediate
Desyrel, Oleptro	trazodone	50–150	Intermediate
Equanil, Miltown	meprobamate	200–400	Intermediate
Unisom	doxylamine	25	Rapid
Lunesta	eszopiclone	2–3	Rapid
Requip	ropinirole	2–4	Rapid
Rozerem	ramelteon	8	Rapid
Silenor	doxepin	3–6	Intermediate
Somnote	chloral hydrate	50mg/kg	Rapid
Xyrem	gamma-hydroxybutyrate/ sodium oxybate	4.5–9 g/night	Rapid

Benzodiazepine receptor agonists (BRAs) have emerged in recent years as the mainstay of sleep medications for the average patient. They are less likely to be abused when compared to standard benzodiazepines. Zaleplon (Sonata) has a rapid onset but may wear off before the patient has had adequate sleep. Zolpidem (Ambien and Ambien CR) is available in immediate-release or sustained-release formulas, allowing for the medication to be released throughout the night; the CR version is less likely to cause the patient to awaken again during the night. A sublingual formulation (Edluar) has been shown to significantly reduce sleep onset time in patients currently taking zolpidem tablets (Staner et al., 2010). Zolpimist, a zolpidem oral spray, is also available. The FDA approved eszopiclone (Lunesta) early in 2005 as a new treatment for insomnia. This novel nonbenzodiazepine sleep aid is indicated for patients with both initial insomnia and those who have trouble sleeping through the night. Doses of 1 mg to 2 mg before bedtime are indicated for patients who have trouble falling asleep, and higher doses of 2 mg to 3 mg are indicated for those with sleep maintenance difficulty. The FDA approved eszopiclone for both short- and long-term treatment of insomnia because it may pose less of an abuse and tolerance risk. These drugs have been labeled to indicate the possibility of rare, but troubling, side effects that may include allergic reaction, facial swelling, sleep driving, and nighttime bouts of eating with no memory of the events (Zammit, 2009).

Barbiturates such as amobarbital (Amytal), phenobarbital (Nembutal), and secobarbital (Seconal) cause sedation and have been used to treat insomnia; however, they are not used much today because they have a narrow therapeutic index, a high potential for abuse, and may interfere with normal sleep cycles.

Melatonin is an endogenous chemical produced in the pineal glad. The levels of melatonin fall with age and may be further depleted if the patient regularly uses aspirin or ibuprofen. Various studies have demonstrated that taking 0.5 mg/day to 3 mg/day of melatonin may reduce the effects of insomnia due to jet lag and shift changes, but side effects include daytime drowsiness, cognitive slowing, and possibly an increase in depression over time (Oxenkrug & Requintina, 2003).

Newer drugs such as a sustained-release formula of melatonin (Circadin) and a melatonin receptor agonist (ramelteon, Rozerem) have been developed in recent years. Sustained-release formulas of melatonin and ramelteon have been shown to be efficacious in treating insomnia, especially phase shifts, jet lag, and sleep onset latency (Hardeland, 2009). Some research has suggested that ramelteon may be an effective alternative to antidepressants in the treatment of generalized anxiety disorder (GAD; Gross, Nourse, & Wasser, 2009). Since these medications are not benzodiazepines and carry no known risk of dependency, they may be a safer choice for those with substance abuse concerns. Little research has been conducted about the safety of long-term use of these sustained-release melatonin agonists and synthetic melatoninergic agonists. Researchers caution against their use in children; adolescents; any patient who has hepatic impairment, autoimmune disorders, or Parkinson's disease; or any patients taking drugs like fluvoxamine (Luvox), which utilizes the cytochrome P450 pathway in the liver, possibly increasing circulating levels of melatonin and ramelteon (Hardeland, 2009; Neubauer, 2009). Sleep researchers at Henry Ford Hospital Sleep Disorders Center in Detroit conducted a one-year open-label study in the use of ramelteon. They concluded that it was well tolerated by patients and improved their sleep onset. The researchers expressed some concern about its effect on endocrine functioning, however, noting a mild, transient increase in prolactin levels in women. They noted no changes in other endocrine functions (Richardson & Wang-Weigand, 2009; Richardson, Zammit, Wang-Weigand, & Zhang, 2009).

Diphenhydramine (Benadryl) or other antihistamine hypnotics may be used to reduce problematic intermittent insomnia. A diphenhydramine dose of 25 mg/day to 50 mg/day is recommended for adult patients. Like most sleep medications, it should not be taken long term, as rebound insomnia may occur. Anticholinergic side effects are, of course, probable with these medications, and both pediatric and geriatric patients should not take diphenhydramine without physician supervision due to increased sensitivity to these side effects.

Suvorexant (Belsomra) is a newer drug that works by inhibiting the activity of orexin (hypocretin), a neuropeptide responsible for wakefulness. This neuropeptide appears to regulate more global sleep–wake systems, including metabolism and circadian rhythm, and it may regulate dopamine, acetylcholine, norepinephrine, and histamine levels. Suvorexant acts as a competitive antagonist for both orexin type 1 and 2 receptors, effectively preventing orexin binding and thus suppressing wakefulness (Patel, Aspesi, & Evoy, 2015).

HOLISTIC TREATMENTS

Various holistic remedies have mixed results. These remedies may include substances such as kava, which has been used by the peoples of the South Pacific for thousands of years. Its action is similar to a sedative-hypnotic because it appears to bind at the GABA receptors. Animal studies have shown that kava acts much like a benzodiazepine (Jullien, 2001). More recently, the FDA, scientists, and others promoting holistic health have stated that kava may increase the risk of liver damage with prolonged use.

Valerian or valerian root has historically been used as a mild sedative, anxiolytic, and antidepressant. Its action is not well understood, but since GABA itself is a component of valerian, scientists and holistic advocates believe that valerian is a source of naturally occurring GABA. However, since GABA crosses the blood–brain barrier poorly, valerian is an unlikely source of GABA that would affect the central nervous system. Since valerian causes sedation, those taking other sedating medications should use it with caution. Valerian contains quercetin, a substance that inhibits the liver cytochrome enzymatic pathway CYP1A2. This inhibiting action could result in other significant drug interactions (Jullien, 2001; Tyler, 1993).

As with all sedative-hypnotic treatments, the clinician must take great caution to correctly identify the type and nature of a patient's sleep difficulties. If medications are used, patients must be educated about typical side effects. Clinicians must use sedating medications with caution when prescribing them for elderly patients, who often become disoriented during the night and might fall and injure themselves. Patients with a history of substance abuse should be carefully screened for their potential to abuse stimulants and to use benzodiazepines excessively.

CASE VIGNETTES

Case 1

CLINICAL HISTORY

Lotus is a 36-year-old Asian American female who recently started a new executive position with an advertising firm. While she loves her new job and the field of advertising, she admits that the new schedule is grueling and that she often doesn't get home until quite late. She has noticed that it is difficult for her to relax before getting to bed and her mind often wanders to the many tasks she needs to complete when she returns to work in the morning. These "racing thoughts" result in significant initial insomnia, causing her to be alert for nearly an hour or more before she is able to fall asleep. When questioned about these symptoms, she claims that she has never seen a therapist before, doesn't consider herself to be anxious or depressed, and has never had a problem with sleeping in the past. There are no worries of money or health-related issues, and she claims to enjoy her job and the people with whom she works. She even does not find these thoughts unpleasant, as she uses the time to plan her next day. She admits that they are just a bit intrusive and that she really needs to wind down and get more rest.

POSTCASE DISCUSSION AND DIAGNOSIS

While Lotus may have a case of adjustment disorder related to starting her new position, it is more likely that she is just attempting to do well in her new duties and is a bit overly diligent. A complete physical, including a sleep study, is suggested to rule out other physical causes. She agreed to limit or eliminate the use of any stimulants in her diet and to follow sleep hygiene suggestions given to her by her family's physician assistant (PA). Since there is no history of mental illness in her family, and she denies feeling depressed or anxious, there is no reason to suggest a more serious mental illness. Although some Asian Americans do minimize their mental health symptoms, Lotus is a third-generation female who does not present with physical symptoms seen more often in first-generation patients with depression or anxiety.

PSYCHOPHARMACOLOGICAL TREATMENT

Since Lotus has no positive history for substance abuse, benzodiazepines could be safely used in the short term; however, it was decided that a benzodiazepine receptor agonist would be a safer choice. She was given 5 mg q.h.s. of zolpidem rather than the extended-release formulation since her insomnia was limited to the first hour or so and did not reoccur throughout the night. In a follow-up appointment with her PA, Lotus reported that her sleep had improved dramatically and that she had more energy during the day. Her sleep study was unremarkable, and her history and results were within normal limits. She agreed to follow up with a mental health professional should the symptoms return or worsen in the future. Her PA agreed to prescribe the drug only for the next three weeks and if the symptoms persist to reassess her condition to avoid any problems with potential drug tolerance or dependency.

Case 2

CLINICAL HISTORY

Jackson is a 20-year-old white male currently enrolled in a four-year college. Jackson states that he has struggled throughout his life to fall asleep consistently, and that this has "come to a head" in recent months due to an early morning class that he occasionally misses due to his erratic sleep schedule. He indicates that while he "wants to fall asleep at a decent hour," he is not consistently tired at night. Instead, Jackson states that he seems to be tired slightly later each night and that this becomes increasingly frustrating and anxiety provoking, leading to some racing thoughts and difficulty staying asleep. Jackson says he's never spoken to a therapist or physician about these symptoms, as he otherwise feels minimal anxiety or feelings of sadness. He says he usually just "resets" himself by "staying up all night and the next day so that [he] can pass out at a reasonable hour the next evening." He states that he drinks minimally, does not use recreational drugs, and is not currently on any prescription medications.

POSTCASE DISCUSSION AND DIAGNOSIS

The pattern and consistency of Jackson's sleep difficulties suggest a Circadian Rhythm Sleep Disorder, Delayed Sleep Phase Type (G47.21), especially in light of Jackson's indication that this has occurred throughout his life and without significant anxiety or depression outside of that directly caused by the sleep disorder. A sleep study is strongly recommended to confirm this diagnosis, and a physical exam is encouraged to rule out any other biological factors. Pending the results of the sleep study, Jackson is encouraged to engage in chronotherapy and is referred out for possible light therapy.

PSYCHOPHARMACOLOGICAL TREATMENT

Jackson's sleep study confirmed a likely Delayed Sleep Phase Disorder, with a shift of approximately 30 minutes per day, consistent with his self-report. Jackson was encouraged to continue with the chronotherapy and provided with a light box for daily light therapy. In addition, he was prescribed 1 mg melatonin q.h.s. and 5 mg p.r.n. of zolpidem. During his follow-up appointment a month later, Jackson reported significant improvement overall. The psychiatrist therefore removed the zolpidem and continued the combination of melatonin, chronotherapy, and light therapy. Jackson agreed to follow up with his psychiatrist and sleep specialist in three months to reassess his condition.

CHAPTER 12

Treatment of Personality Disorders

While there are technically no FDA-approved medications for treating personality disorders, this chapter explores some common helpful medications or combinations of medications used in day-to-day practice for symptom reduction and control.

Topics to be addressed include the following:

- Use of medications for personality disorders
- Tailoring medications to symptom clusters
- Other considerations
- Case vignettes

USE OF MEDICATIONS FOR PERSONALITY DISORDERS

Historically, psychotherapy has been the mainstay of treatment for personality disorders (PDs), as opposed to pharmacotherapy, which has been the primary therapeutic method for the majority of mood disorders. Reich (2002) reports that epidemiological studies have consistently estimated that 10% of the population of the United States has a personality disorder, whereas Grant et al. (2004) puts that estimate closer to 15%. Other researchers have noted a prevalence rate for these disorders in the general population of up to 23% (Sadock, Sadock, & Ruiz, 2017). Psychopharmacological treatment for personality disorders is a fairly new phenomenon in the field of psychopharmacology. Historically, clinicians believed that the use of medications in the treatment of personality disorders would be counterproductive because it would interfere with the psychotherapy, and their use is still debated. Recent authors still argue that psychopharmacology should be avoided in the treatment of PD when possible, in particular borderline personality disorder (Limandri, 2018). Nonetheless, psychopharmacological treatments are now quite common, with recent reports indicating that 90% to 99% of borderline personality disorder (BPD) cases are treated with one or more psychotropic medications (Starcevic & Janca, 2017). As such, the combined use of psychotherapy and psychopharmacological treatments is an important consideration in effective psychotherapeutic treatment.

Most types of psychotherapy have been used in the treatment of personality disorders. Each school of thought provides some understanding of behavior and method of intervention; however, the different schools are not mutually exclusive because they tend to overlap and complement one another. Numerous forms of psychotherapy have been tried, including dynamic, behavioral, cognitive, supportive, and dialectical. As a rule, the best way to approach patients with personality disorders is to use combinations of various orientations. The emphasis should be on teamwork (i.e., doing something *with* the patient, not *to* the patient).

For many years there was an assumption that mood disorders arose from "biological" predispositions and personality disorders from "environmental" issues. Research evidence suggests that personality disorders are a biopsychosocial entity caused by complex interactions of psychosocial and biological factors (New, Triebwassar, & Goodman, 2009). For example, Livesley (2000) notes that twin studies indicate that personality disorder traits are genetically linked about

40% to 60% of the time. The variance is accounted for by specific environmental factors. When reviewing available information on twin studies, adoption studies, twins reared apart, and molecular genetics, researchers found significant evidence that antisocial and aggressive behaviors have genetic influences. Keep in mind that genetic processes need an environment in which to become expressed. Environmental stressors may turn genetic influences on and off across the lifespan (Raine, 2002). New and colleagues (2009) further state that genetic vulnerability appears to place individuals at increased risk for the development of various personality disorders. According to Kaylor (1999), impulsive and violent behavior may stem from brain dysfunction or damage secondary to head trauma, toxic chemical substances, focal lesions of the temporal lobe, low serotonin levels, or other serotonergic dysfunction. Even neuroimaging studies have demonstrated measurable differences in key frontal regions during the memory retention period of a visuospatial working memory test with schizotypal personality disorder when compared to normal controls (Koenigsberg et al., 2005). These complicated interactions between nature and nurture will continue to be the focus of attention for many years to come.

Before considering pharmacotherapy for personality disorders, the clinician must obtain a comprehensive assessment (see Chapter 4 for details). Obtaining a complete psychiatric and medication history is not only important but crucial. The focus is on targeting symptoms and their response to the pharmacotherapy, rather than treating the diagnosis. With the patient's permission, an interview with family members would be helpful in making a personality disorder diagnosis. An assessment of substance abuse or dependence is important and may mimic diagnostic symptoms of a personality disorder. Comorbidity also exists with respect to chemical dependency and personality disorders in a subset of the population. Family history is also valuable and may suggest the existence of biological vulnerabilities for mood disorders, drug and alcohol abuse, and perhaps personality disorders. Furthermore, endocrine, neurological, rheumatological, and metabolic disturbances may present as psychiatric illnesses, including personality or character disorders. Medications prescribed for these medical conditions may have cognitive, behavioral, or affective consequences. Laboratory evaluation, appropriate neuroimaging studies, and an electroencephalogram (EEG) may be necessary in the evaluation to rule out confusing medical symptomatology.

TAILORING MEDICATIONS TO SYMPTOM CLUSTERS

First of all, clinicians need to know that the FDA has not approved any medications for use in personality disorders. With the exception of avoidant personality disorder, there are no specific drugs for specific disorders. Thus, clinicians are basically treating comorbid mood diagnoses and personality disorder *traits*. Their goal is to find medications that can appropriately treat the individual array of symptoms with which a patient presents. Although combinations of various classes of medications may be useful, clinicians should be cautious of polypharmacy.

Most experts define three different symptom clusters for personality disorders, which can prove useful during treatment. The clusters are as follows:

Cluster A. The odd or eccentric cluster
Cluster B. The dramatic, emotional, or erratic cluster
Cluster C. The anxious or fearful cluster

This theoretical construct helps clinicians determine pharmacological treatment options. The three categories generally correspond to the DSM-5 Personality Disorder Clusters A, B, and C. Each cluster will be considered and some recommendations for treatment will be made.

CLUSTER A The odd or eccentric cluster involves psychotic symptoms and a thought disorder that are theoretically at the mild end of the spectrum. Schizotypal personality disorder is a good example of this category. The treatment of choice would be an atypical antipsychotic medication because of the mild psychotic symptoms. As noted in Chapter 8, risperidone (Risperdal) is probably the best place to start; lower dosages are preferred. Reich (2002) recommends using about one quarter to one half of the usual dose that clinicians would use for other schizophrenia-related disorders. If the first antipsychotic fails, the clinician should then try a second atypical agent, such as olanzapine (Zyprexa) or quetiapine (Seroquel). Typical antipsychotics are not recommended because of the risk of tardive dyskinesia.

CLUSTER B The dramatic, emotional, or erratic cluster corresponds to Cluster B in the DSM-5. Impulsivity, aggression, mood lability, self-destructiveness, and suicidality are the main symptoms in this group. Many patients in this cluster also report various somatic complaints. Research has demonstrated the effectiveness and tolerability of duloxetine (Cymbalta) for borderline personality disorder patients who may also present with excessive impulsivity and somatic preoccupation (Bellino, Paradiso, Bozzatello, & Bogetto, 2010). Although these symptoms are most commonly found in borderline personality disorder, they may occur in other forms in the other Cluster B diagnoses. For example, impulsivity and aggression in antisocial personality may present as lying, stealing, and destruction of property. Patients with these symptoms have a major disregard for social norms. In histrionic personality, low frustration tolerance would correlate with this impulsivity and aggressiveness; narcissistic rage expressed in response to criticism would be a good example in that disorder.

    With respect to medications, an SSRI antidepressant would be the most logical place to start; however, recent research suggests that mood stabilizers such as topiramate (Topamax), lamotrigine (Lamictal), and valproate (Depakote), along with atypical antipsychotics such as aripiprazole and olanzapine, would be better choices for mood control than would SSRIs (Lieb, Vollim, Rucker, Timmer, & Stoffers, 2010; Paolini, Mezzetti, Pierri, & Moretti, 2017). SSRIs, when used, should be titrated upward as tolerated to high doses, which are the doses used in obsessive-compulsive disorder. If one SSRI fails, try another. If the patient has a partial response to an SSRI, the clinician might consider augmenting with other medications, such as atypical antipsychotics. Some clinicians may use gabapentin (Neurontin) for anxiety, impulsivity, and sedation in these types of patients. They may use naltrexone (Revia), an opiate antagonist, known to reduce self-harming behaviors when present. As noted previously, combinations of medications may be the most useful.

CLUSTER C The anxious or fearful cluster may be manifested by shyness, diminished ability to function or use opportunities, rejection sensitivity, avoidant behaviors, and anxiety. Initially, an SSRI would be the treatment of choice. A second SSRI should be tried if the first one fails. With Cluster C patients, the clinician could consider a long-acting benzodiazepine such as clonazepam (Klonopin) as an adjunctive treatment option. Other considerations for treatment would be atypical antipsychotics, buspirone (Buspar), gabapentin (Neurontin), and perhaps beta blockers. Some clinicians still use MAOIs to help reduce isolative behaviors and rejection sensitivity. However, their use has declined since the introduction of medications with safer side-effect profiles. If patients have a history of substance abuse, remember to avoid benzodiazepines due to their addictive nature.

OTHER CONSIDERATIONS

The duration of medication treatment with personality disorders is debatable. Treatment trials should last for at least four to six weeks to determine the drug's effectiveness (i.e., adequate trial). Although no patient should be on a medication longer than necessary, the clinician should be mindful that character issues are long term and chronic. If a drug or combination of drugs improves the patient symptomatically and has an acceptable level of side effects, long-term treatment can be justified.

Personality traits and disorders are best conceptualized on a continuum. Hopefully, future research will illuminate the role of biological, psychological, and social factors in each personality disorder. Clinicians may then focus on primary prevention rather than treating the chronic sequelae of these illnesses.

CASE VIGNETTES

Case 1

CLINICAL HISTORY

Cindy is a 21-year-old white female. She has been recently released from a short hospital stay for self-mutilating behavior and threatening suicide. While she managed to finish high school, she has attended more than six different colleges. Her classes start off okay, but then she accuses her professors of not caring about her and claims that her roommates seem to hate her. If she meets and dates a young man, she quickly accuses him of cheating on her and threatens to kill herself to punish him. When questioned about her symptoms, she claims to be depressed and empty, yet her level of anger reaches the point where she screams at others until she cries uncontrollably while accusing everyone of abandoning her in her hour of need. She attempted to get help at the university counseling center, but when she was placed in a therapy group, she dominated it and wouldn't let others talk. When she was confronted by the other group members, she told them all to "go to hell" and walked out of the center never to return. She refused to call her psychologist back because she needed to punish her for not running after her when she left the session. Recently, she sought out another private therapist, but when the therapist refused to allow her to call her cell phone whenever she felt angry or upset, she "fired" the therapist and self-mutilated to feel better. History provided by her parents confirms that Cindy has been exhibiting these behaviors for several years with little treatment success from her past therapists and psychiatrists.

POSTCASE DISCUSSION AND DIAGNOSIS

Cindy clearly has problems with Borderline Personality Disorder (F60.3). She reports chronic feelings of emptiness and anger. She also has a long history of arguing with her parents and siblings, claiming they do not understand or love her. When it gets especially bad, she will stop talking to them for months on end. She has a history of self-mutilation and suicidal ideation.

PSYCHOPHARMACOLOGICAL TREATMENT

While there are no FDA-approved medications for personality disorders per se, her psychiatrists have tried spot treatments with various drugs without success. The main reason for this appeared to be poor compliance on the part of the patient. Cindy agreed to see a new psychiatrist upon discharge from the hospital. At the urging of her family, she agreed to follow her doctor's medication orders and attend a dialectical behavior therapy (DBT) group conducted by a local therapist. She was prescribed Lamictal 25 mg qd for the first week and increased 25 mg each week until she was taking 200 mg per day. After 8 weeks of Lamictal therapy, her psychiatrist added 50 mg of naltrexone to control her urges to cut herself.

Upon follow-up with Cindy one month later, she reported less labile behavior, no cutting behaviors, and much less depression. She was able to maintain herself at school and was attending the DBT group with regularity. Although she still had many personality issues to address in treatment, her behavior was much calmer and less labile.

Case 2

CLINICAL HISTORY

Amed is a 34-year-old, single, Middle Eastern male working as an IT specialist for a large insurance company. He presents for psychotherapy at the suggestion of his manager who thinks that he may be reacting to job stress and that he appears depressed. Amed feels that his job is a little stressful at times, but he does not feel distressed about it, nor has he ever taken a day off in the seven years he has worked for the company. In fact, he reports that he did not take one single day off from his last IT job with another company. Although he appears depressed, he denies any mood issue. He claims to love his job as he states, "Computers are great, and they allow you to explore alternative realities and the boundaries of the universe." Amed reports that he feels that the issue may be that he has no friends at work and others appear to avoid him. When asked why this may be, he only states, "They think I'm weird." When questioned further it was learned that he has a very "animated" office at work. It contains several science fiction action figures. He keeps the lights off so he can view the star-and-planet display he has projected on the ceiling. He is often questioning others about their beliefs in "alternative realities" and insists that he and others are actually part of some type of dual reality where he and the other members of the IT team exist in another galaxy and that his other self may be trying to reach him via misdirected emails disguised as spam. Upon further examination, Amed reports that he never knew his father who his mother divorced when Amed was only 18 months old due to the father's history of mental illness. Amed has an older sister who was diagnosed as schizophrenic when she was 19. Amed denies visual or auditory hallucinations and does not feel that others, including aliens, are out to harm him. His mental status exam was, for the most part, unremarkable. He has never dated and claims that other people sometimes scare him, especially women his age. He offered that on his last job he was advised by HR not to ask personal questions of other employees. This came after an incident during which he asked a female employee what she did with her belly button lint. He offered that he puts his outdoors, as it makes excellent nesting material for birds.

POSTCASE DISCUSSION AND DIAGNOSIS

Amed appears to understand that alternative realities are just theories and that they are not necessarily happening. He maintains that they should be considered as possibilities. He also did not understand why the female coworker was upset by his comments about the belly button lint. He in fact verified that it does make good nesting material, but he had little insight into why someone would find these questions odd and off-putting. Given his history and family background, Amed was diagnosed as Schizotypal Personality Disorder (F21).

PSYCHOPHARMACOLOGICAL TREATMENT

As has already been stated, no medications are approved by FDA for any personality disorder, but in this case, Amed's preoccupation with rather odd thinking and lines of questioning are becoming an occupational issue for him. He was started on a very low dose (1 mg) of brexpiprazole (Rexulti). Low-dose atypical antipsychotics are often helpful for those with this condition, especially if they have a history of mood concerns and a family history of psychotic spectrum illness. Amed responded well to the medication and reported that he felt less anxious around others at work. His manager also thanked him for talking less about the "alternative universe" in staff meetings. Amed now thinks that others are friendlier with him as he smiles more often when he talks with others. While he still thinks about his alternative theories from time to time, he keeps them to himself.

CHAPTER **13**

Treatment of Chemical Dependency and Co-Occurring Conditions

This chapter provides an overview of treatment considerations for people with co-occurring substance abuse conditions. The dopamine hypothesis and relevant treatment issues are explored with helpful diagnostic instruments and pharmacological suggestions for each substance of concern.

Topics to be addressed include the following:

- Co-occurring conditions
- The dopamine hypothesis
- Treatment issues
- Assessment instruments and strategies
- Treatment phases and goals
- Psychopharmacology for dually diagnosed patients
- Summary and treatment reminders
- Case vignettes

CO-OCCURRING CONDITIONS

In many patients presenting with various DSM-5 conditions, clinicians also observe the use and abuse of various substances. These substances may include alcohol and various other illegal drugs, but may also include prescription medications. The use of a substance, even to alter mood or the patient's physical state, is not necessarily problematic unless patients experience detrimental effects on their social and occupational functioning. Clinicians should try to examine the nature and intensity of drug use to determine if patients are compulsive in their use patterns and appear to have little control over the conditions and amounts used. Here the clinician is concerned with the following issues:

1. *Loss of control* (cannot stop or limit drug use)
2. *Tolerance*, or the need to use more and more of the substance to avoid *withdrawal* or to maintain a desired state
3. *Impairment in functioning*, such as failure to work or keep other life obligations

The clinician needs to evaluate these issues even if the patient meets full criteria for a singular diagnosis of substance abuse or dependence per the DSM-5.

Research into the use patterns of patients with co-occurring conditions indicates that substance abuse is a problem for about 61% of those with bipolar disorder, 47% of those with schizophrenia, 39% of those with personality disorders, 33% of those with obsessive-compulsive disorder, and 32% of those with an affective disorder (Regier et al., 1990). In addition, about 50% of bipolar patients seriously abuse alcohol at various points in their lifetime (Azorin et al., 2010). It is not surprising then to learn that the majority of patients who have been treated for a substance abuse condition also meet criteria for another DSM-5 diagnosis.

According to the 2014 National Survey conducted by the Center for Behavioral Health Statistics and Quality (CBHSQ; 2015), more than 27 million people ages 12 and over used an illicit substance in the last 30 days. The largest increase was in the use of marijuana and pain killers. About 22 million met criteria for an official substance use diagnosis. According to the National Survey on Drug Use and Health from the Substance Abuse and Mental Health Services Administration (SAMHSA), 22.5 million people (8.5% of the U.S. population) ages 12 or older needed treatment for an illicit drug or alcohol use problem in 2014. Only 4.2 million (18.5% of those who needed treatment) received any substance use treatment in the same year. Of these, about 2.6 million people received treatment at specialty treatment programs (CBHSQ, 2015).

Although attempting to determine which condition (mental health or substance abuse) came first, the task may be nearly impossible. The clinician who can obtain a good history from the patient or the family may be able to accomplish this task. Current longitudinal research has suggested that chronic drinking may in fact lead to major depression because the drinking behaviors were observed long before reports of a mood disorder (Fergusson, Boden, & Horwood, 2009). The clinician should consider these questions: In the absence of a family or personal history of mental illness, did the patient develop depression after years of abusing alcohol or drugs? After years of struggling with anxiety and panic, did the patient notice that drinking had a calming effect and reduced the number of panic attacks? Did the ADHD teenager start abusing caffeine and speed once he noticed that it allowed him or her to relax and concentrate? Stress and other environmental stimuli are responsible not only for addiction but also for former abusers relapsing (Haass-Koffler & Bartlett, 2012). In addition, chronic drug use over time may lead to the brain being less responsive to natural rewards (Volkow, Wang, Fowler, Tomasi, & Telang, 2011).

In patients with an existing psychological disorder, a co-occurring or dually occurring substance abuse and mental illness disorder exists when the use of a substance exceeds social use. For these patients, treatment for chemical dependency or detoxification (detox) may be needed. Determining the type and scope of treatment is based largely on the nature and intensity of the presenting problems and the particular treatment philosophy employed in the treatment setting. Researchers have long wondered how to improve patient compliance in substance abuse treatment and to increase sobriety. Some believe that increasing patients' positive perceptions of treatment and their level of alliance with their treating clinician are associated with more days of abstinence (Ernst, Pettinati, Weiss, Donovan, & Longabaugh, 2008).

Some researchers believe that chemical addiction is not simply a direct effect of the drug on the brain but, rather, a pathological relationship that a person has with the drug (Schneider & Irons, 2001). Milkman and Sunderwirth (1987) found that *drugs and behaviors* can have addictive effects on the brain. When people pursue gratification, they experience three basic types of neurochemical responses: arousal, satiation, or an increase in preoccupation of the desired object (fantasy). *Arousal* is accompanied by an increase in dopamine and norepinephrine, satiation with GABA, and fantasy with serotonin. Typically, people seeking arousal use drugs that increase arousal (cocaine or amphetamines), or they engage in high-risk behaviors such as gambling; both types of activities increase dopamine and norepinephrine. A sedation and/or *satiation* response could be achieved with excessive food consumption, television watching, video games, or drugs such as benzodiazepines or alcohol. *Fantasy* is often the core issue in sexual addiction. These researchers believe that when a person is addicted, the addiction is in fact to *a set of behaviors involving a drug or an activity*. The behavioral activities themselves can produce chemical changes in the brain similar to those produced by any exogenous drug.

GABA-B receptors are involved in reinforcing actions in the reward centers of the brain—namely, the ventral tegmental area. GABA-B agonists, such as baclofen (a muscle relaxant), may reduce these reinforcing effects, especially for cocaine and alcohol users. (Muzyk, Rivelli, & Gagliardi, 2012; Nutt & Lingford-Hughes, 2008). Some studies, however, did not find that baclofen performed much better than placebo in reducing alcohol consumption or days to relapse (Beraha et al., 2016). N-acetylcysteine (NAC; an antioxidant), along with certain other antibiotics, may be effective in reducing the likelihood of relapsing, especially among cocaine users (a).

THE DOPAMINE HYPOTHESIS

Most drugs of abuse, including cigarettes, increase the concentration of dopamine in the nucleus accumbens and the mesolimbic system (the brain's reward centers). Overstimulation exhausts the dopamine system and causes the brain to reduce both the amount of dopamine available and the receptor sites with which they bind. Most abusers start out seeking the high that comes from drug use; later they use drugs to avoid withdrawal. In withdrawal they experience dysphoria and depression because of an increase in dopamine-3 receptor sites that are craving or looking for dopamine. Much of the psychopharmacology used in the treatment of patients with co-occurring conditions attempts to address depression, anxiety, and craving to increase the patient's chances of a sustained recovery.

TREATMENT ISSUES

While most treatment centers (and the general public) adhere to a zero-tolerance model that emphasizes total abstinence, some researchers believe that the patient could learn harm-reduction techniques leading to nonsymptomatic, responsible use (Marlatt & Witkiewitz, 2002). These researchers cite empirical studies that demonstrate that harm-reduction approaches to alcohol are at least as effective as abstinence-based treatment approaches in reducing alcohol consumption and alcohol-related consequences.

As mentioned, treatment centers tend to have their own unique philosophies about detox and recovery. Some centers adhere to the *traditional moral model*, often utilizing some type of 12-step approach. Others employ more of a *rational-recovery viewpoint*, assuming that patients may not buy into a spiritual or religious reason for their use or recovery. Still other centers consider the disease model that assumes complete abstinence with no return to nonproblematic or social use of any kind.

A good treatment center takes *all* modalities into consideration. It does not assume that the patient is self-medicating a mental health condition or that all of the patient's behaviors are caused by drug use. Neither does the center assume that all patients have chemically addicted brains and can never use a drug again. Typically the treatment center treats both co-occurring issues together and watches to see if after treatment a singular condition reemerges to be treated more aggressively.

ASSESSMENT INSTRUMENTS AND STRATEGIES

Many assessment instruments can be used to assess client readiness for recovery and levels of resistance. The Michigan Alcohol Screening Test (MAST) is a short, 24-item questionnaire in a yes/no format that detects the presence and extent of drinking. A shorter, 13-item version is also available. The Substance Abuse Subtle Screening Inventory (SASSI-4) is a 93-item instrument that measures issues such as openness, chemical dependency predisposition, and defensiveness. It is also available in an Adolescent version (100 items) and a Spanish version. The SASSI-A2 is an adolescent version with 100 items. There is also a Spanish version available. The Substance Abuse Life Circumstance Evaluation (SALCE) contains 98 items and may be helpful in identifying triggers for relapse—for example, the patient's levels of stress. The MacAndrew Alcoholism Scale of the MMPI-2 is helpful in identifying the potential for drug or alcohol abuse in a patient. The Substance Abuse Problem Checklist consists of 377 items and examines problematic areas such as treatment motivation, health problems, personality issues, social relationships, job problems, leisure issues, legal issues, and spirituality. This checklist is helpful in assessing patients who have co-occurring personality disorders and social concerns.

For many clinicians who do not work in chemical dependency settings, substance abuse screening is often determined simply from historical information. In this case, using the CAGE questionnaire is helpful:

1. Have you ever felt that you should *Cut* down on your drinking (or drug use)?
2. Have people *Annoyed* you by criticizing your drinking (or drug use)?
3. Have you ever felt bad or *Guilty* about your drinking (or drug use)?
4. Have you ever had a drink (or used drugs) first thing in the morning (an *Eye* opener) to steady your nerves or get rid of a hangover?

TREATMENT PHASES AND GOALS

In most treatment centers, treatment is achieved in a series of steps or phases of treatment. A typical first phase involves a complete assessment of the patient and his or her situation. Here the clinician obtains the nature and patterns of drug use, as well as related emotions. A detailed history is taken, including the types of drugs abused, dates of use, attempts at treatment, relevant legal or medical problems, and the extent of financial hardships caused by the patient's condition. In determining the nature of drug use, the clinician needs to inquire about the intensity and frequency of the patient's use of drugs. Patients who use drugs on a steady basis may exhibit more antisocial tendencies; patients who are more binge users are more likely to use drugs for self-medication or social lubrication reasons. The clinician will find it helpful to interview spouses, partners, and other family members to learn how they view the patient and his or her level of functioning.

In the second phase of treatment, the clinician attempts to determine the special needs of the dually diagnosed patient. The following questions guide this effort:

1. Does the patient need medically supervised detox?
2. Does the patient need psychotropic medication or a psychiatric evaluation?
3. Does the patient need inpatient observation based on the patient's behaviors or threats?
4. What is the patient's level of resistance?
5. What is the patient's potential for relapse?
6. What, if any, are the environmental issues that affect treatment (i.e., childcare, work, finances, spousal abuse, co-dependency, enabling issues, etc.)?

In the third phase of treatment, the clinician examines the need for using various medications in the treatment of the patient with co-occurring concerns. The clinician should carefully weigh the use of psychotropic medications. In most cases only antidepressants and appropriate antipsychotics should be considered. The use of pain medications and/or anxiolytics should be avoided, except during the initial stages of detox and only when the clinician or prescriber determines that their use outweighs their risks (Sattar & Bhatia, 2003).

PSYCHOPHARMACOLOGY FOR DUALLY DIAGNOSED PATIENTS

This section describes medications and various other substances used in the treatment of dually diagnosed patients with alcohol, opioid, and cocaine dependence along with other addictions. Table 13.1 lists the medications used to treat chemical dependency.

Alcohol Dependence

To date, only four agents are approved by the FDA for the treatment of alcohol abuse: disulfiram (Antabuse), acamprosate (Campral), oral naltrexone (Revia/Depade), and once-monthly

Table 13.1   Medications Used for Chemical Dependency

Trade Name	Generic Name	Typical Dose (mg/day)	Type of Addiction
Antabuse	disulfiram	125–500	Alcohol
Bunavail, Zubzolv	buprenorphine/naloxone	2.1, 4.2, 6.3	Opioid
Campral	acamprosate	2000	Alcohol
Chantix	varenicline	0.5–2	Nicotine
Depade	naltrexone	50	Alcohol
Dolophine	methadone	20–200	Opioid
Kemstro/Lioresal	baclofen	10–80	Alcohol
LAAM	levo-alpha-acetyl-methadol	20–80 (3x/wk)	Opioid
Norpramin	desipramine	150–300	Cocaine
Parlodel	bromocryptine	2.5–15	Cocaine
Probuphine	buprenorphine implant	74.2 (80 mg)	Opioid
Revex	nalmefene	20–80	Alcohol
Revia	naltrexone	50	Alcohol
Ritalin	methylphenidate	15–60	Cocaine
Sanorex/Mazanor	mazindol	1–3	Cocaine
Sublocade	buprenorphine	100–300 mg (monthly)	Opioid
Suboxone	buprenorphine/naloxone	2–16	Opioid
Subutex	buprenorphine	2–16	Opioid
Symmetrel	amantadine	100–400	Cocaine
Topamax	topiramate	25–300	Alcohol
Vivitrol	naltrexone	380 mg/4 weeks	Alcohol
Wellbutrin SR/Zyban	bupropion	150–300	Nicotine
N/A	ibogaine	10–60	Cocaine

injectable naltrexone (Vivitrol). This section will examine these four, as well as the novel uses of other medications used in the treatment of various DSM-5 conditions that now appear to show real promise in the treatment of substance abuse conditions.

1. Disulfiram (Antabuse) is used as a form of aversion therapy because it causes a very unpleasant chemical reaction when patients who use it drink alcohol. Typically, the enzyme acetaldehyde dehydrogenase converts acetaldehyde to harmless acetate, but disulfiram interferes with this process and allows toxic acetaldehyde to accumulate when alcohol is consumed, causing nausea, sweating, and rapid pulse. While not life-threatening to most patients, this medication is not indicated for those who have serious health concerns or for cardiovascular patients. The typical dose is 125 mg/day to 250 mg/day, but doses of up to 500 mg/day may be considered. The clinician should know that this medication can stay in a patient's system for several days after discontinuance, so drug holidays may still lead to chemical reactions in patients who "fall off the wagon." For this reason, disulfiram is most helpful for binge drinkers trying to maintain sobriety. Most patients tolerate this medication without difficulty, but some complain of mild gastrointestinal upset. The clinician might suggest taking the medication with food to avoid this side effect.

Some treatment centers request that the medication be given by a family member to ensure compliance. When the medication is obtained from the pharmacy, the pharmacist will give the patient some other instructions. For example, if disulfiram is used with any alcohol-containing product such as aftershave, mouthwash, or rubbing alcohol, unpleasant rashes or other side effects can result. One may need to look for and use alcohol-free mouthwashes, antiperspirants, and hair gels while using this drug.

2. Naltrexone (Revia, Depade) mimics the action of naturally occurring opiate neurotransmitters in the brain by acting as an opioid receptor antagonist. In animal studies, when opiate antagonists are administered, the animals consumed less alcohol. In human studies, patients reduced their levels of drinking and reported prolonged abstinence. The typical daily dose of naltrexone is 50 mg/day. Side effects may include sedation, nausea, and liver dysfunction. This medication is not indicated for patients with compromised liver functioning because higher doses of naltrexone have been associated with liver toxicity. This medication is best suited to patients who are early in recovery and who are steady users. An extended-release injectable is available (380 mg given IM) and appears to demonstrate clinical efficacy by reducing drinking behaviors by about 49% in studies with chronic steady drinkers and by an overall increase in reported quality of life (Lee et al., 2010; Pettinati, Gastfriend, Dong, Kranzler, & O'Malley, 2008).

3. Similar to naltrexone, nalmefene (Revex) was FDA approved for complete or partial reversal of opioid drug effects (used primarily in the field of anesthesia) and for management of known or suspected opioid overdose (as in an emergency department). However, the use of more quick-acting opioid antagonists such as Narcan is an advantage over longer half-life drugs like nalmefene, especially when patients increase opioid use to overcome the blocking effects of the drug. As with naltrexone, endogenous opioid brain circuits are blocked, thus blocking the dopamine-mediated euphoria. Nalmefene is a mu opioid antagonist with fewer side effects and a longer half-life than naltrexone. While used as a pill form and injectable in Europe for some time, the pill form was never available in the United States. The drug was discontinued completely by the manufacturer in 2008 due to the expense and infrequent use.

4. Acamprosate (Campral) was approved by the FDA in 2004 for use in patients with alcohol dependence. It has been used in Europe for many years. Although the mechanism of action is unknown, researchers believe that acamprosate may facilitate the calming action of GABA at its receptors, while inhibiting glutamate (an excitatory neurotransmitter). In fact, it may restore the normal activity of glutamatergic neurotransmission altered by chronic alcohol exposure (Mason & Heyser, 2010). Acamprosate may also reduce the hyperexcitability associated with alcohol withdrawal and craving. The typical dose is approximately 2000 mg/day.

Other promising medications not approved by the FDA are currently being investigated as treatments for conditions like alcoholism. Topiramate (Topamax) has been shown not only to reduce craving and withdrawal symptoms but also to increase days of abstinence and overall quality of life for alcohol recovery patients (Johnson, 2007; Kenna, Lomastro, Schiesl, Leggio, & Swift, 2009). Some research has shown it to be superior compared to naltrexone in terms of treatment outcome and Alcoholics Anonymous (AA) attendance (Baltieri, Daro, Ribeiro, & de Andrade, 2008). In addition to topiramate, the muscle relaxant baclofen may also be helpful with some patients (Garbutt, 2009). Also, topiramate may be helpful not only in alcohol abuse but also for gambling, overeating, and sex-related addictions by reducing the impulsivity associated with them (Olive, Cleva, Kalivas, & Malcolm, 2012).

The use of benzodiazepines is typically reserved for detox settings and is not recommended for maintenance because of the possibility of developing dependence. Some clinicians find that SSRIs, such as fluoxetine (Prozac) or sertraline (Zoloft), are helpful and may reduce alcohol use, but only in patients with a co-occurring affective disorder. Some research suggests that ondansetron (Zofran), which is used to reduce nausea for cancer patients in chemotherapy and for bulimia nervosa patients, may help reduce the craving for both alcohol and cocaine (Montoya & Vocci, 2008). Although some clinicians have used trazodone for sleep disturbance after alcohol detox, researchers caution that, despite a short-term improvement of sleep quality, trazodone may lead to increased drinking behaviors when it is discontinued (Friedmann et al., 2008).

Opioid Dependence

1. Methadone (Dolophine) is a synthetic opiate that is taken orally (liquid). It produces a minimal high and sedation and has few side effects at therapeutic doses. Although controversial, methadone maintenance programs have helped many heroin users return to work and maintain family obligations. Typical methadone doses range from 20 mg/day to 200 mg/day, depending on the severity of the addiction.

2. L-alpha-acetyl-methadol, or long-acting analog methadone (LAAM), has properties that are similar to methadone, but it has been shown to be superior to methadone in reducing intravenous drug use. Since it has a slower onset of action and a longer half-life, it can be administered only three times per week, rather than daily, as for methadone. Typical doses of LAAM start at 20 mg three times per week and may go up to 80 mg three times per week. This medication may not be indicated for cardiac patients per FDA warnings.

3. Naloxone (Narcan) is used to reverse the effects of an opioid overdose. Medications like naloxone act as antagonists and shorten the withdrawal period, but they also intensify withdrawal. The *ultrarapid detox procedure* uses naloxone in combination with clonidine or other sedatives for a 24-hour detoxification.

4. Buprenorphine (Subutex, Sublocade, Probuphine) is a mixed, opioid agonist–antagonist used as an analgesic. In treatment centers, it is given sublingually at 2 mg/day to 4 mg/day and can be increased to 16 mg/day if needed. Sublocade is an injection given once per month. Probuphine is a buprenorphine implant approved by the FDA in 2016. It can be implanted for up to six months. Advantages of buprenorphine include a milder withdrawal upon discontinuance and less potential for abuse because the agonist effects are diminished at higher doses. This medication is also available as a compound of buprenorphine and naloxone (Suboxone), which has been shown to be more effective than clonidine as a medically supervised withdrawal therapy. Also, because the naloxone part of the medication exerts no clinically significant effect, the opioid agonist effects of buprenorphine predominate. This combination of drugs is much less likely to be abused (Orman & Keating, 2009). It may also show promise as an emergency treatment in cases of heroin overdose (Welsh, Sherman, & Tobin, 2008). It is also available as an oral film (Bunavail), which is placed just inside of the cheek with a starting dose of 2.1 mg/day increased to a target dose of about 8.4 mg/day. As with most medications containing buprenorphine, it's best to avoid other drugs, alcohol, and benzodiazepines unless directed by a healthcare professional. Some SSRIs may have to be avoided as well due to an increased risk of serotonin syndrome.

Longer acting formulations of buprenorphine, such as those that are injected or implanted, may not only decrease use but may increase days of sobriety, as well as eliminate the risk for misuse and diversion (Bouquié et al., 2014; Walsh et al., 2017). Similar studies found that injectable formulations of naltrexone and buprenorphine/naloxone sublingual showed similar effectiveness in reducing use and preventing relapse. Neither was superior to the other (Lee et al., 2018). Clonidine (an antihypertensive medication; see Chapter 7) may be useful in prolonging abstinence from opioids when compared to those using buprenorphine and a placebo (Kowalczyk et al., 2015). Some research suggests that tramadol (an opioid agonist) may be superior to clonidine for medically supervised opioid withdrawal (Dunn, Tompkins, Bigelow, & Strain, 2017). Naltrexone was also found effective for reducing use and craving for those who were methamphetamine dependent (Ray et al., 2015).

Cocaine Dependence

1. Tricyclic antidepressants like desipramine (Norpramin) have shown some promise in reducing cravings and improving abstinence associated with cocaine abuse, even when depression is not present.

2. Bromocriptine (Parlodel), amantadine (Symmetrel), and mazindol (Sanorex/Mazanor) are dopamine agonists given to reduce craving and discomfort in the early stages of cocaine withdrawal.

3. Ibogaine is derived from the root of the African iboga shrub. This botanical substance is an indole alkaloid that helps to mask cocaine and opioid withdrawal, but it is a potent hallucinogen with potential for abuse. Ibogaine was shown to reduce stimulant use in lab animals. It may have some promise as a treatment for stimulant abuse as well (Jullien, 2001). Typical doses range from 10 mg/day to 60 mg/day.

4. Methylphenidate (Ritalin) has been shown to reduce cocaine relapse, especially in patients with ADHD. Typical doses range from 15 mg/day to 60 mg/day (see Chapter 9 for details regarding its use). Methylphenidate and disulfiram show promise as potential treatments, but the effectiveness is optimized depending on genetic polymorphisms in patients (Haile, Kosten, & Kosten, 2009).

5. Buprenorphine (Subutex) is a mixed, opioid agonist–antagonist used as an analgesic. In treatment centers, it is given sublingually at 2 mg/day to 4 mg/day and can be increased to 16 mg/day if needed. Advantages of buprenorphine include a milder withdrawal upon discontinuance and less potential for abuse because the agonist effects are diminished at higher doses (see formulations above).

Other Types of Addiction

Bupropion (Wellbutrin SR and XL/Zyban) has been approved by the FDA for the treatment of nicotine addiction. It has been shown to be more effective than nicotine replacement gums or patches in reducing relapse in smokers (Williams & Hughes, 2003). This result was found to be especially true when a co-occurring depression was present. Nicotine dependence has a high comorbidity, not only with depression but also with conduct disorder and ADHD. The newer drug varenicline (Chantix) has been shown to be twice as effective as sustained-release bupropion, mainly because it actually binds with neuronal nicotinic acetylcholine receptors; thus, nicotine is blocked and cannot activate receptors. It further binds with moderate affinity to the 5HT3 receptor (a pleasure receptor), resulting in a reduction of nicotine as a reinforcer (Tobin, 2007). Tobin cautions about using this medication with patients presenting with mood disorders even though it is not metabolized by the cytochrome P450 system typically utilized by some antidepressants. Changes in mood and behavior have been reported in patients and should be noted when the medication is taken for the first time. Although the use of nicotine replacement in the form of gums or patches is more effective than using nothing at all, the use of bupropion and varenicline appears to be more effective, and with fewer adverse effects (Anthenelli et al., 2016). Tabex (cytisine) is an over-the-counter partial agonist of the nicotinic acetylcholine receptor also used to assist in smoking cessation.

Because SSRIs often reduce sexual appetite, they may offer some hope to people with sexual addiction and compulsivity. Sexual addiction disorders often coexist with chemical dependency and frequently trigger relapse (Schneider & Irons, 2001). This research also mentions that as many as 70% of cocaine addicts are also sexually addicted, and as many as 76% of methamphetamine users consider themselves to be "sexually obsessed."

SUMMARY AND TREATMENT REMINDERS

In the fourth or final phase of treatment, the clinician assesses the patient's progress and the need for paying more attention to either the substance abuse issue or the mental health issue. Clinicians must keep in mind that when treating the primary mental health diagnosis with medications, they must not compromise the patient's chemical dependency issues (i.e., treating an anxiety disorder with benzodiazepines in a patient with a history of alcohol dependence). In this situation, the clinician is likely to see abuse of the benzodiazepines. Another common example is the anxious patient who is trying to remain substance free and presents with a chief complaint of initial insomnia. The patient's physician gives the patient a sedative-hypnotic as a sleep aid only to learn months later that the patient has become dependent on them.

Clinicians also need to be sensitive with respect to patients whom they refer to Alcoholics Anonymous (AA) and Narcotics Anonymous (NA) groups. Most of these groups have little tolerance for people with co-occurring conditions and are likely to hassle them for taking "other drugs" for their condition. The clinician needs to inquire about the group's composition and send patients only to groups that are sensitive to the medication issues.

Preventing a patient's relapse is the key to continued success, and reducing stress is the key to preventing relapse. "Booster" sessions and stress-reduction groups are excellent ideas. While relapse tends to happen in about 50% of all cases, clinicians should have a clear plan for resuming treatment without a heavy emphasis on failure so that patients can rework their program without shame and to strive for full recovery.

CASE VIGNETTES

Case 1

CLINICAL HISTORY

Reggie is a 42-year-old African American male recently referred for outpatient psychotherapy by his PCP. While he is in relatively good health, he admitted to his doctor that he has been drinking alcohol excessively again over the last three months. Reggie had a problem with alcohol when he was in his twenties, but with the help of AA and his first male partner, he was able to cease drinking for the last 19 years. Reggie admits that it has not always been easy for him to abstain, but he is committed to trying again. He has attended AA meetings but has not been able to maintain complete sobriety. On average, he has one or two drinks nearly every evening. His partner, Bob, has a zero-tolerance policy for Reggie's drinking and has moved in with a friend rather than deal with Reggie's promises to stop. Reggie is worried that Bob may not come back. Reggie does not want to end up like his father, who drank himself to death at the age of 56. His father and mother divorced when Reggie was only 15. Reggie's only sister had a serious addiction to benzodiazepines and spent 28 days in a rehab center. She is clean now but also abuses alcohol on occasion.

POSTCASE DISCUSSION AND DIAGNOSIS

Reggie has Alcohol Dependence in Sustained Partial Remission with Moderate Symptoms (F10.20) He clearly shows signs of dependence and abuse as he continues to use alcohol despite the effect it is having on his relationship. He admits that coworkers have commented on his being late to work and that they have noticed alcohol on his breath. He has now taken to chewing gum to mask his alcohol breath and working longer hours to justify his lateness in the morning.

PSYCHOPHARMACOLOGICAL TREATMENT

At the urging of his family doctor and friends, Reggie has agreed to attend 90 meetings in 90 days. He now attends only gay AA meetings so he can feel more comfortable sharing aspects of his relationship with Bob without strange looks or criticism. Reggie also agreed to try Campral at the suggestion of his doctor. Reggie typically dislikes taking any medications, so his dose was started low (1000 mg qd). His dose was slowly raised to 2000 per day, and he reported that he was tolerating it without side effects. Reggie did not immediately crease drinking, but by the end of the first week he reported a tremendous drop in both his interest in alcohol and the enjoyment of drinking while engaging in drinking. He thought at first that he was losing interest in drinking whiskey, so he switched to beer. He later lost interest in beer and reported several days without alcohol. In a follow-up appointment with his PCP after six weeks on the medication, he reported that he celebrated 30 days sober and was on his way to the meeting to get his 30-day chip. He admits he has a long road to a sustained recovery, and he believes that Campral has helped him take the first serious steps and, with Bob's forgiveness, he is taking one day at a time.

Case 2

CLINICAL HISTORY

Brianne is a 29-year-old white female who is recovering from an auto accident that occurred seven months ago. Although immediately after the accident her injuries were not serious or life-threatening, her PCP prescribed her opioids for the pain. While he suggested that she discontinue using them after 30 days and switch to using acetaminophen, she claimed that her pain was still severe. He reluctantly allowed another 15-day refill, but she reported that if she stopped using the opioids her pain would return. When she could no longer get the opioid from her doctor, she feigned a sports injury and managed to get more from urgent care. When she ran out of that supply, she purchased another 60 pills from a friend who had recently had surgery. When this supply ran out, she presented to the ER in severe pain and panic. The ER staff referred her to a detox program.

POSTCASE DISCUSSION AND DIAGNOSIS

Brianne was diagnosed at the opioid treatment center as having Opioid Use Disorder (F11.20). She had been off from work for more than seven months, claiming that her pain was unpleasant and interfered with her ability to function as an IT specialist. She was constantly worried that she would not be able to find opioids and that her pain would get worse. She was unable to limit or cut down on using them on her own.

PSYCHOPHARMACOLOGICAL TREATMENT

Brianne was started on Suboxone 2 mg taken about every four hours. By day 2 she was increased to 16 mg/day. She reported some withdrawal issues, but they were not severe, and with the help of her recovery group, she was able to ride them out. The use of relaxation therapy and hypnosis assisted her with some mild pain issues, and by day 30 of treatment she was discharged without pain and with a commitment to attend an outpatient group therapy program.

CHAPTER 14

Treatment of Comorbidity and Other Disorders

This chapter examines the often complex role of comorbid conditions. All clinicians deal with patients who present with issues such as chronic pain, eating disorders, obesity, and, of course, disorders of impulse control, but few suggestions for treatment are presented in most psychopharmacology texts. Helpful pharmacological considerations are presented here with a rationale for reducing symptoms.

Topics to be addressed include the following:

- Medical and psychiatric comorbidity
- Chronic neuropathic pain
- Eating disorders and obesity
- Disruptive and impulse control disorders
- Case vignettes

Psychiatric disorders exist in real life, not in an isolated system, but rather within the context of other serious medical and psychiatric diagnoses. In addition to looking at the various medical and psychiatric comorbidities, in this chapter we consider other important psychiatric issues. Frequently, these diseases co-occur with multiple other medical illnesses. The common features that bind these topics together are the complexity and sometimes the resistant nature of their treatment. According to Kroenke (2003), unexplained or multiple somatic symptoms are the leading cause of outpatient medical visits and also the predominant reason patients with common mental disorders, such as anxiety and depression, initially present themselves in primary care. Hall & Reynolds (2014) describe depression as among the leading causes of illness-related disability, and it is projected to be the greatest contributor to disease burden by 2030 in high-income countries. They estimate depression prevalence rates among aging populations range between 1% and 3% in the community and 6% and 9% in primary care settings. The accepted term for people with multiple chronic conditions is now *multimorbidity* rather than *comorbidity*, which have been used interchangeably in the past. Comorbidity is best used when there is a specified index condition or where there are defined combinations of conditions (e.g., hypertension and cardiovascular disease) as opposed to multimorbidity where any condition could be included. Multimorbidity is common in clinical practice and is an important problem in most healthcare systems (Smith, Wallace, O'Dowd, & Fortin, 2016).

MEDICAL AND PSYCHIATRIC COMORBIDITY

The complicated interaction between the mind and body may lead to disease processes that are more difficult to treat than individual illnesses themselves. According to Blazer, Steffens, and Busse (2004), depression has been shown to be a risk factor for declines in physical functioning; likewise, declines in physical functioning have been shown to be a risk factor for depression. Attention to psychiatric symptoms among medically ill patients has emerged in general medical settings over the last few decades. Kroenke (2003) reports that patients have at least a twofold greater risk of experiencing a depressive or anxiety disorder if they have a concomitant disease, including cardiovascular disease, neurological disease, cancer, diabetes, HIV, and many other physical disorders. The proportion of primary care patients with a probable depressive and/or anxiety disorder ranges from 33% to 80%; primary care patients also have alarmingly high levels of multimorbidity of depressive, anxiety, and physical disorders. Depression and anxiety among primary care patients contribute to poor compliance with medical advice and treatment, deficits in patient–provider communication, reduced patient engagement in healthy behaviors, and decreased physical well-being (Zhang, Park, Sullivan, & Jing, 2018). Psychiatric comorbidities are important factors that may increase the length of acute medical–surgical inpatient stays, the frequency of medical complications, and the overall mortality (Sadock, Sadock, & Ruiz, 2017). Larsen and Christenfeld (2009) suggest that the high comorbidity between cardiovascular disease and psychiatric disorders may be attributable to a general state of inflexibility (cognitive, emotional, or physiological), leading to rumination, worry, obsessions, low heart rate variability and vagal tone, and extended sympathetic arousal. Furthermore, medical comorbidity in bipolar disorder increases early mortality an average of 9 years for women and 8.5 years for men compared to the general population. More recent studies have also focused on common medical comorbidities and potential pathological pathways (such as oxidative stress and inflammation) that may underlie the link between medical illness and bipolar disorder (Sinha et al., 2018).

Depression often co-occurs with a variety of psychiatric and substance use disorders. In co-occurrence, the presence of both illnesses is frequently unrecognized and, unfortunately, leads to serious and unnecessary negative consequences for patients and families. According to Kupfer and Frank (2003), concurrent depression is present in 13% of patients with panic disorder. With respect to eating disorders, 50% to 75% of patients suffering from anorexia nervosa or bulimia nervosa have a lifetime history of major depressive disorder. These high levels of comorbid diagnoses with depression are also true for substance use disorders (see Chapter 13). When Axis II disorders are considered, dysfunctional personality traits have a negative effect on the outcome of treatment of Axis I disorders (Reich, 2003).

When looking at concurrent medical disease, Lesperance, Frasure-Smith, and Talajic (1996) demonstrated that 40% to 65% of patients who have experienced a myocardial infarction suffer from depression. Large-scale epidemiological studies of patients in the community yield increased relative risks of myocardial infarction and cardiac-related mortality of approximately 1.5 to 2.0 in association with depression (Sadock et al., 2017). In general practice, cancer patients suffer from depression about 25% of the time according to many experts. In patients with neurological diseases (e.g., stroke), researchers suggest that depression occurs in about 25% of cases. Morbidity and mortality continue to increase in connection with the number of medical and/or psychiatric diagnoses (Kupfer & Frank, 2003).

Even in the medical–psychiatric comorbidity context, the treatment of the particular psychiatric diagnosis is very similar to the treatment of the psychiatric problem alone. For example, depression either alone or in the context of a comorbid medical condition should be treated similarly. However, the clinician should use the lowest possible medication dose to treat the disorder, especially when treating multiple conditions with many different pharmacotherapies. Communication among the various prescribers treating the patient's co-occurring conditions is of utmost importance.

The field of psychosomatic medicine is a rapidly evolving and increasingly important area of study. For example, psycho-oncology is a recognized field in which mental health professionals provide consultative services to support cancer patients and their families at all stages of disease, including cancer survivorship (Breitbart & Alici, 2009). Psychoneuroimmunology is another emerging interdisciplinary science that examines the impact of behavior and psychological states on immunity. Biobehavioral factors that show robust associations with markers of inflammation include variables such as diet, smoking, coffee consumption, alcohol consumption, exercise, and sleep disruption (O'Connor & Irwin, 2010). Other current fields of study related to comorbidity include psychocardiology, psychoneuroendocrinology, and functional gastrointestinal disorders.

CHRONIC NEUROPATHIC PAIN

According to the International Association for the Study of Pain, pain is an unpleasant sensory and emotional experience associated with actual or potential tissue damage (Merskey, 1979). The emotional dimension of pain was even noted by Freud in the 1890s (Strachey, 1953). Since pain is neither a purely physiological state nor a purely psychological one, treatment demands a comprehensive, integrated, multidisciplinary plan, as well as clear communication of all findings to the patient. Neuropathic pain has been redefined as "pain arising as a direct consequence of a lesion or disease affecting the somatosensory system" (Jensen et al., 2011; Treede et al., 2008). According to Cruccu and Truini (2017), the prevalence of neuropathic pain in the general population has been estimated at 6.9% to 10.0%. A number of factors, including the aging population, increasing obesity rates, and increased survival of cancer patients being treated with interventions likely to cause neuropathic pain, mean that the prevalence of neuropathic pain is likely to increase in our future. Keep in mind that neuropathic pain can adversely affect patients' overall quality of life, including physical and emotional functioning, and it is associated with substantial societal costs (O'Connor, 2009). The clinician must keep in mind that there is no typical pain patient; individualized treatment is absolutely necessary. Although there are many types of peripheral and central neuropathic pain, postherpetic neuralgia and diabetic peripheral neuropathy are the most common types studied.

Evidence-based guidelines for the pharmacological treatment of chronic neuropathic pain have been published. First-line treatments include tricyclic antidepressants, dual reuptake inhibitors of serotonin and norepinephrine, and calcium channel alpha2-delta ligands (such as gabapentin and pregabalin). Tramadol, capsaicin 8% patches, and lidocaine patches are recommended as second-line treatments that can be considered for initial use in certain clinical circumstances. Cannabinoids, strong opioids, and botulinum toxin type A are considered third-line treatments. Although some of these treatment options are not psychopharmacologic, they are included for completeness (Dworkin et al., 2010; Finnerup et al., 2015; Gilron, Baron, & Jensen, 2015; Moulin et al., 2014). We must keep in mind that although strong opioids are efficacious in the treatment of neuropathic pain, they are not considered to be a first choice because of adverse drug reactions and concerns about abuse, diversion, and addiction (Fornasari, 2017).

Although many chronic pain patients resist psychiatric help, a formal psychiatric consultation is important to clarify the medical diagnoses, screen for psychiatric diagnoses, and identify emotional influences that underlie or exacerbate primary pain. Chronic pain may be a presenting symptom of many of the following psychiatric diagnoses: major depression, generalized anxiety disorder, panic disorder, posttraumatic stress disorder, and substance abuse. Other less common psychiatric diagnoses that may be present in the context of chronic pain include delusional disorders, chronic psychosis, somatoform disorders, and malingering. Over 75% of depressed patients report chronic pain issues (Delgado, 2006). Sansone and Sansone (2008) indicate that patients with pain have a substantially increased risk for depression, from two to five times that of the general population. Furthermore, emotional influences that may affect the experience of pain include unresolved grief; sexual or developmental conflicts; sexual, physical, or emotional abuse; anger at physicians; and even symbolic identification with a loved one (Mufson, 1999).

Chronic pain conditions such as fibromyalgia are especially difficult to treat. Fibromyalgia is different from most other rheumatologic disorders in that it is not due to tissue damage or inflammation per se (Spaeth & Briley, 2009). Häuser, Ablin, Perrot, and Fitzcharles (2017) estimate the prevalence of fibromyalgia to be approximately 2% with a female-to-male ratio of 3:1 in epidemiology studies and of 8:1 to 10:1 in clinical settings. In addition to widespread pain, patients also experience fatigue, cognitive, and sleep disturbances. Many of these patients also present with depression and, increasingly often, with anxiety (Arnold, Crofford, Martin, Young, & Sharma, 2007). Most researchers agree that no one medication best addresses the pain and accompanying mood concerns, but antidepressants are becoming increasingly effective with this group of patients. Although the older TCAs have been shown to be effective, the newer dual-action (serotonin/norepinephrine) inhibitors have been shown to be as effective, without the typical anti-cholinergic side effects (McCleane, 2008; Spaeth & Briley, 2009). Dual-action medications such as venlafaxine, duloxetine, and milnacipran may be more efficacious because norepinephrine and serotonin are two key neurotransmitters in the pain modulation pathway from the basil ganglia. Medications that combine serotonergic and noradrenergic reuptake inhibition may have stronger analgesic effects than agents that inhibit reuptake of either neurotransmitter alone (Mease, 2009). In addition to antidepressants, pregabalin (Lyrica; a calcium channel alpha2-delta ligand) and tramadol (an opioid) are used for pain management in patients with fibromyalgia and neuropathic pain.

From the psychiatric perspective, the treatment of chronic pain and its emotional components relies on medications and various forms of psychotherapy. Antidepressants are probably the most prescribed group of medications because of their effect on improving mood and decreasing anxiety. Tricyclic antidepressants are still widely used in this context, not only for the reasons already mentioned (see Chapter 5), but also for their noradrenergic effects that decrease neuropathic pain. Many pain physicians use amitriptyline (Elavil) in a 25 mg dose at bedtime to help decrease pain, improve sleep, and possibly improve mood. As a class, the SNRIs (serotonin–norepinephrine reuptake inhibitors), such as venlafaxine/desvenlafaxine (Effexor/Pristiq) and duloxetine (Cymbalta), may be more effective than SSRIs in decreasing the somatic symptoms associated with depression and anxiety syndromes (Grothe, Scheckner, & Albano, 2004). Psychotherapeutic options for chronic pain patients include individual, marital, and family therapy to address the underlying dynamic factors. Cognitive-behavioral therapy, hypnosis, and biofeedback are probably the most useful and most practical ways to approach treatment for these complicated and challenging patients.

EATING DISORDERS AND OBESITY

The eating disorders are a complex group of illnesses that are heavily underpinned by psychopathology and are associated with significant medical consequences. These disorders primarily affect young women. Patients who suffer from anorexia nervosa and bulimia nervosa place extraordinary emphasis on weight, shape, and the pursuit of thinness. In addition, binge-eating disorder, which is characterized by episodes of uncontrollable eating, has emerged as a diagnostic entity. Patients with eating disorders tend to have high rates of psychiatric comorbidity and medical complications (Pederson, Roerig, & Mitchell, 2003). Interestingly, recent data indicate that the majority of people with eating disorders are classified under the Eating Disorder Not Otherwise Specified (EDNOS) category, similar to other psychiatric diagnoses that include personality disorders, dissociative disorders, and somatoform disorders (Thomas, Vartanian, & Brownell, 2009). Furthermore, obesity is discussed because of the prominent nature it plays in one's self-concept, as well as societal views of beauty and attractiveness.

Anorexia Nervosa

Anorexia nervosa is characterized by patients' refusal to maintain a normal body weight, along with their intense fear of gaining weight despite being underweight. According to Pederson et al. (2003) and Moore and Bokor (2017), the disorder can lead to serious medical consequences, including osteoporosis, cardiac arrhythmias, and congestive heart failure. Furthermore, psychiatric comorbidities are very common in anorexia nervosa including mood disorders, anxiety disorders, obsessive-compulsive disorder, developmental disorders (e.g., autistic spectrum and attention-deficit hyperactivity disorder), some personality disorders (e.g., borderline), and substance use disorders. Some researchers suggest a positive genetic correlation between anorexia nervosa and schizophrenia (Marucci et al., 2018).

Anorexia nervosa has two distinct phases of the illness: the acute, underweight phase (usually inpatient) and the maintenance, weight-restored phase (usually outpatient). The two phases basically represent different biological entities in that the treatment options differ. In the acute phase of treatment with patients close to emaciation, the treatment plan largely focuses on inpatient care, medically supervised refeeding programs, dietary counseling, and individual, group, and family therapies. Medications play a more significant role in the maintenance, weight-restored phase of treatment. Although anorexia nervosa was defined as a diagnostic entity over a century ago, the absolute etiology underlying the disorder remains elusive (Mitchell, de Zwaan, & Roerig, 2003; Mitchell, Peterson, Myers, & Wonderlich, 2001). Moore and Bokor (2017) report that biologic and environmental factors play a role in the development of anorexia nervosa. Genetic correlations exist between educational attainment, neuroticism, and schizophrenia. Patients with anorexia nervosa have altered brain function and structure, including deficits in dopamine (eating behavior and reward), serotonin (impulse control and neuroticism), differential activation of the corticolimbic system (appetite and fear), and diminished activity among the frontostriatal circuits (habitual behaviors).

A large variety of compounds have been explored in treating anorexia nervosa, including antidepressants, antipsychotics, antihistamines, narcotic antagonists, lithium, and zinc, to name a few. To date, however, there are no FDA-approved medications for anorexia nervosa (Jackson, Cates, & Lorenz 2010). Controlled medication trials in patients with anorexia nervosa are few in number; thus, optimal treatment has yet to be defined. Research has predominantly focused on two drug groups: antidepressants and antipsychotics. Trials of tricyclic antidepressants (TCAs) and fluoxetine (Prozac) have not been shown to offer much benefit for the acute treatment phase. However, a controlled outpatient maintenance trial suggests that patients randomized to fluoxetine gained more weight, had decreased core eating disorder symptoms, and displayed more improvement in mood symptoms compared with the placebo group at the one-year endpoint (Kaye, Nagata, & Weltzin, 2001). Both in terms of stimulating weight gain and in reducing delusional thoughts about food, weight, and shape, pilot studies and case reports have described successful use of atypical antipsychotics such as olanzapine (Zyprexa), risperidone (Risperdal), and aripiprazole (Abilify) in anorexia nervosa patients (Davis & Attia, 2017).

A summary of research conducted on the use of medication for anorexia nervosa before September 2009 appears to conclude that while atypical antipsychotics have been used with this treatment group, only mild evidence of improvement in depression, anxiety, and core eating-disordered psychopathology was found. As a whole, there is insufficient evidence to confirm that atypical antipsychotics enhance weight gain (McKnight & Park, 2010). More recent anorexia nervosa studies have focused on D-cycloserine, dronabinal (synthetic cannabinoid agonist), and hormonal treatments to improve bone density (Davis & Attia, 2017), as well as the ghrelin receptor agonist, oxytocin, testosterone, neuromodulation with transcranial direct current stimulation, repetitive transcranial magnetic stimulation, or deep brain stimulation and rosiglitazone (Lutter, 2017).

Bulimia Nervosa

In contrast to anorexia nervosa, which is relatively rare, bulimia nervosa is more prevalent and affects about 1% to 3% of adolescent and young adult females. Bulimia nervosa patients place great emphasis on body weight and shape, but unlike anorexia nervosa patients, they usually fall within a normal weight range. This disorder is characterized by binge-eating episodes and associated inappropriate compensatory behaviors aimed at preventing weight gain. Medical consequences of bulimia nervosa include dental complications (permanent loss of tooth enamel, increased frequency of caries, and parotid gland swelling), amenorrhea, electrolyte abnormalities, esophageal tears, gastric rupture, and cardiac arrhythmias. The last three medical conditions may be fatal. As with anorexia nervosa, bulimia nervosa patients have high rates of comorbid psychopathology: About 50% have a lifetime diagnosis of depression, about 25% have a lifetime diagnosis of substance abuse or dependence, and about 40% have a personality disorder (Agras, 2001). The cause of bulimia is uncertain, but mounting evidence suggests that genetic factors play an important role (Bulik, Devlin, & Bacanu, 2003). Disturbances in serotonergic systems may play a role in causing bulimia because of the involvement of serotonin in the regulation of food intake. Cultural attitudes toward standards of physical attractiveness are also believed to be contributing causes (Mehler, 2003).

Bulimia nervosa has been more extensively studied than anorexia. Pharmacotherapy with antidepressants results in significant reductions in target eating behaviors such as binge eating and vomiting and associated mood or anxiety disorders. The only FDA-approved treatment for bulimia nervosa is fluoxetine (Prozac) in the dosage range of 60 mg/day to 80 mg/day. Furthermore, studies have consistently shown that cognitive-behavioral therapy (CBT) is the first-line treatment of choice when it is available. Although CBT alone is superior to medication treatment alone, most experts would consider the use of CBT plus an antidepressant to be more effective than either treatment alone (Mitchell et al., 2001). Other medications studied that may be useful in treating bulimia include ondansetron (Zofran), a 5-HT$_3$ antagonist, and topiramate (Topamax), an anticonvulsant mood stabilizer. Topiramate appears to have efficacy in bulimia nervosa as demonstrated by two placebo-controlled studies (McElroy et al., 2009). According to Lutter (2017), emerging treatments for bulimia include cholecystokinin, glucagon-like peptide 1, polypeptide YY, zonisamide (Zonegran), naltrexone (Revia), neuromodulation with repetitive transcranial magnetic stimulation or transcranial direct current stimulation, and lorcaserin (Belviq).

Binge-Eating Disorder

Binge-eating disorder (BED) is characterized by binge-eating patterns similar to those of bulimic patients but without compensatory weight-loss behaviors such as purging episodes or overexercising. The estimated prevalence of BED is 1.5% to 2% in the general population. When looking at obese populations such as those seeking weight-loss assistance programs, the prevalence of BED increases to 8% to 19% (Devlin, 2002). In bariatric surgery programs, Wadden, Sarwer, and Womble (2001) report that approximately 25% of the individuals may have BED. According to Citrome (2017b), 79% of individuals with BED meet criteria for at least one comorbid psychiatric disorders and 49% meet criteria for three or more disorders.

Treatment efforts for BED have included TCAs, SSRIs, anticonvulsants, and anti-obesity medications. Unlike the information available for bulimia nervosa, pharmacological data for treatment of BED are much more preliminary. Cognitive-behavioral therapy appears to be more efficacious than SSRIs in about half of the controlled trials. However, lisdexamfetamine (Vyvanse) was the first medication approved by the U.S. Food and Drug Administration for treatment of BED and is generally reported to be well tolerated and effective. Research has focused on topiramate (Topamax) and sibutramine (Meridia) as future possibilities for decreasing the psychopathology and promoting weight loss (Pederson et al., 2003). Sibutramine (Meridia) is an SNRI, like venlafaxine (Effexor) and duloxetine (Cymbalta). According to Tziomalos, Krassas, and Tzotzas (2009), three placebo-controlled studies have shown sibutramine to reduce body weight and the frequency of binge-eating episodes more than placebo. Topiramate has shown positive results in three placebo-controlled trials, and zonisamide (Zonegran) indicated positive results in one small controlled study in binge-eating disorder with obesity (McElroy et al., 2009). Glucagon-like peptide 1, naltrexone, and neuromodulation with transcranial direct current stimulation are the most recently compounds under investigation (Lutter, 2017).

Obesity

Obesity is another prevalent disease that affects over 60 million Americans today. Approximately 64% of adult Americans are categorized as being overweight (body mass index [BMI] of 25–29.9 kg/m^2) or obese (BMI more than 30 kg/m^2). Obesity is associated with increased mortality and comorbidities such as hypertension, hyperglycemia, dyslipidemia, coronary artery disease, and certain cancers. Obesity is influenced by a myriad of factors, including genetic, developmental, biological, environmental, behavioral, and iatrogenic ones. Historically, obesity was regarded solely as a lifestyle or behavioral disorder; however, current perspectives focus on the complex physiology and its devastating effect on quality of life (Srivastava & Apovian, 2018).

Over the last few decades, fenfluramine (Pondimin), dexfenfluramine (Redux), phenylpropanolamine (an ingredient in over-the-counter nasal decongestants and weight-control drugs), and sibutramine (Meridia) have been withdrawn by the FDA because of severe adverse effects. The medications approved by the FDA as anorectics are the following: phentermine (Adipex-P/Ionamin), orlistat (Xenical), phentermine/topiramate extended release (Qsymia), larcaserin (Belviq), naltrexone sustained release/bupropion sustained release (Contrave), and liraglutide injection (Saxenda). According to Campbell and Mathys (2001), phentermine has been shown to cause 5% to 15% weight loss if given daily or intermittently. The limiting factor with this medication is that it is approved only for short-term use, and tolerance often develops.

Orlistat (Xenical) works as a reversible inhibitor of lipases in the gastrointestinal tract; these inactivated enzymes are unavailable to hydrolyze dietary fat, and thus the fats are not absorbed. Orlistat has an advantage over the other medications in that it is not absorbed systemically, and it may have cholesterol-lowering effects in some patients. Unfortunately, orlistat is less desirable in some patients due to the high incidence of gastrointestinal side effects, and it must be given three times daily with meals (Rao, 2010).

Phentermine/topiramate (Qsymia) is an extended-release combination that was approved by the FDA in 2012. The exact anorexigenic mechanism of topiramate is not well understood, although it is postulated that the effects are mediated through modulation of various neurotransmitters, including the inhibition of voltage-dependent sodium channels, glutamate receptors and carbonic anhydrase and the potentiation of γ-aminobutyrate activity. The combination drug has shown greater potential weight-loss effects than monotherapy alone for each while also reducing adverse effects (Srivastava & Apovian, 2018).

Lorcaserin (Belviq), a 5-hydroxytryptamine receptor 2C (5-HT2c) agonist that acts on anorexigenic neurons in the hypothalamus, was also approved by the FDA in 2012 as an adjunct to a reduced-calorie diet and increased physical activity for chronic weight management in adults with at least one weight-related comorbid condition such as diabetes mellitus, hypertension, hyperlipidemia or sleep apnea. Lorcaserin has specific selectivity towards the 5-HT2c receptor, which alleviates risk associated with prior agents of this class, such as fenfluramine, which was found to have affinity for both 5-HT2A (causing hallucinations) and 5-HT2B receptors (causing cardiac valve insufficiency and pulmonary hypertension). Serotonin has been known to modulate food intake and appetite (Joo & Lee, 2014).

The naltrexone SR/bupropion SR (Contrave) combination was demonstrated in preclinical animal models to function in a synergistic manner. Naltrexone blocks opioid receptor-mediated auto-inhibition, and bupropion selectively inhibits reuptake of dopamine and noradrenaline. Monotherapy of these two drugs has also been used to treat addiction to nicotine (bupropion) and alcohol (naltrexone). Thus, the combination has an effect on CNS reward pathways, food intake and satiety through antagonistic feedback inhibition (Srivastava & Apovian, 2018).

Liraglutide (Saxenda) is a glucagon-like peptide 1 (GLP1) receptor agonist of an incretin-derived hormone that acts through both peripheral and central receptor pathways affecting glucose homeostasis, food intake and satiety. Currently, liraglutide is the only injectable anti-obesity drug (Srivastava & Apovian, 2018).

DISRUPTIVE AND IMPULSE CONTROL DISORDERS

Disruptive, impulse-control, and conduct disorders are conditions involving problems in the self-control of behavior and emotions leading to violating the rights of others or bringing the individual into conflict with authority figures or societal norms. Disorders under this classification include oppositional defiant disorder, conduct disorder, intermittent explosive disorder, kleptomania, and pyromania. Onset of these disorders is usually in childhood or adolescence. Because some of these behaviors may be common in adolescent development, it is important to look at factors such as frequency, persistence, and pervasiveness in comparison with the individual's age, gender, and culture before making an official diagnosis. Common general symptoms of these disorders include a pattern of angry or irritable mood, argumentative or defiant behavior, verbal or physical aggression toward others, bullying or threatening others, initiating physical fights, deliberately damaging property (e.g., setting fires), stealing objects that are not needed for personal use or for their monetary value, and recurring rule defiance (e.g., running away from home or skipping school).

Successful psychopharmacological interventions have been described throughout the literature but are limited to mostly case reports and case series. SSRIs have shown mixed results. An open label trial with naltrexone (a mu-opiate receptor antagonist) reduced urges to steal and stealing behaviors. In another open-label trial, memantine (an NMDA receptor antagonist), also reduced urges to shoplift and associated behaviors (Sadock et al., 2017). Mood stabilizers such as lithium, valproate (Depakote), and topiramate (Topamax) have been successful in some case studies (Dannon, 2003). As mentioned in Chapter 13, opioid-receptor antagonists such as naltrexone (Revia) have been used with the impulse control disorders, resulting in positive outcomes for some, especially for pathological gambling (Leung & Cottler, 2008). For intermittent-explosive disorder, research evidence suggests that mood stabilizers, atypical antipsychotics, beta blockers, alpha-2 agonists, phenytoin (Dilantin), and serotonergic antidepressants may be useful (Coccaro, Lee, & McCloskey, 2014; Olvera, 2002).

Problematic Internet use (PIU) is an ever-growing concern. PIU has been defined as use of the Internet that creates psychological, social, school, and/or work difficulties in a person's life (Beard & Wolf, 2001). Scientific understanding of PIU has lagged behind media attention mainly because of inconsistencies in definitions, disagreement over whether it exists or not, and the variable methodological approaches used in studying it. Despite this, a global body of data unequivocally highlights the Internet's potential to bring about considerable psychological harm (Aboujaoude, 2010). Problems range from inappropriate personal use of the Internet in the workplace and excessive use of online games, pornography, and gambling, to cyberbullying among children and adolescents. SSRIs are recommended treatment for PIU unless there is a manic or hypomanic component (Recupero, 2008). More recently, pharmacological and psychotherapeutic treatments specific to PIU have received limited testing in large, rigorous studies. However, preliminary evidence suggests that both psychotropic medications (escitalopram, naltrexone, and methylphenidate) and cognitive-behavioral therapy may have some utility in the treatment of PIU (Spada, 2014).

Furthermore, problematic mobile phone use is associated with health hazards, such as texting while driving, leading to injury and death, and types of psychopathology, including anxiety and depression. Smartphones can distract drivers (especially young adults) who talk or text on the phone while driving, potentially leading to traffic accidents. Smartphone use is also a distractor among pedestrians while walking or crossing the street, and it is associated with neck and shoulder pain because of one's posture while using that type of phone, as well as hand dysfunction. Mobile phone use in students is associated with poor physical fitness and worse academic performance. Greater problems from use can expose individuals to more hazards or negative effects (Elhai, Dvorak, Levine, & Hall, 2017).

Although we have focused only on medical–psychiatric comorbidity, chronic neuropathic pain, eating disorders, obesity, and disruptive/impulse control disorders, medications may be used with some effectiveness for many other psychiatric diagnoses. Most of these areas of study are based on small case reports or anecdotal evidence from busy clinicians. In conclusion, more randomized controlled trials are needed to evaluate individual and combination treatments for short-term and long-term use.

CASE VIGNETTES

Case 1

CLINICAL HISTORY

Ray is a 32-year-old white male seeing a clinical social worker for the first time for an "anger problem." He was recently arrested for assault after a road rage incident in Los Angeles. It happened at 6:20 in the evening. Ray was in a hurry to get home and catch the Lakers game during the playoffs. He encountered someone driving a bit too slow in the fast lane of the freeway. He couldn't get around the vehicle because of heavy traffic in the other lanes. He used his horn and flashed his lights to no avail. The longer he sat behind this car, the angrier Ray became. Finally, he noticed his exit was coming up so he moved from the fast lane to the right lane, just as the person in front of him did the same. Unfortunately, the car exited at the same exit and was once again traveling slowly in front of Ray. At the first traffic light they came to, Ray pulled up alongside the car and yelled several obscenities at the driver. The driver very calmly gave Ray the finger and started to drive away. Ray sped up and whipped his car in front of the other driver, nearly causing the driver to rear-end him. Ray jumped out of the car, walked over to the other driver's side window and struck the driver twice in the face. Unfortunately for Ray, a California Highway Patrol motorcycle cop witnessed the whole event.

POSTCASE DISCUSSION AND DIAGNOSIS

Ray has no clinical diagnosis per se. He does not meet criteria for Intermittent Explosive Disorder or a mood disorder. He denies use of alcohol or other substances. Although he has no history of domestic violence, he did get into more than one physical altercation with former boyfriends of his current wife of six years. He had one other arrest for assault 10 years ago over a parking spot at a crowded shopping mall.

When questioned about his behavior, Ray admits he shouldn't react to people so harshly, but he claims that "stupid drivers" are his pet peeve. Construction sites and lane closings are sure to set him off. He admits that he has always been a "hothead" and is worried now that he will have a police record.

PSYCHOPHARMACOLOGICAL TREATMENT

In addition to anger management, Ray's clinical social worker arranged for a medication consultation with a local psychiatrist. Ray agreed to try taking a low-dose SSRI to see if it helped him curb his anger. He was started on 10 mg of citalopram (Celexa) every morning. In a follow-up visit with his therapist two weeks later, he reported feeling less tense while driving and less likely to anticipate problems when he encountered a construction site on the freeway. In fact, his wife reported that when they pulled into the grocery store parking lot last week, he didn't seem to mind that someone else got to the last spot before he did. In the past he would have raced to the spot and yelled to the other driver to inform him that the spot was taken. He once got out of the car and waited for the other car to drive away before taking the spot. His wife is so happy that he appears to have become a new "chilled-out" man. Ray is also happy with his progress, noting that he is also less argumentative with others in the workplace.

Case 2

CLINICAL HISTORY

Perlean is a 63-year-old black female who was referred from her family physician for depression over the last six months or so. She has never seen a psychiatrist and reports never having depression in the past. Her current symptoms include low self-esteem, hopelessness, poor appetite with a 20-pound weight loss over the last three months, excessive sleepiness, decreased energy, and no interest in her two grandchildren. Perlean also has diabetes mellitus with significant diabetic neuropathy leading to pain and significant restriction of her usual activities because of this. "I can't even play with my grandchildren anymore because of the depression and pain." She has mentioned this to her family doctor, but he has not explored or prescribed anything for her symptoms. Over the last three months, her life has consisted of sitting in her recliner with intermittent walks to the kitchen and bathroom. Her husband of 40 years has been doing all the housework and caring for her during this time.

POSTCASE DISCUSSION AND DIAGNOSIS

Perlean has a diagnosis of Major Depressive Disorder, Single Episode, Moderate (F.32.1), as well as a diagnosis of chronic neuropathic pain from her diabetes mellitus. Upon interview, she reports a family history of depression with a sister being treated with "Elavil" in the past successfully. She indicates that she feels like her "life is not worth living" but denies active suicide ideation, plan, or intent. Perlean is able to contract for her safety. Her husband reports that she is a "shell of the person she used to be."

PSYCHOPHARMACOLOGICAL TREATMENT

Due to Perlean's comorbid diagnosis of major depressive disorder and neuropathic pain, options for her current treatment include TCAs or SNRIs. Given her family history, Perlean preferred to take the same medication that helped her sister when she struggled with the depression previously. Elavil (amitriptyline) was initiated at 10 mg nightly x 1 week, then increased to 20 mg nightly for the second week. Perlean noticed mild sedation and some dizziness after starting the drug, but this resolved after four days. She did not report any falls or blackouts due to the dizziness. Over the first two weeks of treatment, she was starting to report less pain in her legs and her appetite was definitely better. At her next visit in two weeks, the dose of amitriptyline was increased to 25 mg nightly thereafter. After four weeks on 25 mg nightly, Perlean had more energy and was starting to smile again. Six weeks into her treatment, she was basically back to her "old self" and was enjoying her grandchildren daily.

CHAPTER 15

Case Vignettes: Children

Napoleon

CLINICAL HISTORY

Napoleon is a nine-year-old Hispanic male with a four-year history of behavior problems consisting of hyperactivity, impulsivity, and incorrigibility. He presented to a community mental health clinic for evaluation and treatment. His mother reported that her son had always been extremely moody and had difficulty sitting still, paying attention in school, and following rules. The mother is getting to the point where she cannot manage him anymore, and she may need to look into placement options because his behavior is uncontrollable. During the clinical interview, further details about Napoleon were obtained, including his extremely irritable moods, elevated or euphoric moods, grandiose ideas about the future, severe bouts of depression, distractibility, frequent use of profanity, and sexually inappropriate comments toward females. Napoleon's self-esteem seemed to correlate with his moods, as did his school performance. Napoleon also reported that when he was sad, he heard the voice of the devil who told him that he was no good and should die. On the other hand, when his mood was "really good," Napoleon heard God's voice telling him that he was special.

Napoleon's mother reported that he had always been fairly healthy except for the use of an inhaler at times for asthma. When asked about psychiatric family history, his mother reported that she had some mood swings when she was younger and was hospitalized on two occasions. Although she had taken medications, she was unable to recall the names of the medications or the diagnosis for which she had been treated. Napoleon's maternal grandfather was an alcoholic and went on intermittent binges.

Napoleon's mother recalled that her son had taken medications such as Ritalin and Dexedrine in the past, but they reduced his appetite without any therapeutic benefit. Napoleon has been disruptive in school and was frequently sent home for his bad behavior. However, he has gone weeks or months at a time without any behavioral problems in school.

POSTCASE DISCUSSION AND DIAGNOSIS

Napoleon appears to have some symptoms consistent with ADHD as well as bipolar disorder. When his mother was questioned in more detail, further symptoms emerged, including periods of increased energy and hyperactivity, a decreased need for sleep, grandiose thoughts with hyper-religiosity, increased verbal output (nonpressured speech), and being easily distracted. Following these elevated moods, Napoleon would experience depressed periods characterized by hypersomnia, poor appetite, intermittent voices (mood congruent), low energy, sense of hopelessness, and anhedonia. Given the family's history of bipolar spectrum disorders (the mother's moodiness and the grandfather's binge drinking), Napoleon appears to have Bipolar Disorder, Unspecified (F31.9) and needs immediate treatment. Since suicidality is not present, treatment can be initiated in the outpatient setting with his mother's consent and support. Inpatient treatment may be necessary if Napoleon becomes a danger to himself, a danger to others, and/or unmanageable at home for his mother.

PSYCHOPHARMACOLOGICAL TREATMENT

After an appropriate medical and psychiatric evaluation, Napoleon was started on lithium 150 mg twice daily with a plan to increase as tolerated to a dose of 600 mg/day to 900 mg/day. Lithium was chosen for its tolerability and effectiveness. When starting any psychotropic medication in children, parents must watch the child closely and monitor his or her moods on a daily basis. Prior to starting the lithium, appropriate laboratory testing was done and will be followed per typical protocols.

When Napoleon returned for a follow-up visit 10 days later, he was feeling okay while taking lithium at 600 mg/day. His mother reported that he had been doing much better. He was less impulsive and irritable, his sleeping patterns improved, and his moods were more level or even. Napoleon and his mother agreed to proceed with outpatient medication management and to engage in psychotherapy to address the school and social problems his mood disorder had caused. After approximately one year of treatment, Napoleon was doing well in school with minimal behavioral issues.

Christina

CLINICAL HISTORY

Christina is a 12-year-old African American female who has been in foster care for the last two years because her mother died from HIV/AIDS. She resides with her foster parents (also her legal guardians) and two other foster children who are two and three years younger than she. At the strong encouragement of the Child Protective Services social worker, Christina was brought in for a psychiatric evaluation because she was sleeping *all* the time. Christina reluctantly admitted that she liked to sleep too much and did not like to talk about her emotions. When asked about her mother, she was very distant and aloof but admitted to missing her sometimes. Christina would not discuss the process of losing her mother or the disease that overcame her mother. In passing, the social worker reported that Christina was not doing as well in school lately and had been missing an excessive number of school days because she refused to get up in time to get on the bus. Christina denied ever seeing a therapist previously or taking any psychiatric medications.

Christina's mother contracted HIV from her father who was an intravenous heroin user. He died from HIV/AIDS during Christina's first year of life. Other psychiatric family history was basically unknown. According to the social worker, Christina has no other family involvement or support. Her developmental history was basically normal, although her language was somewhat delayed.

POSTCASE DISCUSSION AND DIAGNOSIS

Christina's symptoms were further explored and revealed the following: experiencing depressed mood, feeling listless, feeling hopeless or helpless, having intermittent thoughts of wanting to die in order to join her mother, having poor appetite with a 10-pound-weight loss over the past month, feeling tired, having difficulty concentrating in school, and showing increased isolative behaviors. Christina was diagnosed with Major Depressive Disorder, Single Episode, Moderate (F32.1), and she needs immediate treatment. Given her thoughts of death, Christina must be carefully evaluated for suicidality. Psychotherapy is strongly recommended to address the enormous changes and losses that she has experienced in her short life. Although the issue of HIV transmission from mother to child should have already been addressed, the clinician needs to investigate and recommend an appropriate workup if necessary.

PSYCHOPHARMACOLOGICAL TREATMENT

Christina was started on escitalopram (Lexapro) 5 mg/day after consent was obtained from her foster parents. After two weeks, she was reevaluated and the medication was increased to 10 mg/day. After four weeks in treatment, she returned to the clinic with much less depression and isolation. She had also started psychotherapy to confront issues in her life. After taking the medication for 10 weeks, Christina's depression had completely remitted and her therapy was progressing appropriately. She was beginning to process the loss of her mother and to look at how it had affected her own young life.

Marky

CLINICAL HISTORY

Marky is an eight-year-old white male who presented to the psychiatrist's office with both of his parents, although they are divorced. He was being brought in for evaluation at the recommendation of his third-grade teacher because he was disruptive in the classroom. His mother, who is the primary caretaker, reported that he is always on the go and has trouble sitting still to do essentially anything. Marky's mother reported, "Everything in his room is in disarray." His father admitted that their son may be a little hyper but sees him as basically just a normal kid. The parents presented a letter from Marky's teacher that raised the following issues: difficulty attending to and following through with tasks, hyperactive in and out of the classroom, difficulty awaiting his turn, highly impulsive, often procrastinates, frequently forgets, constantly daydreams, fights frequently, talks excessively, and so on. Marky has made average grades in school but has the potential to perform much better, according to his teachers. Marky and his parents denied any significant depression, psychotic symptoms, obsessions, compulsions, or suicidality. Marky did admit to some anxiety and tends to worry mostly about the future.

Marky has always been in excellent health and tends to excel athletically. The parents denied any psychiatric family history of mental disorders or substance abuse. When giving the history, the father acknowledged that he also had trouble focusing in school when he was Marky's age. For this reason he tends to see Marky as a normal child. Marky has never used any psychotropic medications in the past.

POSTCASE DISCUSSION AND DIAGNOSIS

Marky clearly meets criteria for Attention Deficit Hyperactivity Disorder, Combined Type (F90.2). After having the parents, teacher, and a family friend complete the Conners Comprehensive Behavior Rating Scales (CBRS), the diagnosis was undisputed. The patient has features of hyperactivity, impulsivity, and inattention. The patient was also seen by his pediatrician, who felt that Marky was healthy and developing normally.

PSYCHOPHARMACOLOGICAL TREATMENT

Marky and his parents agreed to a trial of Dyanavel XR (a liquid brand of amphetamine) starting at 2.5 mg every morning; the medication will be titrated up by 2.5 mg as tolerated every three to five days until Marky has a clinical response or has limiting side effects. A clinical response may be reported by the parents or child or objectively observed by a significant decrease in his CBRS scores for ADHD symptoms. The extended-release (XR) form of the medication was chosen because the medication is given as a single dose only in the morning, which helps improve compliance. Marky preferred the liquid form as he does not like to swallow pills. Psychoeducation and therapy are necessary not only for the patient but also for the family to ensure the best prognosis.

After being on the medication for a few weeks, Marky was functioning much better in school with improved self-confidence in his own abilities. His parents and teachers have noticed significant clinical improvements in his overall attitude, functioning, and demeanor. Marky had experienced no side effects to date from the psychostimulant. Objective measurements from the CBRS showed Marky with lower scores, which correlate with a therapeutic response.

CHAPTER 16

Case Vignettes: Adolescents

Johnny

CLINICAL HISTORY

Johnny is a 16-year-old white male with no previous history of mental or physical illness. He recently presented to his family physician with complaints of depressed mood, loss of energy, poor motivation, and middle insomnia. His parents also mentioned that he had isolated himself from friends and dropped out of soccer. The history and physical showed no significant findings, but Johnny had lost seven pounds since his last physical about a year ago and appeared to be rather apathetic about personal hygiene. Johnny denied drug use, and while not presently suicidal, he did appear to have significant passive-death themes in this conversation.

Johnny's parents appeared to have a good relationship, and they appeared to have no concerns about Johnny's sister, who is two years older than Johnny. His sister had a brief period of depression last year, but it remitted without the need for further treatment. His mother, age 41, had several bouts of depression earlier in her life that resulted in a few years of psychotherapy and a course of antidepressant medication (imipramine) for several years. She claimed to have had no real depression over the last 10 years. Johnny's father, age 45, reported that he occasionally is "down," but he had never felt the need to see a therapist or take medication. He does, however, drink two or more beers each evening when he gets home from work. He claimed that the beer calmed him and helped him sleep. Johnny's maternal grandfather committed suicide when Johnny's mother was three years old.

To date, Johnny has taken no medication and has talked with the school counselor on only three occasions about his depression and slumping grades. The counselor then referred him to his family physician for an assessment and gave him the name of a therapist in the area.

POSTCASE DISCUSSION AND DIAGNOSIS

Johnny appears to have Major Depressive Disorder, Single Episode, Moderate (F32.1). His score of 32 on the Beck Depression Inventory further confirms the presence of depression. He complains of poor motivation, death themes, tearful bouts, difficulty concentrating and remembering, isolative behaviors, and trouble staying asleep at night. At this time, it is not certain if he will have subsequent bouts of depression, but based on the family's history, it is likely. Although Johnny poses no immediate suicide risk, a timely evaluation by a mental health professional is needed. Psychotherapy and medication are indicated. Johnny will see a local counselor at least twice a week for individual sessions and have an immediate medication and psychiatric evaluation with a psychiatrist.

PSYCHOPHARMACOLOGICAL TREATMENT

After the evaluation was completed, Johnny was placed on vortioxetine (Trintellix) 5 mg/day for the first two weeks and then increased to 10 mg/day starting with the third week. This particular medication was selected because of its low overdose profile, low sedation, and its efficacy for facilitating sleep and improving cognition. Johnny will be watched closely by his parents and counselor for any changes in suicidal thoughts or behaviors. Follow-up sessions with the psychiatrist were scheduled in three-week intervals.

Upon follow-up with the counselor and the psychiatrist, Johnny reported that his depression was 80% better and that his grades had returned to normal. He no longer had trouble sleeping, nor was he plagued by thoughts of death or issues with concentration. He had decided to continue to talk with the counselor as needed since it helps him think more clearly and positively.

Jennifer

CLINICAL HISTORY

Jennifer is a 17-year-old Hispanic female who presented with anger, agitation, and antisocial tendencies. She lived with her parents until her father was sent to jail for an auto theft. Her mother, who was unable to support herself and her three children on a farm worker's salary, moved in with her sister and her five children. Jennifer had been in and out of school until she dropped out last year. She has about a sixth-grade achievement level. Her grades have always been poor, especially in reading and math. Jennifer claimed that she spent most of the fifth and sixth grades in the hallway because of her poor behavior. She just cannot seem to listen and sit still long enough for things to stick. Her parents and teachers thought of her as just a headstrong tomboy who had to have the last word.

Jennifer's aunt had taken a strong interest in her behavior and believed that Jennifer should be able to have a decent educational experience. She talked with Jennifer often and believed that she was "hyper and indifferent" to her current situation. Jennifer has spent much too much time with some neighborhood boys who have formed a type of gang with other young boys who have dropped out of the local high school. The neighborhood boys would rather skip school than attend, and their grades were also poor. Jennifer's parents wanted to see her succeed in school but were more concerned that she would ruin her social reputation by hanging out with "bad boys." They never really noticed her hyper behaviors before and just thought she had a lot of youthful energy. They feared she might become like many girls who hang out with such boys and end up dropping out of school, getting into legal trouble, or getting pregnant.

Reviews of Jennifer's academic records showed poor performance and behavior patterns. She spent at least an hour a day in the hallway or in the principal's office when she last attended school last year. While Jennifer had little insight into her behavior, she was aware that school was not one of her favorite places and that she was not doing well there. She maintained that school was "stupid and for geeks." Although she tended to hang out with a rather antisocial crowd, she appeared to be concerned about her family and her other childhood friends. She appeared to have some sense of conscience, as she would not go with boys who planned vandalism or petty crimes. She also was very sensitive to other teens who had trouble learning in school and was often observed talking with them in the cafeteria.

POSTCASE DISCUSSION AND DIAGNOSIS

After extensive conversations with her former teachers, counselor, school psychologist, and social worker and a thorough workup from her family physician and her current psychologist, the team determined that Jennifer demonstrated enough clinical criteria for a diagnosis of Attention Deficit Hyperactivity Disorder, Predominantly Hyperactive Type (F90.1). She was beginning to notice *less* hyperactivity and *more* restlessness with her life and her friends. Her self-esteem was rather low because she realized that her educational skills were poor and her job prospects weak. With her psychologist's help, Jennifer was willing to work toward progress and improvement.

PSYCHOPHARMACOLOGICAL TREATMENT

In addition to her weekly counseling sessions, Jennifer was sent to a psychiatrist who specializes in adult and childhood ADHD. She was initially started on a trial of atomoxetine (Strattera) but showed little response after one month. She was then switched to bupropion (Wellbutrin XL) 300 mg/day and methylphenidate (Ritalin) 15 mg b.i.d. Her psychiatrist was not concerned about stimulant abuse since Jennifer abused no known substances. Jennifer responded well to this regime, as evidenced by self-reports and weekly reports from her psychologist. Subsequent psychological evaluations revealed that Jennifer had better concentration, attention, and retention of learned material.

In a series of follow-up sessions she demonstrated more calmness, less anger and agitation, and a willingness to enroll in a GED program. Her career and vocational tests indicated a strong interest and the ability to assist others in a counseling or teaching capacity. Jennifer hopes to become a teen counselor working with ADHD youth.

Violet

CLINICAL HISTORY

Violet is a 15-year-old female in the ninth grade. She came with her parents to a local mental health center, complaining of intense anxiety and social shyness. The visit was prompted by a rather traumatic school dance. Violet came home early with her friend, Lisa, at Violet's insistence. Violet reported that she was feeling more and more uncomfortable at the dance, and when she mentioned her feelings to Lisa, her friend told her "lighten up" and to stop obsessing about everything. Violet became quite upset and started to cry. Others at the dance gathered around her until school personnel escorted Violet and Lisa from the building. Violet's parents were called, and the two girls were taken home.

Violet is the older of two children. She has an 11-year-old brother who has no apparent mental health concerns. Her parents appeared to be happy and well adjusted with no history of mental illness; however, her mother reported that she was rather anxious herself in high school and college. Violet's mother took nortriptyline (Pamelor) for several years but reported no anxiety problems in recent history.

Both parents claimed that Violet had always been a shy, quiet, and very sensitive little girl. She was always uncomfortable around strangers and other students. In fact, she had a difficult time adjusting to both kindergarten and first grade. Although she is a very pretty girl, Violet avoided social contact with other students, and quickly excused herself when approached by them. Recently, while Violet was visiting at Lisa's home, a few more friends showed up and suggested calling some boys over. Violet became more and more anxious until she excused herself and retreated to Lisa's bedroom. Lisa called Violet's mom, who came to take her home.

Violet is aware that her fears and behaviors are ruining her life. She reported that she feels very inadequate in social situations. Violet is afraid that she will do or say something that will bring attention to her, and others will laugh at her. She also reported feeling very uncomfortable in the girl's shower room at school. Violet will not shower or dress unless the other students have gone. She once became so concerned that others were watching her that she had trouble breathing and felt dizzy.

After a complete physical by her family doctor and an evaluation by the therapist in the clinic, no physical causes for Violet's anxiety were found. She functioned quite well at home and in the presence of people she knew well. School performance was good except when she had to raise her hand or give speeches in front of the class. She appeared to have no other phobias, no history of depression, and no history of trauma or abuse.

POSTCASE DISCUSSION AND DIAGNOSIS

Violet appears to have Social Anxiety Disorder (F40.10). She has always been rather shy and anxious in social situations, but recently her symptoms have worsened. She purposely avoids social situations and the possibilities of social invitations. She once dropped a class because the teacher said the students would have to work in groups. She fears that if her anxieties continue, she will not be able to finish high school or attend college.

PSYCHOPHARMACOLOGICAL TREATMENT

In addition to cognitive-behavioral therapy and social skills training classes, her therapist and parents decided that Violet should try medication. She was first given paroxetine (Paxil) 20 mg/day. She responded very well but reported feeling rather drugged during the day. Her yawning was so pronounced that her teachers excused her from class to sleep in the student lounge. She was then instructed to take the medication before bed, which helped, but sedation and dizziness continued to be a problem. She was then switched to venlafaxine (Effexor XR) starting at 75 mg, after which she showed less sedation and balance issues. She was increased to 150 mg daily.

A follow-up found that Violet was much happier and certainly more social. Once the medication reduced her fears, Violet opened up to the therapist and really worked hard on finding ways to reduce her fears and increase her strengths. The social skills classes increased her self-esteem and allowed her to address her need that everyone must like her.

In a true in vivo test, she attended a school dance recently and actually accepted a boy's invitation to dance. She was quite smitten with him and the two are now dating.

CHAPTER 17

Case Vignettes: Early Adulthood

Stone

CLINICAL HISTORY

Stone is a 23-year-old white male college student who presented to the campus health center with concerns about failing health. Upon further questioning, the patient reported concerns about microwaves, X-rays, and other electromagnetic forces interfering with his decision-making capacity. Although he was initially guarded, Stone confided that he stopped watching television one year ago and stopped listening to the radio six months ago because he felt like "the government" was trying to control his mind. At times, the patient referred to hearing his "mother and father" in his head but refused to elaborate when questioned.

Stone had been attending college for the past four years and had approximately one more year to finish his bachelor's degree in chemistry. Stone remorsefully admitted to drinking and smoking "too much weed" that led to his withdrawal from about half of his classes during his first and second years of college. Stone denied any current use of drugs, but he did admit to having alcohol and weed about once a week with friends. Further assessment of his alcohol history revealed two positive answers out of a possible four on the CAGE Questionnaire. Stone also admitted that when he does have pot, he cannot think straight and tends to skip class. He also reported that he did not date much and preferred to be alone. He casually mentioned having some friends but was reluctant to give any names or reveal anything specific. Despite his initial complaint of failing health, his review of physical systems was basically negative.

Stone denied any significant medical history except for surgery on a broken arm when he was about 15 years old. When questioned about his psychiatric family history, Stone admitted that his maternal grandfather had a "nervous breakdown" and was institutionalized most of his adult life. Stone admitted that his grandfather used to hallucinate and act strangely. He was unsure of the diagnosis. Stone reported that his father drinks too much alcohol and has had one DUI in the past. Stone also denied any particular stressors lately, except for the pressure he was getting from his parents to finish college and get a job.

POSTCASE DISCUSSION AND DIAGNOSIS

According to Stone's history, he appears to have a diagnosis of Paranoid Schizophrenia (F20.0), Alcohol Abuse, Uncomplicated (F10.10), and Cannabis Abuse, Uncomplicated (F12.10). Additional information about Stone revealed few relationships, increasing isolation over the last few years, increasing paranoid delusions, and intermittent auditory hallucinations even at times when he has not been using pot or alcohol. His school performance was average but appeared to be declining overall when compared to his high school years. He was ambivalent about discussing his concerns with others because he feared his health would deteriorate. Stone's use of alcohol and marijuana complicated his presentation but was probably an independent phenomenon. If his substance abuse continues or progresses, his psychotic disorder will likely worsen. Stone's family history most likely indicated that his maternal grandfather had been diagnosed with either schizophrenia or some other psychotic illness. Although he desired to process his thoughts and feelings only in therapy, Stone was not an appropriate candidate due to his subacute psychotic symptoms. At some later time, therapy may be appropriate. Before considering medication, Stone was referred for an appropriate medical and neurological examination.

PSYCHOPHARMACOLOGICAL TREATMENT

Stone was started on aripiprazole (Abilify) 10 mg/day because he felt safe taking a neuromodulator, rather than some of the other atypical neuroleptics. Given his chemistry background, he was suspicious of being prescribed anything he felt was a tranquilizer. After four weeks on the medication, Stone reported very little change in his symptomatology. He appeared to be tolerating the medication well without any side effects. At eight weeks, Stone appeared much more relaxed and focused on completing school rather than being obsessed with his "failing health." When asked about his health at this point, Stone denied having any problems and was even listening to the radio in his car again. Furthermore, at 12 weeks of aripiprazole 10 mg/day, he reported having a "potential" girlfriend in his chemistry class. Since his psychosis was responding to the medication, psychotherapy could now be initiated with the focus on psychoeducation, relapse prevention, and avoidance of substances.

Ava

CLINICAL HISTORY

Ava is a 27-year-old Hispanic-Asian homemaker and mother of a three-year-old daughter. She was accompanied to the clinic by her husband of six years who voiced a complaint of unusual behavior. Ava had been taking walks in the middle of the night when she was unable to sleep, had become fearful of her husband for no apparent reason, and was consuming and hiding alcohol at various places in their home. Her husband reported that Ava did not usually drink alcohol whatsoever because of their religious beliefs. Upon further questioning, Ava revealed that she was six weeks pregnant and the father of the baby was not her husband. Both Ava and her husband were unwilling to reveal much information about the pregnancy except to say that they would remain married and raise the child as their own.

When asked about historical information, Ava said that she had a "strange episode" about seven years earlier when she impulsively took a vacation with a college friend. After drinking excessively for one month, Ava returned to school to learn that she had failed her semester classes. She did not seek any mental health treatment and thought her behavior was just related to "growing up."

With the exception of alcohol, Ava had no history of other drug use. She had never previously taken any psychiatric medications. The psychiatric family history was negative for mood disorders, psychotic disorders, anxiety disorders, and substance use disorders. During the interview, Ava acknowledged other symptoms, including increased energy, moodiness (dysphoria, elation, and irritability), racing thoughts, hearing the voice of God, feeling like she is "God's chosen one," and cleaning excessively at home.

Ava saw her primary care physician who felt she was in good health. The physician advised her not to drink alcohol while she is pregnant because of fetal-alcohol concerns and referred her for follow-up with her OB/Gyn. Ava currently takes a prenatal vitamin only.

POSTCASE DISCUSSION AND DIAGNOSIS

Ava appears to have a diagnosis of Bipolar Disorder, Current Episode Manic Severe with Psychotic Features (F31.2) and Alcohol Abuse, Uncomplicated (F10.10). Her symptoms that support this diagnosis include hyperreligiosity, grandiose delusions, mild paranoia, racing thoughts, decreased need for sleep, increased goal-directed activities, auditory hallucinations, impulsivity, possible hypersexuality, substance use, and poor judgment. Her intermittent alcohol consumption may be a form of self-medication to control her mania. Based on Ava's history, she probably had at least one manic episode previously that went undiagnosed and untreated. In addition to referring Ava for medication evaluation and treatment, the clinician needs to provide psychotherapeutic support to her and her husband and ensure the safety of her daughter. Ava's husband agreed to enlist the support of relatives to provide childcare and support for Ava until she gets back to normal functioning.

PSYCHOPHARMACOLOGICAL TREATMENT

After an appropriate evaluation and review of all options available, Ava and her husband chose to start lithium 300 mg b.i.d. initially, with dosage adjustments over the next few weeks. Because of her psychosis, antipsychotics were discussed, but Ava and her husband decided to wait for now and see how she responds to the lithium. After two weeks of lithium, Ava was sleeping about seven hours per night, had fewer racing thoughts, and was abstinent from alcohol. Her husband reported a significant improvement from his perspective: "My wife is coming back." The lithium was increased to 300 mg t.i.d. at that time; the lithium level subsequently was 0.8 mEq/l, which was therapeutic. In consultation with her OB/Gyn, an ultrasound was done to check for cardiac abnormalities in the fetus because of the lithium exposure. Results were negative, indicating that the fetus was unaffected. Given Ava's alcohol abuse, the possibility of fetal-alcohol effects must be assessed after delivery.

Candy

CLINICAL HISTORY

Candy is a 25-year-old white female who presented for an evaluation at the insistence of her primary care physician because of weight loss. Candy reported that she felt overweight, fat, and disgusted with her appearance. She claimed, "My thighs, stomach, and butt are just too fat. . . . I have to lose more weight, look at me!" Candy acknowledged some depression but tended to minimize it, saying she was fine. She denied any sleep disturbance, energy changes, hopelessness, helplessness, concentration problems, or suicidality. She reported having a "normal" appetite but was very careful to eat only "healthy foods." When asked about stressors, she admitted to some trouble in her marriage but did not elaborate. Candy works as an attorney. She reported that she gets angry at clients and even judges when "things" don't go her way. She exercises daily for approximately one hour, focusing on aerobics and cardiovascular fitness. Her stats are as follows: height 5'8", weight 98 pounds, and BMI 14.9 kg/m^2. According to standard measurements, her BMI is in the 2nd percentile. She mentioned in passing that her doctor was concerned because she has not had a menstrual period for the last two years.

Candy went on to report that she had been obsessed with her weight since her teenage years. She remembered constantly struggling with her parents over control issues such as clothing, school performance, friends, dating, and so on. She denied any significant past medical or psychiatric history, as well as any alcohol or drug abuse. Her psychiatric family history revealed some depression in her mother and maternal grandmother. Candy also stated, "Nobody in my family is fat, and I'm not going to be either." In passing, she reluctantly admitted to sexual abuse in the past but refused to discuss details.

POSTCASE DISCUSSION AND DIAGNOSIS

Candy presents with a diagnosis of Anorexia Nervosa, Restricting Type (F50.01) and may have a secondary diagnosis of mood or affective disorder. She is excessively focused on body image and has an intense fear of gaining weight despite being underweight. She appears to be in the acute phase of the illness, although she has not experienced any medical consequences to date other than her amenorrhea. It is difficult to assess whether Candy has experienced depressive episodes in the past because of her vague history. She does not meet criteria for a specific diagnosis of mood or anxiety disorder at this time. Candy does need appropriate laboratory evaluation to check for electrolyte abnormalities, which could be medically dangerous. An appropriate trial of psychotherapy should be initiated, and the need for inpatient hospitalization should be evaluated.

PSYCHOPHARMACOLOGICAL TREATMENT

Although most data would not suggest treating the acute phase with medications, and while most medications do little to control anorexia, Candy agreed to a trial of fluoxetine (Prozac) 10 mg/day for one week, then 20 mg/day. She understood that the medication may help her mood as well as decrease her core eating-disorder symptoms. The fluoxetine was increased over the next four weeks to 40 mg/day, which she tolerated well without side effects. After approximately six weeks on the fluoxetine, Candy appeared to be less depressed and less obsessed with her weight. Over the subsequent six weeks, her weight increased to 104 pounds, and she appeared to be unconcerned about it. The combination of psychotherapy and medication management has provided Candy with the best possible prognosis. Ongoing psychotherapy, medications, and psychoeducation will be required to maintain her emotional health.

CHAPTER 18

Case Vignettes: Middle Adulthood

Chester

CLINICAL HISTORY

Chester is a 42-year-old white male seeking an evaluation at a university-based treatment center. He decided to consult the experts because he had tried so many other treatments in the past with mixed results. He presented with a history of panic attacks dating back to high school. His first attack came during his senior year when he was not accepted to Princeton University. This rejection was a terrible blow to his self-esteem because his father attended Princeton and expected that both Chester and his brother would also attend. His brother was then in his junior year at Princeton and planning to attend law school when finished.

After Chester's first panic attack in high school, he and his parents consulted their family doctor and a cardiologist who found no reason for the attacks and no heart-related issues. Chester was told to reduce his stress and return if the attacks continued. They did not return, and Chester was accepted to Harvard, an acceptable alternative. In his freshman year, Chester experienced another panic attack while he was sleeping. He consulted the university health services, which once again found no medical reason for the attacks. The staff explained to him that the attacks might be a stress-related condition. An appointment was made for him at the university counseling service, but he did not keep the appointment.

Chester made it through college by using alcohol to self-medicate. He was able to hide most of his drinking from his family and friends until he graduated and met Judy. He and Judy fell in love and married within six months. His drinking became harder to hide, and Judy confronted him after he fell at a neighbor's dinner party where he was very drunk and rather loud. Chester confided in Judy about his panic and fears and how he needs the alcohol to function at home and at work. With Judy's help, he decided to attend AA and seek counseling from a mental health professional.

Chester slowly refrained from drinking but felt increasingly more anxious until he had three panic attacks in one week. He was placed on 2.5 mg of alprazolam (Xanax) by a consulting psychiatrist. He found the medication very helpful and was able to learn how to identify, label, and modify his thoughts in counseling with the use of cognitive therapy. He attended therapy weekly for nearly two years but stopped when he and the therapist felt they had progressed far enough. He continued to take the medication and remained symptom free for over 10 years.

When he was 32 years old, his primary care physician believed that Chester was over his emotional concerns. His physician felt Chester should stop taking the alprazolam, which now had increased from 0.25 mg/day to over 3 mg/day. He still attended AA meetings from time to time but never touched alcohol again. By the second week of his step down from alprazolam, Chester experienced a panic attack while driving home from work. His medication was increased back to 3 mg/day of alprazolam and has remained at this dose for the past year. He attempted to return to therapy but found the principles of therapy were not helping him much this time around. Chester changed therapists, but the next therapist was less versed than the first, adding to his sense of failure.

About a month ago, Chester's 17-year-old son was accepted to Princeton. Although happy for his son, Chester became very depressed and, while shopping with his wife in a grocery store, he experienced an intense panic attack. He is tired of partially effective approaches and desires a more comprehensive form of treatment. He is aware that he now needs to address the concerns in therapy and deal with his reliance on alprazolam.

POSTCASE DISCUSSION AND DIAGNOSIS

Chester has a long history of Panic Disorder Without Agoraphobia Tendencies (F41.0), with secondary, alcohol, and sedative-hypnotic abuse. While he used alcohol to self-medicate early in his life, he abused the benzodiazepine alprazolam later in his life. Both drugs offered some level of immediate relief but did not provide a permanent solution to his concerns.

PSYCHOPHARMACOLOGICAL TREATMENT

Since Chester has such a long and chronic history of panic disorder, it is very likely that he will continue to experience panic, especially if he attempts to reduce his dose of alprazolam. Since cognitively based psychotherapy helped him before, he should try it again. Antidepressants, especially SSRIs, are very helpful in reducing or eliminating panic. Chester will be placed on an SSRI such as fluoxetine (Prozac), sertraline (Zoloft), citalopram (Celexa), or escitalopram (Lexapro), and he will be reevaluated every two weeks to determine drug effectiveness. Concurrently, the alprazolam will be very slowly tapered off in increments of 0.25 mg/week. Good patient education will be needed to help Chester understand that he will not have additional panic attacks once the antidepressant medication takes effect. It is important to remember that selling the idea of reducing the benzodiazepine and starting an SSRI often causes patients with anxiety spectrum disorders to report increases in anxiety and side effects. It is wise to make sure they don't reduce the benzodiazepine too quickly and advise them to try to hold on for at least a month for the initial side effects to subside.

At a five-month follow-up visit, Chester was symptom free and attending counseling twice per month. He continues to take the SSRI but no longer uses benzodiazepines or alcohol for symptom relief. He also attends a group for others with panic disorder called Agoraphobics in Motion.

Sally

CLINICAL HISTORY

Sally is a 47-year-old white female, who worked as a loan officer in a bank. She was married for nearly 20 years when her husband Jack asked her for a divorce. She loved Jack, but she admitted that they had fallen out of love many years ago. They had a very civil divorce when their only daughter, Amy, was a senior in high school. Amy appeared to be the only person in the home who was upset about the divorce, and Sally was there to be supportive. Amy is now in her junior year at a university more than 1,500 miles away. Amy comes home for major holidays, but she spends little time with Sally or with her father, who lives in an apartment in a nearby town. This tends to upset Sally more than Jack, and Sally is trying to understand that college kids would rather spend more time with their old high school friends than with their parents.

After the divorce, Sally started to spend more time with her own parents. They were well into their seventies. While she loved her father, she was closer to her mother. Sally also was an only child, and she often stopped by her parents' home just to check in on them. One Sunday morning Sally received a call from her mother; her father had suffered a heart attack. He was pronounced dead before he arrived at the emergency room. Sally and her mother were devastated, but Sally tried to be strong for her mother. Her mother moved in with Sally, and Sally started to care for her. Sally started spending less and less time with others. She never went out with friends or coworkers; in fact, the only time Sally left the house was to go to work or take her mother on errands.

Sally began to notice that she was isolating more and was growing more depressed. Her sleep had been problematic since her father had died, and it was not getting better. Sally tried to treat the initial insomnia with over-the-counter sleep aids, but they offered only temporary assistance. She would also experience terminal insomnia two to three times per week. Sally was also growing more concerned that she seldom saw or heard from her daughter. She once took a trip to see Amy at the university, but Amy was away on an extended field trip.

When Sally returned from her trip to see Amy, she found that her mother had a very serious cold. When her mother's breathing became labored, Sally took her to a local urgent-care center, and her mother was immediately hospitalized with pneumonia. Her condition continued to decline until she was placed on a respirator. Four days later, Sally's mother died. Sally was overwhelmed with grief. She phoned her daughter, who came home but only stayed until the day of the funeral. Amy claimed that she needed to return to school to prepare for her LSAT exam.

Sally was tearful nearly 24 hours a day. She barely slept, and the sleep remedies offered no relief. She attempted to see her minister, but he referred her to a grief group. She attended meetings for several weeks but found that the grief of others made her worse. Sally attempted to return to work but could not concentrate or do her job well. After more than six months, her grief and loss were still very much with her. She felt that she might need to consult a mental health professional for the first time in her life.

POSTCASE DISCUSSION AND DIAGNOSIS

Sally clearly exhibited all clinical criteria for a major depressive episode, which should be considered in her treatment approach, and she most certainly demonstrated a complicated bereavement. Sally often dreamed of her mother, and once she thought that she heard her mother calling out to her and asking for assistance because she had fallen down the basement steps. Sally raced down the stairs in the middle of the night, only to find that her cat was locked outside and wanted to come in for the night. Sally feels she cannot continue to live in the house because it has too many reminders of her mother. She has basically sealed off the guest room where her mother slept and is afraid to touch her mother's things.

When Sally's father died, she did not have an opportunity to grieve. She had to be strong for her mother and daughter. Sally wanted to be comforted but could not find comfort in her own daughter. Sally had few close friends to confide in, but her bond with her mother was close. When her mother died, the only bond Sally ever really had was broken and lost. She realized that the bond with Amy was weak and unreliable. Sally panicked, thinking about her own vulnerabilities. Who would care for her when she got sick? Who would grieve for her? Did she fail as a mother? Why did her daughter distance herself?

PSYCHOPHARMACOLOGICAL TREATMENT

Sally was evaluated at a comprehensive health and mental care facility. After a complete physical, change-of-life issues were assessed by her gynecologist. Her gynecologist suggested appropriate hormone replacement and referred Sally to a counselor who specialized in grief therapy. Since Sally's depressive symptoms have been severe for so long, she was referred to a psychiatric nurse practitioner for medication. She was placed on 150 mg/day of bupropion XL (Wellbutrin). Although this medication did offer some relief from depression, Sally reported feeling rather agitated during the day, and her sleep disturbances continued. Her bupropion was reduced, and 100 mg of sertraline (Zoloft) was added, which improved her sleep but increased her irritable bowel symptoms. Finally, the sertraline was discontinued and Sally was placed on 50 mg of trazodone (Desyrel) at bedtime. This offered antidepressant action with sedation and helped her sleep through the night.

Upon follow-up three months later, Sally reported feeling much less depressed. Her sleep had returned to normal without disturbing dreams. She felt that she was able to "move on" now and let her mother rest. She continues to take the medication and see the counselor when needed. Sally approached her daughter on her last trip home. Her daughter did not realize just how far they had drifted apart, and Amy vowed to try harder to bridge the gap between them.

Tony

CLINICAL HISTORY

Tony is a 50-year-old Asian male with a long history of severe depression. He is the oldest of three siblings who were raised in the suburbs of Philadelphia. His parents owned a dry cleaning and tailoring business; each family member worked there as well. Tony's family were devout Catholics and expected each child to attend a Catholic school. Tony's parents hoped that he would get a scholarship to Notre Dame or Georgetown University. Tony was a good student and did in fact earn a scholarship to Georgetown.

Tony first noticed his depression at age 14. He was afraid that he was different from other boys because he found other boys attractive. He never mentioned his fear to his parents because the family never really talked about problems in the home. Tony did not want to disrespect his family by talking to an outsider about his concerns, so he kept it to himself. During his years at Georgetown, the depression became quite severe, and Tony had to inform his family about it. As often happens in Asian families, they were disappointed in him for having a mental illness. Tony never did tell them he was gay.

At the insistence of a professor, Tony entered therapy and started taking nortriptyline (Pamelor) for his depression. He showed enough improvement to finish his degree and move to Detroit to start a new job in engineering. Tony functioned fairly well for about six years, until he decided to stop the medication due to weight gain and other side effects. He experienced a serious depressive episode that led to a fairly lengthy hospitalization. Tony was reintroduced to nortriptyline, but this time it would not work. He was finally placed on a heavy dose of trazodone (Desyrel) and 0.5 mg clonazepam (Klonopin) because of his agitation and related anxiety. When he was released, he attended a day hospital for several weeks. Although Tony was functioning fairly well, he believed that he was only 60% better.

The next eight years demonstrated Tony's need for additional medications and increases in medications already in use. He was introduced to various SSRIs as they arrived on the treatment scene, but each offered only moderate effectiveness. Numerous consultations with experts at both Wayne State University and the University of Michigan led to various polypharmacologic approaches. Tony demonstrated only moderate levels of improvement with lithium augmentation and stimulant boosters. He refused to try MAOIs because of their dietary restrictions.

Tony was able to return to work, but he took so much sick time that he was transferred to a less stressful department. The transfer resulted in a pay cut that Tony viewed as a demotion.

After years of psychotherapy, Tony finally felt comfortable with his sexual orientation and decided to tell his family. His sisters were supportive, but his parents were not. They never missed an opportunity to tell him about "change therapies" and the "evils" of a gay lifestyle. Tony stopped returning to Philadelphia to see them. Over time, the rejections had somewhat of a "kindling effect"—that is, these stressors were setting off subsequent bouts of depression that were becoming more severe.

Feeling more comfortable with his gay identity, Tony was able to venture out a bit and meet others. He met a man, and they started to date. This man was very understanding about Tony's chronic depression and tried to help Tony with some of his issues. Since this man had a very accepting family, Tony quickly felt welcomed and accepted by them, but he continued to obsess over the loss of his own family.

Over the next few years, Tony and his partner, Bob, set up housekeeping, but Tony's numerous hospitalizations and leaves from work led him to apply for permanent disability. Tony was granted disability, but unfortunately he spent his time lying around the house and sleeping. He isolated and refused to speak to anyone other than Bob. Except for his sisters, Tony had no contact with his family, who viewed his gayness and his mental illness as a major stigma (not unusual in an Asian family). Both Tony and Bob felt there must be more effective forms of treatment.

POSTCASE DISCUSSION AND DIAGNOSIS

Tony is suffering from Major Depressive Disorder, Recurrent Severe Without Psychotic Features (F33.2). Although he has never been actively suicidal, his chronic depressive episodes have left him feeling that life is not worth living. He does not abuse alcohol or other drugs, and there are no psychotic manifestations to his illness. His homosexuality was rather ego dystonic at first, but Tony appears to have made a healthy adjustment to it in the last few years. The family stressors continue, but Tony is happy with the relationship he has with his sisters and Bob's family.

PSYCHOPHARMACOLOGICAL TREATMENT

Tony had been through a trial of every known TCA, SSRI, SPARI, and heterocyclic. Various stimulant and lithium boosters were not very helpful. A recent augmentation with olanzapine (Zyprexa) and aripiprazole (Abilify) showed little change. He was not willing to consider electroconvulsive therapy (ECT) for fear of memory loss, and his insurance company would not pay for transcranial magnetic stimulation (TMS). Also, due to his limited financial resources, the cost of TMS was not an option. Even though Tony was initially opposed to the use of MAOIs, their use was reevaluated with him. With his psychologist's help, Tony was educated about possible MAOI use and referred to a psychiatrist who informed him of the possible benefits. He reluctantly agreed to try them, and after the appropriate discontinuance period from the other medications, he was started on phenelzine (Nardil), 30 mg/day. Initially his depression worsened after the discontinuance of the other medications, but by the third week on phenelzine, Tony was beginning to improve. His dose was increased to 60 mg/day, and by the sixth week of treatment, he was reporting less daytime sleeping, no tearful bouts, and a much improved affect. Bob reported that Tony was helping him in the yard, asking to see their friends, and joining him for family visits.

The final evaluation came three months after the phenelzine was started. Tony reported no measurable depression. He is not working as an engineer, but he is working three half-days per week in a bookstore and loves his new job. He reported that he and Bob are getting along well. Tony is planning a trip home at Christmas with Bob to see his own parents. He believes that he is ready to talk to them and to confront their issues about his depression and sexual identity.

CHAPTER 19

Case Vignettes: Older Adulthood

Rose

CLINICAL HISTORY

Rose is an 82-year-old white female who presented for a psychiatric evaluation with a referral from her primary care physician. According to Rose, "My doctor was concerned about my memory, but I think it is fine." Rose lives alone in a mobile home with her two cats. She reported that she had no family to help her because they are all deceased. Rose was accompanied to the appointment by a longtime friend who drives her to the store and other appointments. Rose admitted to feeling sad but denied feeling depressed on a consistent basis. She worried about the future now that she was getting old but knew that she would be taken care of one way or another. She stated, "My memory is not as good as it used to be, but I get by okay." She does not drink anymore but used to enjoy an occasional martini with friends. Rose reported some difficulty sleeping but denied any energy disturbance, appetite disturbance, difficulty concentrating, hopeless feelings, helpless feelings, or thoughts of death.

According to her friend, Rose is having significant difficulty with her memory. For example, twice within the past two weeks she had forgotten to turn off the stove after preparing a meal. Rose frequently lost her mail, bills, and Social Security checks, but generally they were just misplaced. In the past six months, Rose's electricity had been shut off once and her water had been shut off twice because of nonpayment. When asked about her finances, Rose reported that everything is fine. She was unable to provide further details even when directly asked. Her friend stated that Rose was forgetting to feed her animals and at times she even forgot to eat. Information from Rose's primary care physician revealed an 18-month history of cognitive decline and various medical diagnoses including hypertension, osteoarthritis, and a previous history of myocardial infarction. She is currently taking an antihypertensive medication, as well as an arthritis medication that has remained unchanged for the last seven years. Her primary care physician also noted that Rose was more forgetful, called him by the wrong name at times, and no longer knew the names of the medications she was taking.

Rose's mental status was essentially unremarkable, but she tended to ignore current events and did not know the names of the U.S. president or vice president. She tended to minimize her deficits saying "Those politicians are no good anyway." She was unable to recall three items after five minutes and failed the three-dimensional drawing test.

POSTCASE DISCUSSION AND DIAGNOSIS

Rose appears to have Major Neurocognitive Disorder due to Alzheimer's Disease with Behavioral Disturbance (F02.81). Her mini-mental status exam (MMSE) is 15/30 (–5 orientation, –2 attention, –2 recall, –2 naming, –2 command, –1 writing sentence, –1 copy). Rose has additional symptoms, including aphasia, apraxia, agnosia, and problems with executive functioning. She has also been evaluated recently by a neurologist who ordered an MRI of the brain that showed moderate atrophy. The neurologist agreed with the dementia diagnosis and did not feel any further workup was necessary. In addition, Rose, who was quite distressed at hearing the diagnosis, needed a referral for psychotherapy to address these issues. Her primary care physician indicated that Rose uses atenolol (Tormin) 50 mg/day for her hypertension, and acetaminophen (Tylenol) 2 pills/day (over-the-counter) for her arthritis.

PSYCHOPHARMACOLOGICAL TREATMENT

Rose was started on memantine (Namenda) 10 mg/day for the first four weeks, then 20 mg/day thereafter. She appeared to tolerate the medication well except for mild sedation. When the dosing was changed from the morning to the evening, the sedation side effect resolved. Her medications were reviewed, and no significant drug interactions between the atenolol, acetaminophen, and memantine were found. Rose was able to continue living in her current environment, but four hours daily of home care assistance were added. This care will help ensure compliance with her medication, adequacy of meals, cleanliness of her home, and so on. Rose allowed her longtime friend and her accountant to take over her finances and pay the monthly expenses.

Rose initially attended psychotherapy sessions weekly, but sessions were tapered to monthly by the end of six months. The individual psychotherapy appeared to help Rose adjust to the enormous changes that were occurring in her life. After six months of treatment with memantine, her MMSE was 16/30. Following one year of treatment, Rose was still living at home, had eight hours of home care daily, and had an average MMSE score of 15/30. Since she is still living independently with the same basic MMSE score, the medication to minimize her cognitive decline has definitely been efficacious.

Anthony

CLINICAL HISTORY

Anthony is a 65-year-old African American male who presented for psychiatric evaluation with his daughter. Anthony revealed that he lost his wife suddenly fifteen months ago after a fatal myocardial infarction. He reported, "We were married for forty years. . . . I don't know what to do now." His daughter reported that nothing had been the same since her mother died. She further mentioned, "My dad has been isolating himself to the point of being a recluse." The patient admitted that the isolation was true, along with other symptoms, including early and middle insomnia, decreased appetite with a 25-pound-weight loss over the past year, decreased energy, poor concentration, and increased forgetfulness. When questioned about suicide, Anthony reported thoughts of wanting to join his wife, but he had no acute suicide plan or intent. He has drunk one glass of red wine daily for the last 20 years without any history of abuse. Because he and his wife used to do almost everything together, Anthony was feeling very lonely and had much survivor's guilt.

Anthony, whose only medication is one aspirin and a multivitamin daily, had been evaluated by his internist and given a good bill of health. He denied any personal history of depression or emotional problems, as well as any in his family. He reported that his daughter and extended family were supportive, but life was just not the same without his wife. Anthony had used spiritual resources that had been somewhat helpful at times, but he seemed to fall back again into the grieving process.

In addition, Anthony reported increasing forgetfulness and memory dysfunction over the past year. There was no pattern or consistency to his cognitive dysfunction. According to him, "Some days I can remember recent things . . . some days I can remember past things." Furthermore, his daughter reported that he had stopped his morning walks and had dropped out of his bowling league.

POSTCASE DISCUSSION AND DIAGNOSIS

Anthony clearly has the diagnosis of Major Depression, Single Episode, Moderate (F32.1). Upon further interview, the patient had significantly worsened over the past three months, since the first anniversary of his wife's death. His depressive episode has been further characterized by anhedonia, isolation, distractibility, hopelessness, helplessness, and worthlessness. In order to evaluate the memory complaints, an MMSE was completed during his initial visit with the score being 27/30 (–1 orientation, –1 attention, –1 recall). His effort on this examination was poor due to his level of depression. He was referred for psychotherapy to help facilitate the grieving process, which was most likely the root of his clinical depression.

PSYCHOPHARMACOLOGICAL TREATMENT

Anthony was started on sertraline (Zoloft) 25 mg/day for the first week, then 50 mg/day thereafter. He had requested this medication after seeing an advertisement on TV. After taking the medication for two weeks, it was unclear whether he was benefiting or not. He reported having no side effects. At that time, the sertraline was increased to 75 mg/day for the third week, then 100 mg/day thereafter. During his next visit, he reported a moderate response to the sertraline 100 mg/day after taking it for two weeks. The only side effect he reported was mild loosening of his bowel movements, which was tolerable. His doctor decided to switch him to vilazodone (Viibryd) 20 mg/day, which he seemed to tolerate better. Anthony engaged in psychotherapy with full remission of his grief and depression and even invited his daughter to a few sessions. At three months in treatment, his MMSE was 30/30, revealing that he was cognitively intact. The initial cognitive dysfunction was due to his depression rather than to any dementia process. Again, the combination of psychotherapy and medication management was helpful in restoring Anthony's previous level of functioning.

Margarita

CLINICAL HISTORY

Margarita is a 70-year-old Hispanic American female who was referred by her primary care physician and managed-care plan for ongoing evaluation and treatment. She stated her chief complaint, insisting "I need my medication, doctor. I can't go without it or I'll get sick again." The patient gave a long psychiatric history with multiple psychiatric hospitalizations dating back to her twenties. She now reported that a man was bothering her, making sexual advances to her, and frequently attempting to have "brain sex" with her. Upon further questioning, she reported hearing his voice at night through the walls in her single-family home. She got rather upset, angry, and paranoid that this was happening to her and frequently called the police for help. She stated, "The police don't even try to help me anymore. They say that he is not real." Margarita went on to report "strange sensations" on her skin when she was out in public (e.g., grocery store or bank) and related these sensations to men looking at her amorously. She has siblings and other relatives but refuses contact with them, saying they are "cursed." The patient also reported a history of depression and moodiness with one previous suicide attempt by overdose about 15 years ago.

Margarita is currently taking chlorpromazine (Thorazine) 500 mg/day, diazepam (Valium) 30 mg/day, imipramine (Tofranil) 100 mg/day, and chloral hydrate (Noctec) 500 mg/day. She also takes antihypertensive medication, an oral agent for her diabetes, and an inhaler for her emphysema. She reported that she has been on this psychiatric medication regimen for years with marginal functioning. She had a history of alcohol abuse when she was in her thirties and forties and reported that the alcohol helped decrease her mood swings.

Her psychiatric family history revealed that her paternal grandmother was institutionalized in a sanitarium, and her maternal aunt had depression with multiple suicide attempts. The family had no history of substance abuse. Margarita's social history revealed that she was different from her peers even in her teens. She attempted college but dropped out because she could not concentrate and focus on her work. Although she had never been employed, she had been financially supported by a trust fund from her father, who was a wealthy businessman in Mexico.

POSTCASE DISCUSSION AND DIAGNOSIS

Margarita has the diagnosis of Schizoaffective Disorder, Bipolar Type (F25.0). Observation of her during the interview revealed mild to moderate tardive dyskinesia of the face and upper extremities, resulting from years of exposure to the typical neuroleptics. She appeared very isolated and lonely, which was most likely the result of her chronic psychiatric disability. Although Margarita never had a clear manic episode, she had experienced mixed mood states that were indicative of the bipolar type of the diagnosis. Medication changes could be extremely helpful in decreasing her psychotic mood symptoms.

PSYCHOPHARMACOLOGICAL TREATMENT

After developing some trust with the patient over a few weeks, Margarita's psychiatrist adjusted her medications to an alternative regimen that should be more helpful. The chlorpromazine 500 mg/day was replaced gradually by risperidone (Risperdal) 3 mg/day to 4 mg/day for her psychotic symptoms, which seemed to be the most bothersome at this time. Subsequently, the diazepam and chloral hydrate were tapered slowly over a period of six to eight weeks. Topiramate (Topamax) was a logical alternative to replace these two medications, given Margarita's mood instability, insomnia, and anxiety. After these changes were implemented, the imipramine was reevaluated and tapered to reduce her polypharmacy regimen. She should not be given benzodiazepines because of her history of alcohol abuse and because it presents a slip/fall risk.

After six months of treatment, Margarita was taking risperidone 3 mg/day and topiramate 200 mg/day without any significant side effects. She still had some unusual thoughts and concerns, but she was functioning much better on a daily basis with an improved quality of life. The tardive dyskinesia was still present at the same mild level, but it should not worsen with this atypical antipsychotic drug regimen. The medication Valbenazine may be considered if the tardive dyskinesia symptoms worsen.

APPENDIX

Table of Psychotropic Medications

Abbreviations used in the table include the following:

5-HT (serotonin)
CNS (central nervous system)
DA (dopamine)
EPS (extrapyramidal symptoms)
GABA (gamma-aminobutyric acid)
H (histamine)
M (muscarinic)
NE (norepinephrine)
NMS (neuroleptic malignant syndrome)
ODT (orally disintegrating tablet)
TRPV1 (transient receptor potential vaniloid 1 receptor)
TD (tardive dyskinesia)
VMAT2 (vesicular monoamine transporter-2)
XR (extended release)
WBC (white blood count)

Generic Name (Drug Class)	Trade/Brand Name	Mechanism of Action	Typical Dose (Mg/Day)	Most Common Side Effects
acamprosate (anti-alcohol)	Campral	GABA receptor modifier	2,000–3,000	Diarrhea, dyspepsia, headache, nausea, vomiting, rash
alprazolam (antianxiety)	Xanax, Xanax XR	Increases GABA	0.25–4	Poor coordination, dizziness, sedation, weakness, memory dysfunction, depression, lethargy
amantadine (antiparkinsonian)	Symmetrel	DA agonist	100–300	Nausea, dizziness, insomnia, dry mouth, constipation, confusion, fatigue, anxiety
amitriptyline (antidepressant)	Elavil	5-HT reuptake inhibition, NE reuptake inhibition	150–300	Sedation, weight gain, dry mouth, blurry vision, constipation, urinary retention, sexual dysfunction, orthostatic hypotension, dizziness
amoxapine (antidepressant)	Asendin	NE reuptake inhibition, 5-HT reuptake inhibition	150–400	Sedation, weight gain, dry mouth, blurry vision, constipation, urinary retention, sexual dysfunction, orthostatic hypotension, dizziness
amphetamine (psychostimulant)	Adderall, Adderall XR, Mydayis	NE and DA reuptake inhibition, promotes NE and DA release	5–60/12.5–50	Insomnia, anorexia, weight loss, irritability, tachycardia, agitation, abdominal pain, headache, dry mouth, increased psychosis, asthenia, fever, infection, growth retardation (children), tics
amphetamine ODT (psychostimulant)	Adzenys XR-ODT	NE and DA reuptake inhibition, promotes NE and DA release	3.1–18.8	Insomnia, anorexia, weight loss, irritability, tachycardia, agitation, abdominal pain, headache, dry mouth, increased psychosis, asthenia, fever, infection, growth retardation (children), tics
amphetamine oral suspension (psychostimulant)	Dyanavel XR	NE and DA reuptake inhibition, promotes NE and DA release	2.5–20	Insomnia, anorexia, weight loss, irritability, tachycardia, agitation, abdominal pain, headache, dry mouth, increased psychosis, asthenia, fever, infection, growth retardation (children), tics
amphetamine sulfate (psychostimulant)	Evekeo, Adzenys XR-ODT, Dyanavel XR Oral Suspension	NE and DA reuptake inhibition, promotes NE and DA release	2.5–40/ 12.5–18.8/ 2.5–5	Insomnia, anorexia, weight loss, irritability, tachycardia, agitation, abdominal pain, headache, dry mouth, increased psychosis, asthenia, fever, infection, growth retardation (children), tics

(continued)

Generic Name (Drug Class)	Trade/Brand Name	Mechanism of Action	Typical Dose (Mg/Day)	Most Common Side Effects
aripiprazole (antipsychotic)	Abilify, Abilify Discmelt, Abilify MyCite, Ability Injection, Ability Maintena	D2 and 5-HT1A partial agonist, 5-HT2A and alpha-1 antagonist	10–30 (9.75 mg injection; 300–400 mg/month)	Nausea, vomiting, headache, insomnia, somnolence, dizziness, akathisia, abnormal vision, orthostatic hypotension, NMS, TD, hyperglycemia, leukopenia, tremor, constipation, lethargy (injection-site reactions for injectable forms)
aripiprazole lauroxil (antipsychotic)	Aristada	D2 and 5-HT1A partial agonist, 5-HT2A and alpha-1 antagonist	441–1,064 mg/month	Nausea, vomiting, headache, insomnia, somnolence, dizziness, akathisia, abnormal vision, orthostatic hypotension, NMS, TD, hyperglycemia, leukopenia, tremor, constipation, lethargy, injection-site reactions
armodafinil (antinarcolepsy)	Nuvigil	DA reuptake inhibition	150–250	Headache, nausea, dizziness, insomnia, anxiety, dry mouth, diarrhea, rash
asenapine (antipsychotic)	Saphris	5-HT 1A/1B/2A/2B/2C/5/6/7 antagonism, D1-4 antagonism, alpha-1/2 antagonism, H1-2 antagonism	10–20	Akathisia, oral hypoesthesia, somnolence, dizziness, EPS, increased weight, NMS, TD, orthostatic hypotension, leukopenia, QT-interval prolongation, hyperprolactinemia, insomnia, constipation, headache, cognitive and motor impairment, hyperglycemia
atomoxetine (anti-ADHD)	Strattera	NE reuptake inhibition	40–100	Aggression, irritability, somnolence, vomiting, dyspepsia, nausea, fatigue, decreased appetite
baclofen (anti-alcohol)	Kemstro, Lioresal	CNS depressant (muscle relaxer)	10–80	Dizziness, weakness, fatigue, confusion, headache, insomnia, hypotension, nausea, constipation, urinary frequency,
benztropine (anticholinergic)	Cogentin	Anticholinergic	2–6	Tachycardia, nausea, constipation, confusion, dry mouth, urinary retention, blurry vision
brexpiprazole (antipsychotic)	Rexulti	5-HT1A, D2, and D3 partial agonist; 5-HT2A, 5-HT2B, 5-HT7, α1A, α1B, α1D, and α2C receptors antagonist	1–4	Akathisia, restlessness, weight gain, somnolence
bromocriptine (antiparkinsonian)	Parlodel	DA agonist	2.5–15	Dizziness, nausea, vomiting, dry mouth, poor appetite, abdominal pain, diarrhea, dyspepsia, constipation

Drug (class)	Brand names	Mechanism	Dosage	Side effects
buprenorphine (antiopioid)	Subutex Sublocade (injection) Probuphine (implant)	Partial agonist at muopioid receptor, antagonist at kappa-opioid receptor	2–16, 100–300 monthly, 74.2 (80 mg)	Nausea, vomiting, constipation, liver dysfunction, respiratory depression (injection-site reactions for injections, implant-site reactions for implants)
buprenorphine/ naloxone (antiopioid)	Suboxone, Bunavail, Zubsolv	Mixed opioid agonist-antagonist/opioid antagonist	2–16/0.5–4, 2.1–6.3/0.3–1, 1.4–5.7/0.36–1.4	Nausea, vomiting, constipation, liver dysfunction, respiratory depression, acute withdrawal syndrome
bupropion (antidepressant)	Wellbutrin, Wellbutrin SR (Zyban), Wellbutrin XL, Aplenzin	NE reuptake inhibition, DA reuptake inhibition	75–450/ 100–400/ 150–450	Insomnia, dizziness, headache, dry mouth, nausea, decreased appetite, constipation, agitation/nervousness, seizure
buspirone (antianxiety)	Buspar	5-HT1A agonist, moderate D2 agonist	5–40	Dizziness, insomnia, nervousness, dry mouth, drowsiness, nausea, headache, fatigue
capsaicin patch (analgesic)	Qutenza	TRPV1 receptor channel agonist Receptor agonist	1 patch	Application-site erythema, application-site pain, application-site pruritus, application-site papules
carbamazepine (mood stabilizer)	Tegretol, Tegretol XR, Carbatrol, Equetro	Inhibition of sodium channels	600–1,200	Nausea, vomiting, diplopia, dizziness, poor coordination, drowsiness, anemia, rash, liver dysfunction, fatigue, low WBCs
cariprazine (antipsychotic)	Vraylar	D2 and 5-HT1A partial agonist, 5-HT2A antagonism	1.5–6	EPS, akathisia, dyspepsia, vomiting, somnolence, restlessness
chloral hydrate (sedative-hypnotic)	Noctec, Somnote	CNS depressant	500–1,000	Drowsiness, dizziness, rash, confusion, restlessness, amnesia, irritability
chlordiazepoxide (antianxiety)	Librium	Increases GABA	15–40	Poor coordination, dizziness, sedation, weakness, memory dysfunction, depression, lethargy

(continued)

Generic Name (Drug Class)	Trade/Brand Name	Mechanism of Action	Typical Dose (Mg/Day)	Most Common Side Effects
chlordiazepoxide/ amitriptyline (antianxiety)	Limbitrol	Increases GABA, 5-HT reuptake inhibition, NE reuptake inhibition	30–60/75–150	Poor coordination, dizziness, sedation, weakness, memory dysfunction, depression, lethargy, weight gain, dry mouth, blurry vision, constipation, urinary retention, sexual dysfunction, orthostatic hypotension
chlorpromazine (antipsychotic)	Thorazine	D2 antagonism	200–600	Sedation, weight gain, dry mouth, dizziness, poor coordination, EPS, photosensitivity, lethargy, blurry vision, constipation, seizures, tachycardia, weakness, NMS, gynecomastia, leukopenia, hyperglycemia, hyperlipidemia, QT-interval prolongation
citalopram (antidepressant)	Celexa	5-HT reuptake inhibition	10–60	Nausea, diarrhea, dry mouth, anorexia, weight gain, sexual dysfunction, tremor, restlessness, anxiety/nervousness, insomnia, dizziness, headache
clomipramine (antidepressant)	Anafranil	5-HT reuptake inhibition, NE reuptake inhibition	100–250	Sedation, weight gain, dry mouth, blurry vision, constipation, urinary retention, sexual dysfunction, orthostatic hypotension, dizziness
clonazepam (antianxiety, mood stabilizer)	Klonopin, Klonopin Wafers	Increases GABA	0.5–4	Poor coordination, dizziness, sedation, weakness, memory dysfunction, depression, lethargy
clonidine (anti-ADHD, antianxiety)	Catapres, Catapres Patch, Kapvay	Central alpha agonist	0.1–0.3/0.1–0.4	Drowsiness, dizziness, constipation, sedation, weakness, fatigue, agitation, nausea, vomiting, sexual dysfunction, myalgias, arthralgias, hypotension
clorazepate (antianxiety)	Tranxene	Increases GABA	15–60	Poor coordination, dizziness, sedation, weakness, memory dysfunction, depression, lethargy
clozapine (antipsychotic)	Clozaril, Fazaclo, Versacloz	D4 antagonism, alpha 2 antagonism, H1 antagonism, 5-HT antagonism	400–600	Agranulocytosis, eosinophilia, seizures, myocarditis, dizziness, tachycardia, tremor, hyperglycemia, fever, weight gain, sedation, salivation, sweating, constipation, headache, orthostatic hypotension, hyperglycemia, hyperlipidemia, QT-interval prolongation
cytisine (anti-smoking)	Tabex	Cholinergic agonist	1.5–9	Nausea, vomiting, dizziness, tachycardia, muscle weakness

Drug (class)	Brand	Mechanism	Dose	Side effects
desipramine (antidepressant)	Norpramin	NE reuptake inhibition	150–300	Sedation, weight gain, dry mouth, blurry vision, constipation, urinary retention, sexual dysfunction, orthostatic hypotension, dizziness
desvenlafaxine (antidepressant)	Pristiq	NE reuptake inhibition, 5-HT reuptake inhibition	50–100	Nausea, dizziness, insomnia, hyperhidrosis, constipation, somnolence, decreased appetite, anxiety, sexual dysfunction, vomiting
deutetrabenazine (anti-TD)	Austedo	VMAT2 reversible inhibitor	12–48	Somnolence, diarrhea, dry mouth, fatigue, nasopharyngitis, insomnia
dexmethylphenidate (psychostimulant)	Focalin, Focalin XR	NE reuptake inhibition, DA reuptake inhibition, promotes NE and DA release	5–40	Insomnia, anorexia, weight loss, irritability, tachycardia, agitation, abdominal pain, headache, dry mouth, increased psychosis, asthenia, fever, infection, growth retardation (children), tics
dextroamphetamine (psychostimulant)	Dexedrine, Dexedrine Spansules, Dextrostat	NE reuptake inhibition, DA reuptake inhibition, promotes NE and DA release	5–60	Insomnia, anorexia, weight loss, irritability, tachycardia, agitation, abdominal pain, headache, dry mouth, increased psychosis, asthenia, fever, infection, growth retardation (children), tics
diazepam (antianxiety)	Valium	Increases GABA	5–40	Poor coordination, dizziness, sedation, weakness, memory dysfunction, depression, lethargy
diphenhydramine (antiparkinsonian)	Benadryl	Antihistamine	25–50	Sedation, dry mouth, dizziness, nausea, nervousness, headache
disulfiram (anti-alcohol)	Antabuse	Acetaldehyde dehydrogenase antagonist	250–500	Drowsiness, fatigue, headache, sexual dysfunction, rash, psychotic-like reactions, liver dysfunction
donepezil (antidementia)	Aricept	Cholinesterase inhibitor	5–10	Nausea, vomiting, insomnia, diarrhea, muscle cramps, fatigue, anorexia,
doxepin (antidepressant)	Sinequan, Adapin	NE reuptake inhibition, 5-HT reuptake inhibition	150–300	Sedation, weight gain, dry mouth, blurry vision, constipation, urinary retention, sexual dysfunction, dizziness, orthostatic hypotension
doxepin sedative	Silenor	NE reuptake inhibition, 5-HT reuptake inhibition	3–6	Sedation, weight gain, dry mouth, blurry vision, constipation, urinary retention, sexual dysfunction, dizziness, orthostatic hypotension

(continued)

Generic Name (Drug Class)	Trade/Brand Name	Mechanism of Action	Typical Dose (Mg/Day)	Most Common Side Effects
doxylamine (sedative)	Unisom	Antihistamine	25	Sedation, dry mouth, dizziness, nausea, nervousness, headache
droperidol (antipsychotic)	Inapsine	D2 antagonism	2.5–15	Sedation, weight gain, dry mouth, dizziness, poor coordination, EPS, NMS, lethargy, blurry vision, seizures, constipation, tachycardia, weakness, gynecomastia, leukopenia, hyperglycemia, hyperlipidemia, QT-interval prolongation
duloxetine (antidepressant)	Cymbalta	NE reuptake inhibition, 5-HT reuptake inhibition	20–60	Nausea, hypertension, anorexia, dizziness, somnolence, insomnia, dry mouth, nervousness, sexual dysfunction, sweating
escitalopram (antidepressant)	Lexapro	5-HT reuptake inhibition	5–20	Nausea, diarrhea, dry mouth, anorexia, weight gain, sexual dysfunction, tremor, restlessness, anxiety/nervousness, insomnia, dizziness, headache
estazolam (sedative-hypnotic)	Prosom	Increases GABA	2–4	Sedation, dizziness, falling, lethargy, disorientation, amnesia
eszopiclone (sedative-hypnotic)	Lunesta	Selective modulation of GABA receptor complex	2–3	Daytime drowsiness, dizziness, falls, amnesia, unpleasant taste
fenfluramine (antiobesity)	Pondimin	Sympathomimetic amine anorectic	15–30	pulmonary hypertension, regurgitant cardiac valvular disease, palpitation, tachycardia, elevated blood pressure, ischemic events, overstimulation, restlessness, dizziness, insomnia, euphoria, dysphoria, tremor, headache, psychosis, dry mouth, unpleasant taste, diarrhea, constipation, urticaria, impotence, changes in libido
fluoxetine (antidepressant)	Prozac, Sarafem, Prozac Weekly	5-HT reuptake inhibition	20–80/ 90 (weekly)	Nausea, diarrhea, dry mouth, anorexia, weight gain, sexual dysfunction, tremor, restlessness, anxiety/nervousness, insomnia, dizziness, headache
fluoxetine, olanzapine (antidepressant, antipsychotic)	Symbyax	Inhibition of 5-HT reuptake/DA and 5-HT2 antagonism	6–12/25–50	See fluoxetine and olanzapine

Drug (class)	Brand name	Mechanism	Dose	Side effects
fluphenazine (antipsychotic)	Prolixin, Prolixin Decanoate	D2 antagonism	2–20/25–50 every 2 weeks	Sedation, weight gain, dry mouth, dizziness, poor coordination, EPS, NMS, lethargy, blurry vision, seizures, constipation, tachycardia, weakness, gynecomastia, leukopenia, hyperglycemia, hyperlipidemia, QT-interval prolongation
flurazepam (sedative-hypnotic)	Dalmane	Increases GABA	15–30	Sedation, dizziness, falling, lethargy, disorientation, amnesia
fluvoxamine (antidepressant)	Luvox	5-HT reuptake inhibition	50–300	Nausea, diarrhea, dry mouth, anorexia, weight gain, sexual dysfunction, tremor, restlessness, anxiety/nervousness, insomnia, dizziness, headache
gabapentin (mood stabilizer)	Neurontin	Enhances GABA	300–3,600	Dizziness, somnolence, edema, weight gain, diplopia, headache, agitation, nausea, tremors
galantamine (antidementia)	Reminyl	Cholinesterase inhibitor	16–24	Nausea, vomiting, asthenia, sweating, dizziness, headache, diarrhea, anorexia, insomnia
guanfacine (anti-ADHD)	Tenex	Central alpha-2A agonist	0.5–3	Drowsiness, dizziness, constipation, sedation, weakness, fatigue, agitation, nausea, vomiting, sexual dysfunction, myalgias, arthralgias, hypotension
guanfacine extended release (anti-ADHD)	Intuniv	Central alpha-2A agonist	1–4	Somnolence, sedation, abdominal pain, dizziness, hypotension/decreased blood pressure, dry mouth, constipation, headache, fatigue
halazepam (antianxiety)	Paxipam	Increases GABA	60–160	Poor coordination, dizziness, sedation, weakness, memory dysfunction, depression, lethargy
haloperidol (antipsychotic)	Haldol, Haldol Decanoate	D2 antagonism	2–20/100–300 every month	Sedation, weight gain, dry mouth, dizziness, poor coordination, EPS, NMS, lethargy, blurry vision, seizures, constipation, tachycardia, weakness, gynecomastia, leukopenia, hyperglycemia, hyperlipidemia, QT-interval prolongation

(continued)

Generic Name (Drug Class)	Trade/Brand Name	Mechanism of Action	Typical Dose (Mg/Day)	Most Common Side Effects
hydroxyzine (antianxiety)	Vistaril, Atarax	Antihistamine	50–150	Confusion, irritability, dry mouth, constipation, dizziness, blurry vision, sedation
iloperidone (antipsychotic)	Fanapt	5-HT2A antagonism, D2 and D3 antagonism, alpha-1 and alpha-2 antagonism	12–24	Dizziness, dry mouth, fatigue, nasal congestion, orthostatic hypotension, somnolence, tachycardia, increased weight, nausea, leukopenia, hyperglycemia, hyperlipidemia, QT-interval prolongation, NMS, EPS
imipramine (antidepressant)	Tofranil	5-HT reuptake inhibition, NE reuptake inhibition	150–300	Sedation, weight gain, dry mouth, blurry vision, constipation, urinary retention, sexual dysfunction, orthostatic hypotension, dizziness
isocarboxazid (antidepressant)	Marplan	5-HT reuptake inhibition, NE reuptake inhibition, DA reuptake inhibition	10–40	Nausea, insomnia, drowsiness, dry mouth, increased appetite, dizziness, headache, irritability, nervousness, weakness, sexual dysfunction, muscle twitching/cramps, constipation, weight gain, hypertensive crisis
Lorcaserin (antiobesity)	Belviq	5-HT2C receptor agonist	10–20	Headache, dizziness, fatigue, nausea, dry mouth, constipation, hypoglycemia, back pain, cough
L-alpha-acetyl-methadol (methadone maintenance)	LAAM, Orlaam	Synthetic opioid agonist	20–80 three times weekly	Feelings of unreality, hallucinations, hives, itching, rash, sweating, restlessness, nausea, vomiting, dizziness, sedation, muscle twitching, depression, QT-interval prolongation, Torsades de pointes, cardiac arrest
lamotrigine (mood stabilizer)	Lamictal, Lamictal XR, Lamictal ODT	Inhibition of sodium channels, presynaptic modulation of glutamate release	200–400	Nausea, vomiting, dizziness, diplopia, poor coordination, somnolence, headache, toxic rash
levomilnacipran (antidepressant)	Fetzima	NE reuptake inhibition, 5-HT reuptake inhibition	40–120	Nausea, constipation, hyperhidrosis, heart rate increase, erectile dysfunction, tachycardia, vomiting, and palpitations
lidocaine patch (analgesic)	Lidoderm	Local anesthetic	1 patch	application-site blisters, bruising, burning sensation, depigmentation, dermatitis, discoloration, edema, erythema, exfoliation, irritation, papules, petechiae, pruritus, vesicles, abnormal sensation

Drug	Brand	Mechanism	Dose	Side effects
liraglutide subcutaneous injection (antiobesity)	Saxenda	Glucagon-like peptide-1 (GLP-1) receptor agonist	0.6–3	Nausea, hypoglycemia, diarrhea, constipation, vomiting, headache, decreased appetite, dyspepsia, fatigue, dizziness, abdominal pain, increased lipase
lisdexamfetamine (anti-ADHD)	Vyvanse	Prodrug of dextroamphetamine	30–70	Decreased appetite, dizziness, dry mouth, irritability, insomnia, upper abdominal pain, nausea, vomiting, decreased weight, diarrhea, fatigue, irritability, feeling jittery, anorexia, headache, anxiety, insomnia, tics
lithium carbonate or lithium citrate (mood stabilizer)	Lithobid, Eskalith CR	Enhances 5-HT, increases or decreases NE, blocks DA supersensitivity, alters second messengers	600–1,200	Anorexia, dry mouth, nausea, vomiting, diarrhea, drowsiness, muscle weakness, decreased coordination, fatigue, lethargy, tremor, arrhythmias, polyuria, polydipsia, renal dysfunction, thyroid dysfunction, alopecia, rash, edema, increased appetite, weight gain
lorazepam (antianxiety)	Ativan	Increases GABA	1–6	Poor coordination, dizziness, sedation, weakness, memory dysfunction, depression, lethargy
loxapine (antipsychotic)	Loxitane	D2 antagonism	20–100	Sedation, weight gain, dry mouth, dizziness, poor coordination, EPS, photosensitivity, lethargy, blurry vision, constipation, seizures, tachycardia, weakness, NMS, gynecomastia, leukopenia, hyperglycemia, hyperlipidemia, QT-interval prolongation
lurasidone (antipsychotic)	Latuda	D2, 5-HT2A and 5-HT7 antagonist, α2a and α2c antagonist, partial agonist 5-HT1A	40–160	Akathisia, headache, insomnia, nausea, somnolence, EPS, NMS
maprotiline (antidepressant)	Ludiomil	5-HT reuptake inhibition	150–225	Sedation, weight gain, dry mouth, blurry vision, constipation, urinary retention, sexual dysfunction, orthostatic hypotension, dizziness
mazindol (anticocaine)	Sanorex, Mazanor	NE reuptake inhibition, DA reuptake inhibition, promotes NE and DA release	1–3	Constipation, dizziness, dry mouth, headache, irritability, nausea, vomiting, restlessness, abdominal cramps, insomnia

(continued)

159

Generic Name (Drug Class)	Trade/Brand Name	Mechanism of Action	Typical Dose (Mg/Day)	Most Common Side Effects
memantine (antidementia)	Namenda, Namenda XR	NMDA antagonists	10–20/7–28	Fatigue, pain, dizziness, hypertension, nausea, insomnia, flulike symptoms, edema, anxiety, anorexia, arthralgias, diarrhea, poor coordination, agitation, urinary incontinence, urinary tract infection
memantine/donepezil (anti-dementia)	Namzaric	NMDA antagonists	7/10; 14/10; 21/10; 28/10	Fatigue, pain, dizziness, hypertension, nausea, vomiting, insomnia, flulike symptoms, edema, anxiety, anorexia, arthralgias, diarrhea, poor coordination, agitation, urinary incontinence, urinary tract infection, anorexia, muscle cramps
Meprobamate (sedative-hypnotic)	Equanil, Miltown	GABA agonist	200–400	Drowsiness, ataxia, dizziness, slurred speech, headache, vertigo, euphoria, weakness, vomiting, diarrhea, numbness, tingling
mesoridazine (antipsychotic)	Serentil	D2 antagonism	50–400	Sedation, weight gain, dry mouth, dizziness, poor coordination, EPS, photosensitivity, lethargy, blurry vision, constipation, seizures, tachycardia, weakness, NMS, gynecomastia, leukopenia, hyperglycemia, hyperlipidemia, QT-interval prolongation
methamphetamine (psychostimulant)	Desoxyn	NE reuptake inhibition, DA reuptake inhibition, promotes NE and DA release	5–30	Insomnia, anorexia, weight loss, irritability, tachycardia, agitation, abdominal pain, headache, dry mouth, hypertension, increased psychosis, twitching
methadone (methadone maintenance)	Dolophine	Synthetic opioid agonist	20–100	Feelings of unreality, hallucinations, hives, itching, rash, sweating, restlessness, nausea, vomiting, dizziness, sedation, muscle twitching, depression
methylphenidate (psychostimulant)	Ritalin, Ritalin SR, Ritalin LA, Metadate CD, Metadate ER, Methylin, Concerta, Aptensio XR, Quillivant XR, QuilliChew ER, Cotempla XR-ODT	NE reuptake inhibition, DA reuptake inhibition, promotes NE and DA release	10–60/ 8.6–51.8	Insomnia, anorexia, weight loss, irritability, tachycardia, agitation, abdominal pain, headache, dry mouth, increased psychosis, asthenia, fever, infection, growth retardation (children), tics, crying, nausea, vomiting, nasal congestion

Drug (class)	Brand	Mechanism	Dose	Adverse effects
methylphenidate transdermal system (anti-ADHD)	Daytrana	NE reuptake inhibition, DA reuptake inhibition, promotes NE and DA release	12.5–37.5 cm^2	Application-site reactions, insomnia, anorexia, weight loss, irritability, tachycardia, agitation, abdominal pain, headache, dry mouth, increased psychosis, asthenia, fever, infection, growth retardation (children), tics, crying, nausea, vomiting, nasal congestion
milnacipran (anti-fibromyalgia)	Savella	NE reuptake inhibition, 5-HT reuptake inhibition	100–200	Serotonin syndrome, heart rate increased, seizures, hepatotoxicity, discontinuation syndrome, abnormal bleeding, nausea, constipation, headache, dizziness, insomnia, hot flush, hyperhidrosis, vomiting, palpitations, dry mouth
mirtazapine (antidepressant)	Remeron, Remeron Soltabs	Central presynaptic alpha-2 autoreceptor antagonist, H1 antagonist, moderate alpha-1 antagonist, moderate muscarinic antagonist	15–45	Sedation, weight gain, increased appetite, dry mouth, constipation, dizziness, asthenia
modafinil (antinarcolepsy)	Provigil	DA reuptake inhibition	200–400	Headache, nausea, nervousness, rhinitis, diarrhea, back pain, insomnia, dizziness, dyspepsia
molindone (antipsychotic)	Moban	D2 antagonism	20–100	Sedation, weight gain, dry mouth, dizziness, poor coordination, EPS, photosensitivity, lethargy, blurry vision, constipation, seizures, tachycardia, weakness, NMS, gynecomastia, leukopenia, hyperglycemia, hyperlipidemia, QT-interval prolongation
N-acetyl-cysteine (anti-cocaine)	N/A	Glutamate modulator	1,200–2,400	Nausea, vomiting, diarrhea, constipation
nalmefene (anti-alcohol)	Revex	Opioid antagonist	20–80	Liver dysfunction, constipation, irritability, increased thirst, dizziness, rash, chills, anorexia
naloxone (antiopioid)	Narcan	Opioid antagonist	0.4–2	Acute withdrawal syndrome, agitation, hallucinations, flushing, dyspnea, hypotension, hypertension, arrhythmias

(continued)

Generic Name (Drug Class)	Trade/Brand Name	Mechanism of Action	Typical Dose (Mg/Day)	Most Common Side Effects
naltrexone (anti-alcohol)	Revia, Depade	Opioid antagonist	50	Liver dysfunction, constipation, irritability, increased thirst, dizziness, rash, chills, anorexia, nausea, fatigue, anxiety, insomnia
naltrexone (anti-alcohol)	Vivitrol	Opioid antagonist	380 mg/4 wks	Injection-site reactions, eosinophilic pneumonia, nausea, headache, asthenia, dizziness, insomnia, pharyngitis, diarrhea, vomiting
naltrexone, bupropion (antiobesity)	Contrave	Opioid antagonist, NE reuptake inhibition, DA reuptake inhibition	8–32/90–360	Liver dysfunction, constipation, irritability, in-creased thirst, dizziness, rash, chills, anorexia, nausea, fatigue, anxiety, insomnia, headache, vomiting, dry mouth, diarrhea agitation/nervousness, seizure
nefazodone (antidepressant)	Serzone	5-HT2A antagonist	100–500	Dizziness, blurry vision, headache, dry mouth, nausea, constipation, agitation, increased appetite, drowsiness, weakness, liver toxicity
nortriptyline (antidepressant)	Pamelor, Aventyl	NE reuptake inhibition, 5-HT reuptake inhibition	75–125	Sedation, weight gain, dry mouth, blurry vision, constipation, urinary retention, sexual dysfunction, orthostatic hypotension, dizziness
olanzapine (antipsychotic)	Zyprexa, Zyprexa Zydis, Zyprexa IM	5-HT2A and 5-HT2C antagonism, D1–D4 antagonism, M1–M5 antagonism, H1 antagonism, alpha-1 antagonism	10–20 (5–10 mg IM)	Weight gain, increased appetite, constipation, agitation, dizziness, dry mouth, sedation, abnormal gait, back pain, speech disorder, amnesia, tremor, weakness, leukopenia, hyperglycemia, hyperlipidemia, EPS, NMS, cognitive and motor impairment, seizures, hyperprolactinemia, orthostatic hypotension
olanzapine (antipsychotic)	Zyprexa Relprev	5-HT2A and 5-HT2C antagonism, D1–D4 antagonism, M1–M5 antagonism, H1 antagonism, alpha-1 antagonism	150 mg/2 wks 405 mg/4 wks	See olanzapine + injection-site reactions
onabotulinumtoxin A (analgesic)	Botox	acetylcholine release inhibitor, neuromuscular blocking agent	360 unites/ 3 months	neck pain, headache, pain in extremity, dysphagia, upper respiratory infection, increased cough, flu syndrome, back pain, rhinitis, injection-site pain and hemorrhage, nonaxillary sweating, pharyngitis

Drug (class)	Brand name	Mechanism	Dose	Side effects
ondansetron (anticraving)	Zofran	5-HT3 antagonist	8–24	Diarrhea, headache, constipation, rash, dizziness, dry mouth, drowsiness
orlistat (antiobesity)	Xenical	Reversible lipase inhibitor in GI tract	360	Oily spotting or stool, flatus, fecal urgency, increased defecation, fecal incontinence
oxazepam (antianxiety)	Serax	Increases GABA	30–120	Poor coordination, dizziness, sedation, weakness, memory dysfunction, depression, lethargy
oxcarbazepine (mood stabilizer)	Trileptal	Inhibition of sodium channels, modulation of calcium channels	600–1,500	Dizziness, somnolence, diplopia, nausea, vomiting, headache, ataxia, abnormal vision, abdominal pain, tremor
paliperidone (antipsychotic)	Invega	D2 antagonism, 5-HT2 antagonism, alpha-1 and alpha-2 antagonism, H1 antagonism	3–12	EPS, tachycardia, akathisia, somnolence, dyspepsia, constipation, increased weight, nasopharyngitis, headache, leukopenia, hyperglycemia, hyperlipidemia, QT-interval prolongation, NMS
paliperidone palmitate (antipsychotic)	Invega Sustenna, Invega Trinza	D2 antagonism, 5-HT2 antagonism, alpha-1 and alpha-2 antagonism, H1 antagonism	39–234 mg/month, 273–819 mg/month	See paliperidone + injection-site reactions
paroxetine (antidepressant)	Paxil, Paxil CR	5-HT reuptake inhibition	20–50/25–75	Nausea, diarrhea, dry mouth, anorexia, weight gain, sexual dysfunction, tremor, restlessness, anxiety/nervousness, insomnia, dizziness, headache
pemoline (psychostimulant)	Cylert	"DA mechanisms"	37.5–112.5	Liver dysfunction, agitation, seizures, insomnia, anorexia, weight loss
perphenazine (antipsychotic)	Trilafon	D2 antagonism	8–64	Sedation, weight gain, dry mouth, dizziness, poor coordination, EPS, photosensitivity, lethargy, blurry vision, constipation, seizures, tachycardia, weakness, NMS, gynecomastia, leukopenia, hyperglycemia, hyperlipidemia, QT-interval prolongation

(continued)

Generic Name (Drug Class)	Trade/Brand Name	Mechanism of Action	Typical Dose (Mg/Day)	Most Common Side Effects
perphenazine/ amitriptyline (antianxiety)	Triavil	D2 antagonism, 5-HT reuptake inhibition, NE reuptake inhibition	5–6–16/75–200	Sedation, weight gain, dry mouth, dizziness, poor coordination, EPS, photosensitivity, lethargy, blurry vision, constipation, seizures, tachycardia, weakness, NMS, gynecomastia, urinary retention, sexual dysfunction, leukopenia, hyperglycemia, hyperlipidemia, QT-interval prolongation
phenelzine (antidepressant)	Nardil	5-HT reuptake inhibition, NE reuptake inhibition, DA reuptake inhibition	30–90	Nausea, insomnia, drowsiness, dry mouth, increased appetite, dizziness, headache, irritability, nervousness, weakness, sexual dysfunction, muscle twitching/cramps, constipation, weight gain, hypertensive crisis
phentermine (antiobesity)	Adipex-P, Ionamin	NE reuptake inhibition, DA reuptake inhibition, promotes NE and DA release	37.5–75	Insomnia, anorexia, weight loss, irritability, tachycardia, agitation, abdominal pain, headache, dry mouth, increased psychosis, asthenia, fever, infection, growth retardation (children)
phentermine-topiramate (antiobesity)	Qsymia	NE reuptake inhibition, DA reuptake inhibition, promotes NE and DA release, increases GABA, blocks glutamate receptors	3.75–15/23–92	Insomnia, anorexia, weight loss, irritability, tachycardia, agitation, abdominal pain, headache, dry mouth, increased psychosis, asthenia, fever, infection, paresthesia, dizziness, dysgeusia, insomnia, constipation, dry mouth, poor coordination, speech problems, memory dysfunction, abnormal vision, nervousness, confusion, cognitive dulling
pimavanserin antipsychotic	Nuplazid	5-HT2A and 5-HT2C antagonist	34	Peripheral edema, confusional state, hallucinations, urinary tract infection, fatigue, prolonged QT interval, gait disturbance
pimozide (antipsychotic)	Orap	D2 antagonism	1–10	Sedation, weight gain, dry mouth, dizziness, poor coordination, EPS, lethargy, NMS, blurry vision, seizures, constipation, tachycardia, weakness, gynecomastia
pindolol (anti-anxiety)	Visken	Nonselective beta blocker	10–60	Anxiety, lethargy, bradycardia, hyperhidrosis, visual disturbance, claudication, cold extremities, hypotension, syncope, tachycardia, weight gain, diarrhea, vomiting, wheezing, impotence, excess urination, burning eyes

Drug (class)	Brand name	Mechanism	Dose	Side effects
pramipexole (antiparkinsonian)	Mirapex	DA agonist	1.5–4.5	Nausea, dizziness, somnolence, insomnia, constipation, confusion, asthenia, hallucinations, edema, sedation, headache
prazepam (antianxiety)	Centrax	Increases GABA	20–60	Poor coordination, dizziness, sedation, weakness, memory dysfunction, depression, lethargy
pregabalin (analgesic)	Lyrica	Voltage-gated calcium channels (increases GABA transport)	150–450	Dizziness, somnolence, dry mouth, edema, blurred vision, weight gain, abnormal thinking, asthenia, ataxia, nausea, tremor, headache, vertigo
propranolol (antianxiety, antiparkinsonian)	Inderal, Inderal LA	Nonselective beta blocker	20–80	Bradycardia, rash, hypotension, dizziness, depression, weakness, bronchospasm, fatigue, sexual dysfunction, insomnia, alopecia
protriptyline (antidepressant)	Vivactil	NE reuptake inhibition, 5-HT reuptake inhibition	15–60	Sedation, weight gain, dry mouth, blurry vision, constipation, urinary retention, sexual dysfunction, orthostatic hypotension, dizziness
quazepam (sedative-hypnotic)	Doral	Increases GABA	7.5–15	Sedation, dizziness, falling, lethargy, disorientation, amnesia
quetiapine (antipsychotic)	Seroquel, Seroquel XR	5-HT1A and 5-HT2 antagonism, D1 and D2 antagonism, H1 antagonism, alpha-1 and alpha-2 antagonism	300–600	Sedation, dizziness, dry mouth, asthenia, constipation, headache, liver dysfunction, weight gain, dyspepsia, orthostatic hypotension, EPS, NMS, leukopenia, hyperglycemia, hyperlipidemia
ramelteon (sedative-hypnotic)	Rozerem	Melatonin receptor agonist	8	Somnolence, dizziness, fatigue, nausea, headache
risperidone (antipsychotic)	Risperdal, Risperdal M-tab	D2 antagonism, 5-HT2 antagonism, alpha-1 and alpha-2 antagonism, H1 antagonism	3–6	Somnolence, EPS, weight gain, anxiety, restlessness, insomnia, dizziness, constipation, nausea, rhinitis, rash, tachycardia, sexual dysfunction, NMS, leukopenia, hyperglycemia, hyperlipidemia, QT-interval prolongation, TD, hyperprolactinemia, orthostatic hypotension, cognitive and motor impairment, seizures, dysphagia, priapism

(continued)

Generic Name (Drug Class)	Trade/Brand Name	Mechanism of Action	Typical Dose (Mg/Day)	Most Common Side Effects
risperidone (antipsychotic)	Risperdal Consta	D2 antagonism, 5-HT2 antagonism, alpha-1 and alpha-2 antagonism, H1 antagonism	25–50 mg/2 wks	See risperidone + injection-site reactions
rivastigmine (antidementia)	Exelon	Cholinesterase inhibitor	6–12	Nausea, vomiting, asthenia, sweating, dizziness, headache, diarrhea, anorexia, insomnia
rivastigmine transdermal system (antidementia)	Exelon Patch	Cholinesterase inhibitor	4.6–9.5 mg/ 24 hrs	Application-site reactions, nausea, vomiting, asthenia, sweating, dizziness, headache, diarrhea, anorexia, insomnia
ropinirole (antiparkinsonian)	Requip	Dopamine agonist	0.75–3	Excessive drowsiness, syncope, bradycardia, hypotension, hallucinations, fatigue, nausea, headache, vomiting, dyspepsia, constipation, increased sweating, asthenia, confusion abdominal pain, abnormal vision, leg edema
selegiline (antidepressant)	Eldepryl	5-HT reuptake inhibition, NE reuptake inhibition, DA reuptake inhibition	10–20	Nausea, hallucinations, insomnia, dizziness, confusion, poor balance, agitation, syncope, hypertensive crisis (higher doses)
selegiline transdermal system (antidepressant)	EMSAM	5-HT reuptake inhibition, NE reuptake inhibition, DA reuptake inhibition	6–12 mg/24 hrs	Application-site reactions, nausea, hallucinations, insomnia, dizziness, confusion, poor balance, agitation, syncope, hypertensive crisis (higher doses), diarrhea, constipation
sertraline (antidepressant)	Zoloft	5-HT reuptake inhibition	50–200	Nausea, diarrhea, dry mouth, anorexia, weight gain, sexual dysfunction, tremor, restlessness, anxiety/nervousness, insomnia, dizziness, headache
sodium oxybate/gamma-hydroxy-butyrate (anti-narcolepsy)	Xyrem	CNS depressant	4.5–9.0 gm/night	Seizure, respiratory depression, confusion, headache, nausea, dizziness, nasopharyngitis, somnolence, vomiting, urinary incontinence
suvorexant (sedative)	Belsomra	Orexin antagonist	5–20	Somnolence, headache, abnormal dreams, dry mouth, cough, upper respiratory tract infection

Drug (class)	Brand	Mechanism	Dose (mg)	Side effects
tacrine (antidementia)	Cognex	Cholinesterase inhibitor	40–160	Abdominal pain, anxiety, agitation, poor coordination, constipation, depression, diarrhea, dizziness, fatigue, flushing, headache, insomnia, dyspepsia, liver dysfunction, muscle pain, anorexia, nausea, rash, sedation
temazepam (sedative-hypnotic)	Restoril	Increases GABA	15–30	Sedation, dizziness, falling, lethargy, disorientation, amnesia
tetrabenazine (anti-TD)	Xenazine	Vesicular monoamine transporter 2 (VMAT) inhibitor	12.5–50	Sedation, somnolence, fatigue, insomnia, depression, akathisia, anxiety, nausea
thioridazine (antipsychotic)	Mellaril	D2 antagonism	200–600	Sedation, weight gain, dry mouth, dizziness, poor coordination, EPS, photosensitivity, lethargy, blurry vision, constipation, seizures, tachycardia, weakness, NMS, gynecomastia, leukopenia, hyperglycemia, hyperlipidemia, QT-interval prolongation
thiothixene (antipsychotic)	Navane	D2 antagonism	5–30	Sedation, weight gain, dry mouth, dizziness, poor coordination, EPS, NMS, lethargy, blurry vision, seizures, constipation, tachycardia, weakness, gynecomastia, leukopenia, hyperglycemia, hyperlipidemia, QT-interval prolongation
tiagabine (mood stabilizer)	Gabitril	Increases GABA	8–16	Dizziness, asthenia, somnolence, nausea, nervousness, abdominal pain, decreased concentration, tremor, poor coordination
topiramate (mood stabilizer)	Topamax	Increases GABA, blocks glutamate receptors	100–500	Somnolence, fatigue, dizziness, decreased weight, poor coordination, speech problems, memory dysfunction, abnormal vision, paresthesia, nervousness, confusion, cognitive dulling, headache
tranylcypromine (antidepressant)	Parnate	5-HT reuptake inhibition, NE reuptake inhibition, DA reuptake inhibition	20–60	Nausea, insomnia, drowsiness, dry mouth, increased appetite, dizziness, headache, irritability, nervousness, weakness, sexual dysfunction, muscle twitching/cramps, constipation, weight gain, hypertensive crisis

(continued)

Generic Name (Drug Class)	Trade/Brand Name	Mechanism of Action	Typical Dose (Mg/Day)	Most Common Side Effects
trazodone (antidepressant)	Desyrel, Oleptro	5-HT2A and 5-HT2C antagonism, alpha-1 antagonism	50–400	Somnolence/sedation, vision blurred, dizziness, constipation, priapism, headache, dry mouth, nausea, fatigue
triazolam (sedative-hypnotic)	Halcion	Increases GABA	0.25–0.5	Sedation, dizziness, falling, lethargy, disorientation, amnesia
trifluoperazine (antipsychotic)	Stelazine	D2 antagonism	5–30	Sedation, weight gain, dry mouth, dizziness, poor coordination, EPS, NMS, lethargy, blurry vision, seizures, constipation, tachycardia, weakness, gynecomastia, leukopenia, hyperglycemia, hyperlipidemia, QT-interval prolongation
trihexyphenidyl (anticholinergic)	Artane	Anticholinergic	5–15	Tachycardia, nausea, constipation, confusion, dry mouth, urinary retention, blurry vision
trimipramine (antidepressant)	Surmontil	NE reuptake inhibition, 5-HT reuptake inhibition	150–300	Sedation, weight gain, dry mouth, blurry vision, constipation, urinary retention, sexual dysfunction, orthostatic hypotension, dizziness
valbenazine (anti-TD)	Ingrezza	VMAT2 reversible inhibitor	40–80	Somnolence akathisia, vomiting, arthralgia
valproate or valproic acid (mood stabilizer)	Depakote, Depakote ER, Stavzor	Inhibition of sodium and/or calcium channels, increases GABA, reduces glutamate	500–2,000	Nausea, vomiting, diarrhea, weight gain, abdominal pain, flatulence, edema, rash, drowsiness, tiredness, liver dysfunction, alopecia
varenicline (anti-smoking)	Chantix	Nicotinic acetylcholine receptor agonist	0.5–2	Angioedema, serious skin reaction, nausea, abnormal dreams, constipation, flatulence, vomiting, headache, agitation/hostility, suicide ideation
venlafaxine (antidepressant)	Effexor, Effexor XR	NE reuptake inhibition, 5-HT reuptake inhibition	50–300/75–300	Nausea, hypertension, anorexia, dizziness, somnolence, insomnia, dry mouth, nervousness, sexual dysfunction, sweating
verapamil (mood stabilizer)	Verelan PM, Covera-HS, Isoptin SR	Calcium channel antagonist	200–400	Constipation, nausea, headache, infection, dizziness, edema, liver dysfunction, arrhythmias, rash, hypotension, fatigue

Drug (class)	Brand name	Dose (mg)	Mechanism	Side effects
vilazodone (antidepressant)	Viibryd	20–40	Serotonin transport inhibitor, 5-HT1A receptor partial agonist	Diarrhea, nausea, vomiting, insomnia
vortioxetine (antidepressant)	Trintellix	5–20	5-HT reuptake inhibition, serotonin modulator	Nausea, constipation, vomiting
zaleplon (sedative-hypnotic)	Sonata	5–10	Selective modulation of GABA receptor complex	Daytime drowsiness, dizziness, falls, amnesia
ziprasidone (antipsychotic)	Geodon	80–160	D2 antagonism, 5-HT2 antagonism, H1 antagonism, alpha-1 antagonism	Nausea, agitation, rash, EKG abnormality, asthenia, orthostatic hypotension, anorexia, arthralgias, anxiety, tremor, rhinitis, abnormal vision, EPS, NMS, leukopenia, hyperglycemia, hyperlipidemia, QT-interval prolongation
zolpidem (sedative-hypnotic)	Ambien, Edluar, Zolpimist, Ambien CR, Intermezzo	5–10	Selective modulation of GABA receptor complex	Daytime drowsiness, dizziness, falls, amnesia
zonisamide (mood stabilizer)	Zonegran	200–400	Inhibition of sodium and/or calcium channels, facilitates DA and 5-HT neurotransmission	Somnolence, anorexia, weight loss, dizziness, headache, nausea, agitation, mental slowing

GLOSSARY

acetaldehyde dehydrogenase. An enzyme that converts acetaldehyde to harmless acetate.

acetylcholine. In the central nervous system, this neurotransmitter is thought to play a role in memory, learning, behavioral arousal, attention, mood, and rapid-eye movement activity during sleep. In the peripheral nervous system, acetylcholine is found at synapses where the nerve terminals meet skeletal muscles, causing excitation leading to muscle contraction.

acetylcholinesterase inhibitors. Medications that increase intra-synaptic acetylcholine levels and produce moderate symptomatic improvement in Alzheimer's disease.

action potential. Produced in a neuron when the resting potential becomes less negative or depolarized. It is mediated by voltage-dependent ion channels that transmit the essential cellular information for that neuron's function.

adequate dose. The dose recommended in the package labeling of a medication, indicating what is typically prescribed.

adequate treatment trial. A time period of a minimum of four weeks and a maximum of six weeks before making a major change in the treatment regimen because the patients' response to medication may be delayed.

agonist. A drug that increases the action of a neurotransmitter at its receptor site.

akathisia. A common subacute side effect that may be experienced as inner restlessness, anxiety, or agitation.

antagonist. A drug that prevents an action of a neurotransmitter at its receptor site.

anticonvulsants (anti-seizure medication). A variety of medication used for the treatment of epileptic seizures, bipolar disorder, and other psychiatric conditions.

atypical antipsychotic medication. Second-generation antipsychotic drugs used to treat psychiatric conditions.

axon. A cylindrical, tubelike tail of a neuron that transmits information from the soma to its terminal buttons and ultimately to other neurons or cells.

barbiturates. Medications such as Nembutal and Seconal used in the treatment of anxiety that are very sedating and habit forming.

benzodiazepines. Sedative-hypnotic medications used in the treatment of anxiety and other psychiatric conditions.

bradykinesia. A decrease in movement and spontaneity.

bruxism. A condition in which the patient grinds his/her teeth during sleep.

chloride ion channels. Tiny gateways or receptor sites found on the surface of cells. These are opened or activated by various neurotransmitters.

cholinergic. Relating to nerve cells that utilize acetylcholine as their neurotransmitter.

cross-titration. Gradual decrease or tapering of a drug dose while gradually increasing the dose of a second drug or agent.

dehydroepiandrosterone (DHEA). A steroid secreted by the adrenal gland and the testes that is a precursor to testosterone and estrogen.

dendrites. The branchlike part of the neuron that collects chemical messages via its molecular receptor sites from nearby cells. The surface of the dendrite is also referred to as the "postsynaptic membrane."

depolarization. Results from an increase in the permeability of a cell's membrane, resulting in an action potential.

depression treatment protocol. Procedural steps used in the treatment of depressive illness.

discontinuation syndrome. Various symptoms experienced after the discontinuation of medication. These are not typically dangerous, although they may mimic withdrawal symptoms.

dopamine. A biogenic amine neurotransmitter involved in behavioral regulation, movement, learning, mood, attention, and the reward cycle of addiction.

dopaminergic. Pertaining to the action or function of dopamine.

endogenous substances. Substances that come from within the body, such as endorphins, insulin, and adrenaline.

electrocardiogram (ECG or EKG). A record of the heart's integrated action currents, often obtained in a routine physical or cardiac workup.

electroconvulsive therapy (ECT). A series of treatments involving the application of electrical current to the brain of an anesthetized patient. This induces a seizure to bring about an improvement in mood/psychotic states.

electroencephalogram (EEG). A record of brain-wave activity, which is analyzed during a nocturnal polysomnogram or neurologic exam.

epinephrine (adrenalin). A neurotransmitter, primarily of the peripheral nervous system, that regulates the fight-or-flight response.

exocytosis. The process by which neurotransmitters are released from a cell.

exogenous substances. Substances that are produced outside the body and introduced into the body in some manner.

extrapyramidal symptoms (EPS). Side effects typically found with many medications, including neuroleptics. These may include bradykinesia, parkinsonism, akathisia, and/or tardive dyskinesia.

first-pass metabolism. In the body, the set of reactions in which orally absorbed medications first encounter the liver, where some of the drug is metabolized and then delivered to the target organ.

ginkgo biloba. A tree extract said to relieve mild depression and increase memory and concentration.

glutamatergic. Pertaining to the action or function of glutamate.

half-life. The average time required to eliminate one-half of a drug's concentration from the body.

hyperdopaminergic hypothesis. The concept that too much dopamine may be causing psychotic symptoms.

hyperpolarization. A process that occurs after an action potential when the cell briefly becomes more polarized, or hyperpolarized, as it returns to a relaxed state.

ion. An atom with either a positive or negative electrical charge.

lipid solubility. A characteristic of a drug that determines how easily it may cross a cell membrane. Drugs that are said to be "lipophilic" are more likely to cross the blood-brain barrier.

loading dose. The practice of introducing a drug into the body at high doses in order to obtain a certain desired response, as opposed to starting with a low dose and gradually increasing.

mania treatment protocol. Procedural steps used in the treatment of the manic phase of bipolar illness.

mixed dementia. Dementia that may be caused by a combination of two neuropathological processes, which may occur together. For example, Alzheimer's disease and vascular dementia occurring together would be referred to as mixed dementia.

monoamine oxidase inhibitors (MAOIs). Medications that inhibit the enzyme that breaks down certain neurotransmitter substances and renders them ineffective.

mood stabilizers. A variety of psychiatric medications used to treat mood disorders characterized by intense and sustained mood shifts. Lithium and anticonvulsant medications are examples of mood stabilizers.

neuron. The morphologic and functional unit in the nervous system involved in the transmission of chemical messages to facilitate a thought, action, or behavior. It consists of four basic parts: the soma, dendrites, axon, and terminal buttons.

nocturnal polysomnogram (NPSG). A sleep study, which is conducted at night in a sleep laboratory under the supervision of a neurologist or a sleep specialist. This test is also referred to as a polysomnograph (PSG) and is used to diagnose sleep disorders.

nonsteroidal anti-inflammatory drugs (NSAIDs). Medications typically used to decrease inflammation and pain that may decrease the risk of Alzheimer's disease in some patients.

noradrenergic. Pertaining to the action or function of norepinephrine.

norepinephrine. A biogenic amine neurotransmitter, which is primarily excitatory in the central nervous system. It is involved in attention, arousal, mood, and sleep regulation.

obstructive sleep apnea (OSA). A condition characterized by obstructed airways during sleep, resulting in loud snoring, gasping, awakening throughout the night, and periods when breathing stops (apnea).

overlap and taper. The practice of continuing the same dose of one drug while gradually increasing a second drug to a therapeutic level and then tapering the first.

pharmacodynamics. The process of how drugs affect receptors sites, send signals, and cause neurochemical changes, i.e., what the drug does to the body.

pharmacokinetics. The process of drug administration, absorption, distribution, metabolism, and elimination, i.e., what the body does to the drug.

placebo response. A demonstrated physical response that occurs when a placebo is taken.

potentiation. A process that occurs when one drug enhances the effect of another drug. For example, stimulants and antidepressants.

protein binding. A process in which drugs bind to proteins in the bloodstream, which may reduce the amount of a drug that is actually available to act at a target site based on the size of the bound protein substance. A substance that has high protein binding is not available in the bloodstream to act on its target. Some substances like albumin that have large molecular weight may bind to a drug and interfere with the action of the drug at the target; i.e., they may interfere with the transport of the drug through small capillary junctions.

protein kinases. A secondary messenger activated within the postsynaptic membrane by a neurotransmitter to alter neuronal functions.

psychostimulants. Stimulating medications (i.e., amphetamines and methylphenidate) used primarily for enhancing the efficacy of antidepressants and in the treatment of ADHD.

rebound phenomenon. The observation that after sleep deprivation, patients spend additional time in stages 3, 4, and REM in their next sleep period.

resting potential. The electrical potential of the neuron in the unexcited or relaxed state. The average electrical difference between the inside and the outside of the cell is about 70 millivolts (mV). Typically referred to as –70 mV (the outside is more negative than the inside).

reuptake. A process that signals the end of the action potential; some of the neurotransmitter substance is taken back into the terminal button after exocytosis.

S-adenosyl-L-methionine (SAM-E). A naturally occurring endogenous substance produced by the body and synthesized from food and essential B vitamins. Lower levels have been found in depressed patients. It is available as a synthesized dietary supplement that may increase serotonin and norepinephrine levels.

satiation. A sensation of fullness that can be achieved with excessive food consumption, television watching, video gaming, or drugs like benzodiazepines or alcohol.

selective serotonin reuptake inhibitors (SSRIs). Medications that block the reuptake of serotonin back into the presynaptic cell.

serotonergic. Pertaining to the action or function of serotonin.

serotonin. A neurotransmitter in the central nervous system involved in the inhibition of obsessive thinking and compulsive behaviors, mood regulation, eating and sleeping patterns, and pain regulation.

signal transduction. The process by which a neurotransmitter binds to a receptor site, changing electrical and chemical characteristics within the cell.

soma. The physical cell body that contains the vital parts of the cell, including the nucleus, mitochondria, and other substances in the cytoplasm (the space inside the neuron).

St. John's wort. A plant found to have medicinal properties that may help to control mild to moderate levels of depression.

synapse. A physical gap or space between the terminal buttons (presynaptic cell), and the dendrites of the next neuron (postsynaptic cell). The synapse can be between a terminal button and a dendrite or between the terminal button and the soma.

synergism. A process that occurs when one drug significantly enhances the effect of another drug, for example, alcohol and sedatives.

tardive dyskinesia. A potentially chronic side effect of antipsychotic medications. Symptoms may include involuntary abnormal movements of the tongue, lips, neck, limbs, and/or trunk.

terminal button. Found at the ends of the branches of the axon, this structure contains stored sacs of neurotransmitters substance.

therapeutic dose. The concentration or dose of a drug required to achieve the desired response.

therapeutic index. The difference between a drug's therapeutic level and its toxic level.

tolerance. Condition in which a patient needs to acquire and use greater amounts of a drug to achieve the original desired effect.

toxic rash. Associated with Stevens-Johnson syndrome, a potentially life-threatening skin rash that may require medical attention.

treatment refractory. Applied to an illness when a patient fails to respond to three or more psychotropic medications.

tricyclic antidepressants (TCAs). First-generation antidepressant medications that prevent the reuptake of neurotransmitter substances back into the presynaptic cell.

typical antipsychotic medications. First-generation antipsychotic drugs used to treat psychosis and agitated mood states (mania, agitation, and schizophrenia).

ultrarapid detox. A detoxification procedure conducted under anesthesia that utilizes naloxone in combination with other sedatives for an intense 24-hour detoxification.

upper airway resistance syndrome. A milder form of obstructive sleep apnea. The patient is unable to keep airways open during sleep, and the airway narrows or collapses, leading to gasping or awakening throughout the night.

vascular dementia. Dementia occurring from disease related to the brain's vascular system.

withdrawal. Characteristic symptoms that emerge when a drug is abruptly discontinued after heavy and prolonged use, for example, alcohol.

ADDITIONAL READINGS

Ables, A., & Baughman, O. (2003). Antidepressants: Update on new agents and indications. *American Family Physician, 67,* 547–554.

Aisen, P. S. (2002). The potential of anti-inflammatory drugs for the treatment of Alzheimer's disease. *Lancet Neurology, 1*(5), 279–284. Review.

Allen, M., Currier, G., Hughes, D., Reyes-Harde, M., & Docherty, J. (2001). Treatment of behavioral emergencies. *Postgraduate Medicine,* May, Special Report.

American Psychiatric Association Clinical Resources. Practice guideline for the treatment of patients with eating disorders. www.psych.org/

Antai-Otong, D. (2001). *Psychiatric emergencies: How to accurately assess and manage the patient in crisis.* Eau Claire, WI: PESI Healthcare, LLC.

Arnold, L. (2008). Management of fibromyalgia and comorbid psychiatric disorders. *Journal of Clinical Psychiatry, 69*(suppl 2), 14–19.

Barkin, R., Schwer, W., & Barkin, S. (1999). Recognition and management of depression in primary care: A focus on the elderly. A pharmacologic overview of the selection process among the traditional and new antidepressants. *American Journal of Therapeutics, 7,* 205–226.

Bays, H. (2004). Current and investigational antiobesity agents and obesity therapeutic treatment targets. *Obesity Research, 12*(8), 1197–2211.

Bergh, C., Ejderhamn, J., & Sodersten, P. (2003). What is the evidence basis for existing treatments of eating disorders? *Current Opinion in Pediatrics, 15,* 344–345.

Briley, M. (2004). Clinical experience with dual action antidepressants in different chronic pain syndromes. *Human Psychopharmacology: Clinical and Experimental, 19,* 21–25.

Buelow, G., Hebert, S., & Buelow, S. (2000). *Psychotherapist's resource on psychiatric medications* (2nd ed.). Belmont, CA: Brooks-Cole.

Caccia, S., Pasina, L., & Nobili, A. (2010). New atypical antipsychotics for schizophrenia: Iloperidone. *Drug Design, Development and Therapy, 4,* 33–48.

Carvajal, G., Garcia, D., Sanchez, S., Velasco, M., Rueda, D., & Lucena, M. (2002). Hepatotoxicity associated with the new antidepressants. *Journal of Clinical Psychiatry. 63*(suppl 2), 135–137.

Doody, R. (2003). Current treatments for alzheimer's disease: Cholinesterase inhibitors. *Journal of Clinical Psychiatry, 64*(suppl 9), 11–17.

Evans, K. (1990). *Dual diagnosis: Counseling the mentally ill substance user.* New York: Guilford Press.

Gitlin, M. (1996). *The psychotherapist's guide to psychopharmacology* (2nd ed.). New York: The Free Press.

Gold, L. (2003). Psychopharmacologic treatment of depression during pregnancy. *Current Woman's Health Reports, 3,* 236–241.

Grant, J., Kim, S., & Potenza, M. (2003). Advances in the pharmacological treatment of pathological gambling. *Journal of Gambling Studies, 19*(1), 85–109.

Grant, J., & Potenza, M. (2004). Impulse control disorders: Clinical characteristics and pharmacological management. *Annals of Clinical Psychiatry, 16*(1), 27–34.

Grant, J., Won, K., Hollander, E., & Potenza, M. (2008). Predicting response to opiate antagonists and placebo in the treatment of pathological gambling. *Psychopharmacology, 200*(4), 521–527.

Halpern, A., & Mancini, M. (2003). Treatment of obesity: An update on anti-obesity medications. *Obesity Research, 4*(1), 25–42.

Hayashida, M., & Nakane, Y. (1999). Algorithm for the treatment of acute psychotic episodes. *Psychiatry and Clinical Neurosciences, 53*(suppl), S3–S7.

International Association for the Study of Pain. Definition of pain. http://www .iasp-pain.org//AM/Template.cfm? Section=Home

Janicak, P., Davis, J., Preskorn, S., & Ayd, F. (1993). *Principles and practice of psychopharmacotherapy.* Baltimore: Williams and Wilkins.

Kasckow, J. (2002). Cognitive enhancers for dementia: Do they work? *Current Psychiatry, 1*(3), 22–28.

Kelly, K., & Zisselman M. (2000). Update on electroconvulsive therapy (ECT) in older adults. *Journal of the American Geriatrics Society, 48*(5), 560–566.

Kennedy, S., Lam, R., Cohen, N., Ravindran, A., & CANMAT Depression Work Group. (2001). Clinical guidelines for the treatment of depressive disorders IV: Medications and other biological treatments. *The Canadian Journal of Psychiatry, 46,* 38S–58S

Kramer, P. (1993). *Listening to prozac.* New York: Penguin.

Leon, A. C., Solomon D. A., Mueller T. I., Endicott J., Rice J. P., Maser J. D., ... Keller M. B. (2003). A 20-year longitudinal observational study of somatic antidepressant treatment effectiveness. *American Journal of Psychiatry, 160*(4), 727–733.

Lewis, M. (2002). *Child and adolescent psychiatry: A comprehensive textbook* (3rd ed.). Philadelphia: Lippincott Williams & Wilkins.

Mintzer, J. (2001). Underlying mechanisms of psychosis and aggression in patients with Alzheimer's disease. *Journal of Clinical Psychiatry, 62*(suppl 21), 23–25.

Mintzer, J. (2003). The search for better noncholinergic treatment options for Alzheimer's disease. *Journal of Clinical Psychiatry, 64*(suppl 9), 18–22.

Nace, E. (1992). Emerging concepts in dual diagnosis. *The Counselor, 10,* 10–13.

Nelson, C., Thase M. E., Trivedi M. H., Fava M., Han J., Van Tran Q., ... Berman R. M. (2009). Safety and tolerability of adjunctive aripiprazole in major depressive disorder: A pooled post hoc analysis. *Primary Care Companion Journal of Clinical Psychiatry, 11*(6), 344–352.

Nieoullon, A. (2002). Dopamine and the regulation of cognition and attention. *Progress in Neurobiology, 67,* 53–83.

Padwal, R., Li, S., & Lau, D. (2003). Long-term pharmacotherapy for obesity and overweight. *Cochrane Database of Systemic Reviews, 4,* CD004094

Pearlstein, T. (2000). Antidepressant treatment of posttraumatic stress disorder. *Journal of Clinical Psychiatry, 61*(suppl 7), 40–43.

Perrot, S., Dickenson, A., & Bennett, R. (2008). Fibromyalgia: Harmonizing science with clinical practice considerations. *Pain Practice, 8*(3), 177–189.

Pietrzak, R., Ladd, G., & Petry, N. (2003). Disordered gambling in adolescents: Epidemiology, diagnosis, and treatment. *Paediatric Drugs, 5(9),* 583–595.

Preston, J., & Johnson, J. (2004). *Psychopharmacology made ridiculously simple* (5th ed.). Miami, FL: Medmaster, Inc.

Preston, J., O'Neal, J., & Talaga, M. (2002). *Handbook of clinical psychopharmacology for therapists* (3rd ed.). Oakland, CA: New Harbinger Publications, Inc.

Pridmore, S., Oberoi, G., & Harris, N. (2001). Psychiatry has much to offer for chronic pain. *Australian and New Zealand Journal of Psychiatry, 35,* 145–149.

Pryse-Phillips, W., Sternberg, S., Rochon, P., Naglie, G., Strong, H., & Feightner, J. (2001). The use of medications for cognitive enhancement. *Canadian Journal of Neurological Sciences, 28*(suppl 1), 108–114.

Sachs, G., Koslow, C., & Ghaemi, S. (2000). The treatment of bipolar depression. *Bipolar Disorders, 2,* 256–260.

Sachs, G., Printz, D., Kahn, D., Carpenter, D., & Docherty, J. (2000). Medication treatment of bipolar disorder 2000. *A Postgraduate Medicine Special Report,* 1–104.

Sachs, G., & Rush, J. (2003). Response, remission, and recovery in bipolar disorders: What are the realistic treatment goals? *Journal of Clinical Psychiatry, 64*(suppl 6), 18–22.

Sajatovic, M. (2003). Treatment of mood and anxiety disorders: Quetiapine and aripiprazole. *Current Psychiatry Reports, 5,* 320–326.

Schatzberg, A., & Nemeroff, C. (2004). *Textbook of psychopharmacology* (3rd ed.). Washington DC: American Psychiatric Press.

Sekula, L., DeSantis, J., & Gianetti, V. (2003). Considerations in the management of the patient with comorbid depression and anxiety. *Journal of the American Academy of Nurse Practitioners, 15*(1), 23–33.

Sheehan, D. (2001). Attaining remission in generalized anxiety disorder: Venlafaxine extended release comparative data. *Journal of Clinical Psychiatry, 62*(suppl 19), 26–31.

Singh, Y., & Singh, N. (2002). Therapeutic potential of kava in the treatment of anxiety disorders. *CNS Drugs, 16*(11), 731–743.

Sood, E., Pallanti, S., & Hollander, E. (2003). Diagnosis and treatment of pathological gambling. *Current Psychiatry Reports, 5*(1), 9–15.

Stahl, S. (1997). *Psychopharmacology of antidepressants.* London: Martin Dunitz.

Stahl, S. (2001). *Essential psychopharmacology of depression and bipolar disorder.* New York: Cambridge University Press.

Suppes, T., Dennehy E. B., Swann A. C., Bowden C. L., Calabrese J. R., Hirschfeld R. M., ... Shon S. P. (2002). Report of the Texas Consensus Conference Panel on medication treatment of bipolar disorder 2000. *Journal of Clinical Psychiatry, 63*(4), 288–299.

Swift, R. (2001). The pharmacotherapy of alcohol dependence: Clinical and economic aspects. *The Economics of Neuroscience, 3*(12), 62–66.

Swift, R. (2003). Topiramate for the treatment of alcohol dependence: Initiating abstinence. *Lancet, 361*(9370), 1666–1667.

Tosini, G., Ferguson, I., & Tsubota, K. (2016). Effects of blue light on the circadian system and eye physiology. *Molecular Vision, 22,* 61–72.

U.S. Food and Drug Administration. Proposed medication guide. www.fda.gov/

Walsh, K., & McDougle, C. (2001). Trichotillomania. Presentation, etiology, diagnosis, and therapy. *American Journal of Clinical Dermatology, 2*(5), 327–333.

Weiss, L. (1992). *Attention deficit disorders in adults.* Dallas, TX: Taylor Publishing.

Wenk, G. (2003). Neuropathologic changes in Alzheimer's disease. *Journal of Clinical Psychiatry, 64*(suppl 9), 7–10.

REFERENCES

Aboujaoude, E. (2010). Problematic Internet use: An overview. *World Psychiatry*, 9, 85–90.

Abulseoud, O., Miller, J., Wu, J., Choi, D., & Holschneider, D. (2012). Ceftriaxone upregulates the glutamate transporter in medial prefrontal cortex and blocks reinstatement of methamphetamine seeking in a condition place preference paradigm. *Brain Research*, *1456*, 14–21.

Adler, L., & Chua, H. (2002). Management of ADHD in adults. *Journal of Clinical Psychiatry*, *63*(Suppl. 12), 29–35.

Adler, L., Goodman, D., Weisler, R., Hamdani, M., & Roth, T. (2009). Effect of lisdexamfetamine dimesylate on sleep in adults with attention-deficit/hyperactivity disorder. *Behavioral and Brain Functions*, *5*(34).

Adler, L., Reingold, L., Morrill, M., & Wilens, T. (2006). Combination pharmacotherapy for adult ADHD. *Current Psychiatry Reports*, 8, 409–415.

Advokat, C., Comaty, J., & Julien, R. (2014). *Julien's primer of drug action* (13th ed.). New York, NY: Worth Publishers.

Agras, W. (2001). The consequences and costs of the eating disorders. *Psychiatric Clinics of North America*, *24*, 371–379.

Aisen, P. (2002). The potential of anti-inflammatory drugs for the treatment of Alzheimer's disease. *Lancet Neurology*, *1*(5), 279–284.

Albucher, R., & Liberzon, I. (2002). Psychopharmacological treatment in PTSD: A critical review. *Journal of Psychiatric Research*, *36*, 355–367.

Alzheimer's Association. (2013). *2013 Alzheimer's disease facts and figures.* www.alz.org

Amann, B., Pantel, J., Grunze, H., Vieta, E., Colom, F., Gonzalez-Pinto, A., … Hampel, H. (2009). Anticonvulsants in the treatment of aggression in the demented elderly: An update. *Clinical Practice and Epidemiology in Mental Health*, *5*, 14–21.

Amaresha, A., & Venkatasubramanian, G. (2012). Expressed emotion in schizophrenia: An overview. *Indian Journal of Psychological Medicine*, *34*(1), 12–20.

American Association of Suicidology. (2014). Depression and suicide risk. www.suicidology.org

Antelmi, E., Benedetti, F., Pizza, F., Filardi, M., Vandi, S., Liguori, R., … Plazzi, G. (2017). REM sleep-related episodes in children with narcolepsy type 1 after treatment with sodium oxybate. *Sleep Medicine*, *40*, e263. http://doi.org/10.1016/j.sleep.2017.11.770

Anthenelli, R., Benowitz, N., West, R., St Aubin, L., McRae, T., Lawrence, D., … Evins, A. (2016). Neuropsychiatric safety and efficacy of varenicline, bupropion, and nicotine patch in smokers with and without psychiatric disorders (EAGLES): A double-blind, randomised, placebo-controlled clinical trial. *Lancet*, *387*(10037), 2507–2520.

Anxiety and Depression Association of America. (2017). Clinical practice review for major depressive disorder. www.adaa.org

Arnold, L., Crofford, L., Martin, S., Young, J., & Sharma, U. (2007). The effect of anxiety and depression on improvements in pain in a randomized, controlled trial of pregabalin for treatment of fibromyalgia. *Pain Medicine*, *8*(8), 633–638.

Arnold, V., Feifel, D., Earl, C., Yang, R., & Adler, L. (2012). A 9-week, randomized, double-blind, placebo-controlled, parallel-group, dose-finding study to evaluate the efficacy and safety of modafinil as treatment for adults with ADHD. *Journal of Attention Disorders*, *18*(2), 133–144. http://doi.org/10.1177/1087054712441969

Asnis, G., & Henderson, M. (2015). Levomilnacipran for the treatment of major depressive disorder: A review. *Neuropsychiatric Disease and Treatment*, *11*, 125–135.

Aviram, R., Rhum, M., & Levin, F. (2001). Psychotherapy of adults with comorbid attention deficit/hyperactivity disorder and psychoactive substance abuse disorder. *Journal Psychotherapy Practice Research*, *10*, 179–186.

Azorin, J., Bowden, C., Garay, R., Perugi, G., Vieta, E., & Young, A. (2010). Possible new ways in the pharmacological treatment of bipolar disorder and comorbid alcoholism. *Neuropsychiatric Disease and Treatment*, 6, 37–46.

Baethge, C. (2002). Long-term treatment of schizoaffective disorder: Review and recommendations. *Pharmacopsychiatry*, *36*, 45–56.

Baltieri, D., Daro, F., Ribeiro, P., & de Andrade, A. (2008). Comparing topiramate with naltrexone in the treatment of alcohol dependence. *Addiction*, *103*, 2035–2044.

Bandelow, B., Sher, L., Bunevicius, R., Hollander, E., Kasper, S., Zohar, J., & Möller, H. (2012). Guidelines for the pharmacological treatment of anxiety disorders, obsessive-compulsive disorder and posttraumatic stress disorder in primary care. *International Journal of Psychiatry in Clinical Practice*, *16*, 77–84.

Barkley, R. (2002). Psychosocial treatments for attention-deficit/hyperactivity disorder in children. *Journal of Clinical Psychiatry*, *63*(Suppl. 12), 36–43.

Barlow, D. H., & Durand, M. V. (2005). *Abnormal psychology: An integrative approach* (4th ed.). London: Thomson-Wadsworth.

Barlow, G., & Herbert, S. (1995). Counselor's resource on psychiatric medications: Issues of treatment and referral. Pacific Grove, CA: Brooks/Cole.

Barnett, J., & Smoller, J. (2009). The genetics of bipolar disorder. *Neuroscience*, *164* (1), 331–343.

Bartels, C., Wagner, M., Wolfsgruber, S., Ehrenreich, H., & Schneider, A. (2017). Impact of SSRI therapy on risk of conversion from mild cognitive impairment to Alzheimer's dementia in individuals with previous depression. *American Journal of Psychiatry*, *175*(3), 232–241. doi.org/10.1176/appi.ajp.2017.17040404

Baune, B. (2008). New developments in the management of major depressive disorder and generalized anxiety disorder: Role of quetiapine. *Neuropsychiatric Disease and Treatment*, *4*(6), 1181–1192.

Beard, K., & Wolf, E. (2001). Modification in the proposed diagnostic criteria for Internet addiction. *Cyberpsychology & Behavior*, *4*(3), 377–383.

Beesdo, K., Hartford, J., Russell, J., Spann, M., Ball, S., & Wittchen, H. (2009). The short- and long-term effect of duloxetine on painful physical symptoms in patients with generalized anxiety disorder: Results from three clinical trials. *Journal of Anxiety Disorders*, *23*(8), 1064–1071.

Bell, J. (2008). Propranolol, post-traumatic stress disorder and narrative identity. *Journal of Medical Ethics: Journal of the Institute of Medical Ethics*, *34*(11), 1–4.

Bellino, S., Paradiso, E., Bozzatello, P., & Bogetto, F. (2010). Efficacy and tolerability of duloxetine in the treatment of patients with borderline personality disorder: A pilot study. *Journal of Psychopharmacology*, *24*(3), 333–339.

Bemporad, J. (2001). Aspects of psychotherapy with adults with attention deficit disorder. *Annals of the New York Academy of Science*, *931*, 302–309.

Bentley, S., Pagalilauan, G., & Simpson, S. (2014). Major depression. *Medical Clinics of North America*, 98, 981–1005.

Beraha, E., Salemink, E., Goudriaan, A., Bakker, A., de Jong, D., Smits, N., … Wiers, R. (2016). Efficacy and safety of high-dose baclofen for the treatment of alcohol dependence: A multicentre, randomised, double-blind controlled trial. *European Neuropsychopharmacology*, *26*, 1950–1959.

Berk, M., Copolov, D., Dean, O., Lu, K., Jeavons, S., Schapkaitz, I., … Bush, A. (2008). N-acetyl cysteine for depressive symptoms in bipolar disorder: A double blind randomized placebo-controlled trial. *Biological Psychiatry*, *64*(6), 468–475.

Berger, W., Mendlowicz, M., Marques-Portella, C., Kinrys, G., Fontenelle, L., Marmar, C., & Figueira, I. (2009). Pharmacologic alternatives to antidepressants in posttraumatic stress disorder: A systematic review. *Progress in Neuropsychopharmacology and Biological Psychiatry*, *33*(2), 169–180.

Berlin, R. (2017). Update on medications for PTSD. *The Carlat Report*, *15*, 12, 1–7.

Bezchlibnyk-Butler, K., & Jeffries, J. (2002). *Clinical handbook of psychotropic drugs*. Seattle, WA: Hogrefe & Huber.

Bishara, D., & Taylor, D. (2009). Asenapine monotherapy in the acute treatment of both schizophrenia and bipolar I disorder. *Neuropsyhicatric Disease and Treatment*, *5*, 483–490.

Blazer, D., Steffens, D., & Busse, E. (2004). *Textbook of geriatric psychiatry* (3rd ed.). Washington, DC: American Psychiatric Publishing, Inc.

Bloomfield, H., Nordfors, M., & McWilliams, P. (1996). *Hypericum and depression*. Los Angeles, CA: Prelude Press.

Boeve, B., Silber, M., & Ferman, T. (2002). Current management of sleep disturbance in dementia. *Current Neurology and Neuroscience Reports*, *2*, 169–177.

Bouquié, R., Wainstein, L., Pilet, P., Mussini, J., Deslandes, G., Clouet, J., … Victorri-Vigneau, C. (2014). Crushed and injected buprenorphine tablets: Characteristics of princeps and generic solutions. *PLoS ONE*, *9*(12), e113991. doi:10.1371/journal.pone.0113991

Bourin, M., & Lambert, O. (2002). Pharmacotherapy of anxious disorders. *Human Psychopharmacology*, *17*, 383–400.

Bowden, C. (2001). Novel treatments for bipolar disorder. *Expert Opinion on Investigational Drugs*, *10*(4), 661–671.

Breitbart, W., & Alici, Y. (2009). Psycho-oncology. *Harvard Review of Psychiatry*, *17*(6), 361–376.

Bright, G. (2008). Abuse of medications employed for the treatment of ADHD: Results from a large-scale community survey. *Medscape Journal of Medicine*, *10*(5), 111.

Brooks, S., & Kushida, C. (2002). Recent advances in the understanding and treatment of narcolepsy. *Primary Psychiatry*, *9*(8), 30–34.

Buchanan, R. W., Javitt, D. C., Marder, S. R., Schooler, N. R., Gold, J. M., McMahon, R. P., … Carpenter, W. T. (2007). The Cognitive and Negative Symptoms in Schizophrenia Trail (CONSIST): The efficacy of glutamatergic agents for negative symptoms and cognitive impairments. *American Journal of Psychiatry*, *164*(10), 1593–1602

Bulik, C., Devlin B., & Bacanu, S. (2003). Significant linkage on chromosome 10p in families with bulimia nervosa. *American Journal of Human Genetics*, *72*, 200–207.

Bushnell, G., Stürmer, T., Gaynes, B., Pate, V., & Miller, M. (2017). Simultaneous antidepressant and benzodiazepine new use and subsequent long-term benzodiazepine use in adults with depression, United States, 2001-2014. *JAMA Psychiatry*, *74*(7), 747–755. doi:10.1001/jamapsychiatry.2017.1273

Campbell, M., & Mathys, M. (2001). Pharmacologic options for the treatment of obesity. *American Journal of Health-System Pharmacy*, *58*(14), 1301–1308.

Caraci, F., Leggio, G., Salomone, S., & Drago, F. (2017). New drugs in psychiatry: Focus on new pharmacological targets. *F1000Research*, *6*(F1000 Faculty Rev), 397.

Carlson, N. (2004). *Physiology of behavior* (8th ed.). Boston, MA: Allyn and Bacon.

Center for Behavioral Health Statistics and Quality (CBSHQ). (2015). *2014 National Survey on Drug Use and Health: Detailed Tables*. Rockville, MD: Substance Abuse and Mental Health Services Administration.

Chamberlain, S., Muller, U., Blackwell, A., Robbins, T., & Sahakian, B. (2006). Noradrenergic modulation of working memory and emotional memory in humans. *Psychopharmacology*, *188*(4), 397–407.

Chang, K., Wagner, C., Garrett, A., Howe, M., & Reiss, A. (2008). A preliminary functional magnetic resonance imaging study of prefrontal-amygdalar activation changes in adolescents with bipolar depression treated with lamotrigine. *Bipolar Disorders*, *10*(3), 426–431.

Chen, J., Zhao, L., Liu, Y., Fan, S., & Xie, P. (2017). Comparative efficacy and acceptability of electroconvulsive therapy versus repetitive transcranial magnetic stimulation for major depression: A systematic review and multiple-treatments meta-analysis. *Behavioural Brain Research*, *320*, 30–36.

Choi, Y. (2009). Efficacy of treatments for patients with obsessive-compulsive disorder: A systematic review. *Journal of the American Academy of Nurse Practitioners*, *21*(4), 207–213.

Cipriani, A., Furukawa T., Salanti G., Geddes J., Higgins J., Churchill R., … Barbui C. (2009). Comparative efficacy and acceptability of 12 new-generation antidepressants: A multiple-treatments meta-analysis. *Lancet*, *373*(9665), 746–758.

Citrome, L. (2017a). Long-acting injectable antipsychotics update: Lengthening the dosing interval and expanding the diagnostic indications. *Expert Review of Neurotherapeutics, 17*(10), 1029–1043. doi:10.1080/14737175. 2017.1371014

Citrome, L. (2017b). Binge-eating disorder and comorbid conditions: Differential diagnosis and implications for treatment. *Journal of Clinical Psychiatry, 78*(Suppl. 1), 9–13.

Citrome, L. (2016). Schizophrenia relapse, patient considerations, and potential role of lurasidone. *Patient Preference and Adherence, 10*, 1529–1537.

Coccaro, E., Lee, R., & McCloskey, M. (2014). Validity of the new A1 and A2 criteria for DSM-5 intermittent explosive disorder. *Comprehensive Psychiatry, 55*, 260–267.

Cohen, L. (1997). Rational drug use in the treatment of depression. *Pharmacotherapy, 17*, 45–61.

Craddock, N., & Jones, I. (1999). Genetics of bipolar disorder. *Journal of Medical Genetics, 36*, 585–594.

Cruccu, G., & Truini, A. (2017). A review of neuropathic pain: From guidelines to clinical practice. *Pain and Therapy, 6*(Suppl. 1), S35–S42.

Cruz, M. (2017). Pimavanserin (Nuplazid): A treatment for hallucinations and delusions associated with Parkinson's disease. *Pharmacy and Therapeutics, 42*(6) 368–371.

Cukor, J., Spitalnick, J., Difede, J., Rizzo, A., & Rothbaum, B. (2009). Emerging treatments for PTSD. *Clinical Psychology Review, 29*(8), 715–726.

Cummings, J., Emre, M., Aarsland, D., Tekin, S., Dronamraju, N., & Lane, R. (2010). Effects of rivastigmine in Alzheimer's disease patients with and without hallucinations. *Journal of Alzheimer's Disease, 20*(1), 301–311.

Czeisler, C., Walsh, J., Wesnes, K., Arora, S., & Roth, T. (2009). Armodafinil for treatment of excessive sleepiness associated with shift work disorder: A randomized controlled study. *Mayo Clinic Proceedings, 84*(11), 958–972.

Daniel, D., Zimbroff, D., Potkin, S., Reeves, K., Harrigan, E., & Lakshiminarayan, M. (1999). Ziprasidone 80 mg/d and 160 mg/d in the acute exacerbation of schizophrenia and schizoaffective disorder: A 6-week placebo-controlled trial.

Ziprasidone study group. *Neuropsychopharmacology, 20*, 491–505.

Dannon, P. (2003). Topiramate for the treatment of kleptomania: A case series and review of the literature. *Clinical Neuropharmacology, 26*(1), 1–4.

Darreh-Shori, T., & Jelic, V. (2010). Safety and tolerability of transdermal and oral rivastigmine in Alzheimer's disease and Parkinson's disease dementia. *Expert Opinion Drug Safety, 9*(1), 167–176.

Davidson, J. (2003). Pharmacotherapy of social phobia. *Acta Psychiatrica Scandinavic, 108*, 65–71.

Davis, H., & Attia, E. (2017). Pharmacotherapy of eating disorders. *Current Opinion in Psychiatry, 30*, 452–457.

Davies, P., & Maloney, A. J. (1976). Selective loss of central cholinergic neurons in Alzheimer's disease. *Lancet, 2*, 1403.

Deberdt, W., Lipkovich, I., Heinloth, A. N., Liu, L., Kollack-Walker, S., Edwards, S. E., . . . Hardy, T. A. (2008). Double-blind, randomized trial comparing efficacy and safety of continuing olanzapine versus switching to quetiapine in overweight or obese patients with schizophrenia or schizoaffective disorder. *Therapeutics and Clinical Risk Management, 4*(4), 713–720.

Delgado, P. (2006). Serotonin noradrenaline reuptake inhibitors: New hope for the treatment of chronic pain. *International Journal of Psychiatry in Clinical Practice, 10*(Suppl. 2), 16–21.

Devlin, M. (2002). Psychotherapy and medication for binge eating disorder. Abstract Plenary Session, International Conference on Eating Disorders, April 25–28, Boston, MA.

Di Forti, M., Lappin, J., & Murray, R. (2007). Risk factors for schizophrenia: All roads lead to dopamine. *European Neuropsychopharmacology: The Journal of the European College of Neuropsychopharmacolgy, 17*(2), 101–107.

Doghramji, K. (2003). When patients can't sleep. *Current Psychiatry, 2*, 40–50.

Dunn, K., Tompkins, D., Bigelow, G., & Strain, E. (2017). Efficacy of tramadol extended-release for opioid withdrawal: A randomized clinical trial. *JAMA Psychiatry, 74*(9), 885–893.

Dworkin, R., O'Connor, A., Audette, J., Baron, R., Gourlay, G., Haanpää, M., . . . Wells, C. (2010). Recommendations for

the pharmacological management of neuropathic pain: An overview and literature update. *Mayo Clinic Proceedings, 85*(Suppl. 3), S3–14.

Elhai, J., Dvorak, R., Levine, J., & Hall, B. (2017). Problematic smartphone use: A conceptual overview and systematic review of relations with anxiety and depression psychopathology. *Journal of Affective Disorders, 207*, 251–259.

Emilsson, B., Gudjonsson, G., Sigurdsson, J., Baldursson, G., Einarsson, E., Olafsdottir, H., & Young, S. (2011). Cognitive behaviour therapy in medication-treated adults with ADHD and persistent symptoms: A randomized controlled trial. *BMC Psychiatry, 11*(1), 116. http://doi.org/10.1186/1471-244X-11-116

Ernst, D., Pettinati, H., Weiss, R., Donovan, D., & Longabaugh, R. (2008). An intervention for treating alcohol dependence: Relating elements of medical management to patient outcomes with implication for primary care. *Annals of Family Medicine, 6*(5), 435–440.

Feldman, H., Gauthier, S., Hecker, J., Vellas, B., Subbiah, P., & Whalen, E. (2001). Donepezil: MSAD Study Investigators Group. A 24-week, randomized, double-blind study of donepezil in moderate to severe Alzheimer's disease. *Neurology, 57*(4), 613–620.

Fergusson, D. M., Boden, J. M., & Horwood, L. J. (2009). Tests of causal links between alcohol abuse or dependence and major depression. *Archives of General Psychiatry, 66*(3), 260–266.

FDA. (2018). https://www.fda.gov/drugs/drugsafety/postmarketdrugsafetyinformationforpatientsandproviders/ucm161679.htm

Findling, R., Childress, A., Krishnan, S., & McGough, J. (2008). Long-term effectiveness and safety of lisdexamfetamine dimesylate in school-aged children with attention-deficit/hyperactivity disorder. *European Neuropsychoparmacology, 18*(4), 614–620.

Finnerup, N., Attal, N., Haroutounian, S., McNicol, E., Baron, R., Dworkin, R., . . . Wallace, M. (2015). Pharmacotherapy for neuropathic pain in adults: Systematic review, meta-analysis and updated NeuPSIG recommendations. *Lancet Neurology, 14*(2), 162–173.

Fornasari, D. (2017). Pharmacotherapy for neuropathic pain: A review. *Pain and Therapy, 6*(Suppl. 1), S25–S33.

Fowler, J., Bettinger, T., & Argo, T. (2008). Paliperidone extended-release tablets for the acute and maintenance treatment of schizophrenia. *Clinical Therapeutics: The International Peer-Reviewed Journal of Drug Therapy, 30*(2), 231–248.

Fox, C., Crugel, M., Maidment, I., Auestad, B., Coulton, S., Treloar, A., ... Livingston, G. (2012). Efficacy of memantine for agitation in Alzheimer's dementia: A randomised double-blind placebo controlled trial. *PLoS One, 7*(5):e35185. doi: 10.1371/journal.pone.0035185.

Frankel, J., & Schwartz, T. (2017). Brexpiprazole and cariprazine: Distinguishing two new atypical antipsychotics from the original dopamine stabilizer aripiprazole. *Therapeutic Advances in Psychopharmacology, 7*(1) 29–41.

Freire, R. C., Amrein, R., Mochcovitch, M. D., Dias, G. P., Machado, S., Versiani, M., ... Nardi, A. (2017). A 6-year post-treatment follow-up of panic disorder patients: Treatment with clonazepam predicts lower recurrence than treatment with paroxetine. *Journal of Clinical Psychopharmacology, 37*(4), 429–434.

Friedmann, P., Rose, J., Swift, R., Stout, R., Millman, R., & Stein, M. (2008). Trazodone for sleep disturbance after alcohol detoxification: A double-blind, placebo-controlled trial. *Alcoholism: Clinical & Experimental Research, 32*(9), 1652–1660.

Frye, M., & Salloum I. (2006). Bipolar disorder and comorbid alcoholism: Prevalence rate and treatment considerations. *Bipolar Disorders, 8*(6), 677–685.

Garbutt, J. (2009). The state of pharmacotherapy for the treatment of alcohol dependence. *Journal of Substance Abuse Treatment, 36*(1), 15–23.

Gauthier, S., Feldman, H., Schneider, L., Wilcock, G., Frisoni, G., Hardlund, J., ... Wischik, C. (2016). Efficacy and safety of tau-aggregation inhibitor therapy in patients with mild to moderate Alzheimer's disease: A randomized controlled, double-blind, parallel-arm, phase 3 trial. *The Lancet, 388*(10062), P2873–2884. doi:10.1016/S0140-6736(16)31275-2

Geddes, J., Calabrese, J., & Goodwin, G. (2009). Lamotrigine for treatment of bipolar depression: Independent meta-analysis and meta-regression of individual patient data from five randomized trials. *British Journal of Psychiatry, 194*(1), 4–9.

Gilron, I., Baron, R., & Jensen, T. (2015). Neuropathic pain: Principles of diagnosis and treatment. *Mayo Clinic Proceedings, 90*(4), 532–545.

Gitlin, M., & Frye, M. (2012). Maintenance therapies in bipolar disorders. *Bipolar Disorders, 14* (Suppl. 2), 51–65.

Goldberg, R. (2002). Management of behavioral complications of dementia. *Medicine and Health/Rhode Island, 85*(9), 281–285.

Goldman, R. (2010). ADHD stimulants and their effect on height in children. *Canadian Family Physician, 56*, 145–146.

Goodwin, F. (2002). Rationale for long-term treatment of bipolar disorder and evidence for long-term lithium treatment. *Journal of Clinical Psychiatry, 63* (Suppl. 10), 5–12.

Gorman, J. (2002). Treatment of generalized anxiety disorder. *Journal of Clinical Psychiatry, 63*(Suppl. 8), 17–23.

Grant, B., Hasin, D., Stinson, F., Dawson, D., Chou, S., Ruan, W., & Pickering, R. (2004). Prevalence, correlates, and disability of personality disorders in the United States. *Journal of Clinical Psychiatry, 65*(7), 948–958. http://doi.org/10.4088/JCP.v65n0711

Gray, S., Dublin, S., Yu, O., Walker, R., Anderson, M., Hubbard, R., ... Larson, E. (2016). Benzodiazepine use and risk of incident dementia or cognitive decline: Prospective population based study. *British Medical Journal, 2*(352), i90. https://doi.org/10.1136/bmj.i90

Gross, P., Nourse, R., & Wasser, T. (2009). Ramelteon for insomnia symptoms in a community sample of adults with generalized anxiety disorder: An open label study. *Journal of Clinical Sleep Medicine, 5*(1), 28–33.

Grossberg, G. (2003). Diagnosis and treatment of Alzheimer's disease. *Journal of Clinical Psychiatry, 64*(Suppl. 9), 3–6.

Grothe, D., Scheckner, B., & Albano, D. (2004). Treatment of pain syndromes with venlafaxine. *Pharmacotherapy, 24*(5), 621–629.

Grunze, H., Schlosser, S., & Walden, J. (2000). New perspectives in the acute treatment of bipolar depression. *World Journal of Biological Psychiatry, 1*, 129–136.

Haass-Koffler, C., & Bartlett, S. (2012). Stress and addiction: Contribution of the corticotropin releasing factor (CRF) system in neuroplasticity. *Frontiers in Molecular Neuroscience, 5*, 1–13.

Haile, C., Kosten, T., & Kosten, T. (2009). Pharmacogenetic treatments for drug addiction: Cocaine, amphetamine and methamphetamine. *American Journal of Drug and Alcohol Abuse, 35*(3), 161–177.

Hall, C., & Reynolds, C. (2014). Late-life depression in the primary care setting: Challenges, collaborative care, and prevention. *Maturitas, 79*(2), 147–152.

Hansen, R., Gaynes, B., Thieda, P., Gartlehner, G., De Veaugh-Geiss, A., Krebs, E., & Lohr, K. (2008). Prevention of major depressive disorder relapse and recurrence with second-generation antidepressants: A systematic review and meta-analysis. *Psychiatric Services, 59*(10), 1121–1130.

Hardeland, R. (2009). New approaches in the management of insomnia: Weighing the advantages of prolonged-release melatonin and synthetic melatoninergic agonists. *Neuropsychiatric Disease and Treatment, 5*, 341–354.

Häuser, W., Ablin, J., Perrot, S., & Fitzcharles, M. (2017). Management of fibromyalgia: Key messages from recent evidence-based guidelines. *Polish Archives of Internal Medicine, 127*(1), 47–56.

Henderson, D., Fan, X., Copeland, P., Sharma, B., Borba, C., Boxill, R., ... Goff, D. (2009). Aripiprazole added to overweight and obese olanzapine-treated schizophrenia patients. *Journal of Clinical Psychopharmacology, 29*(4), 165–169.

Henry, M., Fishman, J., & Youngner, S. (2007). Propranolol and the prevention of post-traumatic stress disorder: Is it wrong to erase the "sting" of bad memories? *The American Journal of Bioethics, 7*(9), 12–20.

Herrmann, N., & Gauthier, S. (2008). Diagnosis and treatment of dementia: 6. Management of severe Alzheimer disease. *Canadian Medical Association Journal, 179*(12), 1279–1287.

Hezel, D., Beattie, K., & Stewart, S. (2009). Memantine as augmenting agent for severe pediatric OCD. *American Journal of Psychiatry, 166*(2), 237.

Hollon, S., DeRubeis, R., Fawcett, J., Amsterdam, J., Shelton, R., Zajecka, J., … Gallop, R. (2014). Effect of cognitive therapy with antidepressant medications vs antidepressants alone on the rate of recovery in major depressive disorder: A randomized clinical trial. *JAMA Psychiatry, 71*(10), 1157–1164.

Hood, S., Norman, A., Hince, D., Melichar, J., & Hulse, G. (2014). Benzodiazepine dependence and its treatment with low dose flumazenil. *British Journal of Clinical Pharmacology, 77*(2), 285–294.

Hoque, R., & Chesson, A. (2010). Pharmacologically induced/exacerbated restless legs syndrome, periodic limb movements of sleep, and REM behavior disorder/REM sleep without atonia: Literature review, qualitative scoring, and comparative analysis. *Journal of Clinical Sleep Medicine, 6*(1), 79–83.

Howard, K., Kopta, M., Krause, M., & Orlinsky, D. (1986). The dose response relationship in psychotherapy. *American Psychologist, 41*, 159–164.

Howland, R. (2009). Prescribing psychotropic medications during pregnancy and lactation: Principles and guidelines. *Journal of Psychosocial Nursing and Mental Health Services, 47*(5), 19–23.

Insel, T. (1992). Toward a neuroanatomy of obsessive-compulsive disorder. *Archives of General Psychiatry, 49*, 739–744.

Jackson, C., Cates, M., & Lorenz, R. (2010). Pharmacotherapy of eating disorders. *Nutrition in Clinical Practice, 25*(2), 143–159.

Jaturapaptporn, D., Isaac, M., Kareem, N., McCleery, J., & Tabet, N. (2012). Aspirin, steroidal and non-steroidal anti-inflammatory drugs for the treatment of Alzheimer's disease. *Cochrane Database of Systematic Reviews, 2.* doi:10.1002/14651858. CD006378. pub2

Jenike, M. (2001). An update on obsessive-compulsive disorder. *Bulletin of the Menninger Clinic, 65*(1), 4–25.

Jensen, T., Baron, R., Haanpää, M., Kalso, E., Loeser, J., Rice, A., & Treede, R. (2011). A new definition of neuropathic pain. *Pain, 152*, 2204–2205.

Johnson, B. (2007). Update on neuropharmacological treatments for alcoholism: Scientific basis and clinical findings. *Biochemical Pharmacology, 75*(1), 34–56.

Joo, J., & Lee, K. (2014). Pharmacotherapy for obesity. *Journal of Menopausal Medicine, 20*, 90–96.

Jullien, R. (2001). *A primer of drug action* (9th ed.). New York, NY: Worth Publishers.

Kahn, R., Sommer, I. E., Murray, R. M., Meyer-Lindenberg, A., Weinberger, D. R., Cannon, T. D., … Insel, T. R. (2015). Schizophrenia. *Nature Reviews: Disease Primers, 1,* 15,067. doi:10.1038/nrdp.2015.67

Kalmbach, D. A., Arnedt, J. T., Swanson, L. M., Rapier, J. L., & Ciesla, J. A. (2017). Reciprocal dynamics between self-rated sleep and symptoms of depression and anxiety in young adult women: A 14-day diary study. *Sleep Medicine, 33*, 6–12. http://doi.org/10.1016/j.sleep.2016.03.014

Kane, J., Leucht, S., Carpenter, D., & Docherty, J. (2003). Introduction: Methods, commentary, and summary. *Journal of Clinical Psychiatry, 64* (Suppl. 12), 1–100.

Kaye, W., Nagata, T., & Weltzin, T. (2001). Double-blind placebo-controlled administration of fluoxetine in restricting and purging-type anorexia nervosa. *Biological Psychiatry, 49*, 644–652.

Kaylor, L. (1999). Antisocial personality disorder: Diagnostic, ethical, and treatment issues. *Issues in Mental Health Nursing, 20*, 247–258.

Kelly K., & Zisselman M. (2000). Update on electroconvulsive therapy (ECT) in older adults. *Journal of the American Geriatric Society, 48*(5), 560–566.

Kendell, R. E., & Adams, W. (1991). Unexplained fluctuations in the risk for schizophrenia by month and year of birth. *British Journal of Psychiatry, 158*, 758–763.

Kenna, G., Lomastro, T., Schiesl, A., Leggio, L., & Swift, R. (2009). Review of topiramate: An antiepileptic for the treatment of alcohol dependence. *Current Drug Abuse Reviews, 2*(2), 135–142.

Keshavan, M., Lawler, A., Nasrallah, H., & Tandon, R. (2017). New drug developments in psychosis: Challenges, opportunities and strategies. *Progress in Neurobiology, 152*, 3–20.

Khan, A., & Macaluso, M. (2009). Duloxetine for the treatment of generalized anxiety disorder: A review. *Neuropsychiatric Disease and Treatment, 5*, 23–31.

Klein, E., Kreinin, I., Chistyakov, A., Koren, D., Mecz, L., Marmur, S., … Feinsod, M. (1999). Therapeutic efficacy of right prefrontal slow repetitive transcranial magnetic stimulation in major depression: A double-blind controlled study. *Archives of General Psychiatry, 56*(4), 315–320.

Kneeland, R., & Fatemia, S. (2013). Viral infection, inflammation and schizophrenia. *Progress in Neuro-Psychopharmacology & Biological Psychiatry, 42*, 35–48.

Koenigsberg, H., Buchsbaum, M., Buchsbaum, B., Schneiderman, J., Tang, C., New, A., … Siever, L. (2005). Functional MRI of visuospatial working memory in schizotypal personality disorder: A region-of-interest analysis. *Psychological Medicine, 35*(7), 1019–30.

Kollins, S. (2003). Comparing the abuse potential of methylphenidate versus other stimulants: A review of available evidence and relevance to the ADHD patient. *Journal of Clinical Psychiatry, 64*(Suppl. 11), 14–18

Kollins, S. H. (2008). A qualitative review of issues arising in the use of psychostimulant medications in patients with ADHD and co-morbid substance use disorders. *Current Medical Research and Opinion, 24*(5), 1345–1357. http://doi.org/10.1185/030079908X280707

Kopelowicz, A., Baker, R., Zhao, C., Brewer, C., Lawson, E., & Peters-Strickland, T. (2017). A multicenter, open-label, pilot study evaluating the functionality of an integrated call center for a digital medicine system to optimize monitoring of adherence to oral aripiprazole in adult patients with serious mental illness. *Neuropsychiatric Disease and Treatment, 13*, 2641–2651.

Kordon, A., Wahl, K., Koch, N., Zurowski B., Anlauf, M., Vielhaber, K., … Hohagen, F. (2008). Quetiapine addition to serotonin reuptake inhibitors in patients with severe obsessive compulsive disorder: A double-blind, randomized, placebo-controlled study. *Journal of Clinical Psychopharmacology, 28*(5), 550–554.

Kowalczyk, W., Phillips, K., Jobes, M., Kennedy, A., Ghitza, U., Agage, D., ... Preston, K. (2015). Clonidine maintenance prolongs opioid abstinence and decouples stress from craving in daily life: A randomized controlled trial with ecological momentary assessment. *The American Journal of Psychiatry, 172*(8), 760–767.

Kratochvil, C., Milton, D., Vaughan, B., & Greenhill, L. (2008). Acute atomoxetine treatment of younger and older children with ADHD: A meta-analysis of tolerability and efficacy. *Child and Adolescent Psychiatry and Mental Health, 2*(25).

Kratochvil, C., Vaughan, B., Harrington, M., & Burke, W. (2003). Atomoxetine: A selective noradrenaline reuptake inhibitor for the treatment of attention-deficit/hyperactivity disorder. *Expert Opinions in Pharmacotherapy, 4*(7), 1165–1174.

Kreyenbuhl, J., Buchanan, R., Dickerson, F., & Dixon, L. (2010). The Schizophrenia Patient Outcomes Research Team (PORT): Updated treatment recommendations 2009. *Schizophrenia Bulletin, 36*(1), 94–103.

Kroenke, K. (2003). Patients presenting with somatic complaints: Epidemiology, psychiatric co-morbidity and management. *International Journal of Methods in Psychiatric Research, 12*(1), 34–43.

Kupfer, D., & Frank, E. (2003). Comorbidity in depression. *Acta Psychiatrica Scandinavica, 108*(Suppl. 418), 57–60.

Lam, R., Levitt, A., Levitan, R., Michalak, E., Cheung, A., Morehouse, R., ... Tam, E. (2016). Efficacy of bright light treatment, fluoxetine, and the combination in patients with nonseasonal major depressive disorder: A randomized clinical trial. *JAMA Psychiatry, 73*(1), 56–63.

Lambert, M., Conus, P., Lambert, T., & McGorry, P. (2003). Pharmacotherapy of first-episode psychosis. *Expert Opinions in Pharmacotherapy, 4*(5), 717–750.

Larsen, B., & Christenfeld, J. (2009). Cardiovascular disease and psychiatric comorbidity: The potential role of perseverative cognition. *Cardiovascular Psychiatry and Neurology, 79*, 1–8.

Larson, E., Yaffe, K., & Langa, K. (2013). New insights into the dementia epidemic. *New England Journal of Medicine, 369*, 2275–2277. doi:10.1056/NEJMp1311405

Le Bars, P., Katz, M., Berman, N., Itil, T., Freedman, A., & Schatzberg, A. (1997). A placebo-controlled, double-blind, randomized trial of an extract of ginkgo biloba for dementia. North American EGb Study Group. *Journal of the American Medical Association, 278*(16), 1327–1332.

Lee, J., Grossman, E., DiRocco, D., Truncali, A., Hanley, K., Stevens, D., ... Gourevitch, M. (2010). Extended-release naltrexone for treatment of alcohol dependence in primary care. *Journal of Substance Abuse Treatment, 39*(1), 14–21.

Lee, J., Nunes, E., Novo, P., Bachrach, K., Bailey, G., Bhatt, S., ... Rotrosen, J. (2018). Comparative effectiveness of extended-release naltrexone versus buprenorphine-naloxone for opioid relapse prevention (X:BOT): A multi-centre, open-label, randomised controlled trial. *Lancet, 391*, 309–318.

Leon, F., Ashton, A., D'Mello, D., Dantz, B., Hefner, J., Matson, G., ... Winsberg, B. (2003). Depression and comorbid medical illness: Therapeutic and diagnostic challenges. *The Journal of Family Practice,* Suppl:S19–S33.

Lesperance, F., Frasure-Smith, N., & Talajic, M. (1996). Major depression before and after myocardial infarction: Its nature and consequences. *Psychosomatic Medicine, 58*, 99–110.

Leung, K., & Cottler, L. B. (2008). Treatment of pathological gambling. *Current Opinion in Psychiatry, 22*, 69–74.

Lieb, K., Vollim, B., Rucker, G., Timmer, A., & Stoffers, J. (2010). Pharmacotherapy for borderline personality disorder: Cochrane systematic review of randomized trials. *British Journal of Psychiatry, 196*(1), 4–12.

Limandri, B. J. (2018). Psychopharmacology for borderline personality disorder. *Journal of Psychosocial Nursing & Mental Health Services, 56*(4), 8–11.

Lindesay, J. (1991). Phobic disorders in the elderly. *British Journal of Psychiatry, 159*, 531–541.

Lipsey, M., & Wilson, D. (1993). The efficacy of psychological, educational, and behavioral treatment. *American Psychologist, 48*, 1181–1209.

Livesley, W. (2000). A practical approach to the treatment of patients with borderline personality disorder. *The Psychiatric Clinics of North America, 23*(1), 211–232.

Lockhart, I., Mitchell, S., & Kelly, S. (2009). Safety and tolerability of donepezil, rivastigmine and galantamine for patients with Alzheimer's disease: Systematic review of the real world evidence. *Dementia and Geriatric Cognitive Disorders, 28*, 389–403.

Lohoff, F. (2010). Overview of the genetics of major depressive disorder. *Current Psychiatry Reports, 12*(6), 539–546.

Lopez, O., Becker, J., Wahed, A., Saxton, J., Sweet, R., Wolk, D., ... Dekosky, S. (2009). Long term effects of the concomitant use of memantine with cholinesterase inhibition in Alzheimer disease. *Journal of Neurology, Neurosurgery and Psychiatry, 80*(6), 600–607.

Lourenco, M., & Kennedy, S. (2009). Desvenlafaxine in the treatment of major depressive disorder. *Neuro-psychiatric Disease and Treatment, 5*, 127–136.

Lutter, M. (2017). Emerging treatments in eating disorders. *Neurotherapeutics, 14*, 614–622.

Makris, N., Seidman, L., Valera, E., Biederman, J., Monuteaux, M., Kennedy, D., ... Faraone, S. (2010). Anterior cingulate volumetric alterations in treatment-naïve adults with ADHD: A pilot study. *Journal of Attention Disorders, 13*(4), 407–413. http://doi.org/10.1177/1087054709351671

Malhi, G., Mitchell, P., & Salim, S. (2003). Bipolar depression: Management options. *CNS Drugs, 17*(1), 9–25.

Malhi, G., Gessler, D., & Outhred, T. (2017). The use of lithium for the treatment of bipolar disorder: Recommendations from clinical practice guidelines. *Journal of Affective Disorders, 217*, 266–280.

Marcos, G., Santabárbara, J., Lopez-Anton, R., De-la-Cámara, C., Gracia-García, P., Lobo, E., ... Lobo, A. ZARADEMP Workgroup. (2015). Conversion to dementia in mild cognitive impairment diagnosed with DSM-5 criteria and with Petersen's criteria. *Acta Psychiatrica Scandinavica, 133*(5), 378–385. doi:10.1111/acps.12543

Marino, J., & Caballero, J. (2008). Paliperidone extended-release for the treatment of schizophrenia. *Pharmacotherapy,* *28*(10), 1283–1298.

Marlatt, G.A., & Witkiewitz, K. (2002). Harm reduction approaches to alcohol use: Health promotion, prevention, and treatment. *Addictive Behaviors, 27*, 867–886.

Marucci, S., Ragione, L., De Iaco, G., Mococci, T., Vicini, M., Guastamacchia, E., & Triggiani, V. (2018). Anorexia nervosa and comorbid psychopathology. *Endocrine, Metabolic & Immune Disorders Drug Targets, 18*, 316–324.

Martínez-Cengotitabengoa, M., & González-Pinto, A. (2017). Nutritional supplements in depressive disorders. *Actas Españolas de Psiquiatría, 45*(Suppl. 1), 8–15.

Mason, B., & Heyser, C. (2010). The neurobiology, clinical efficacy, and safety of acamprosate in the treatment of alcohol dependence. *Expert Opinion on Drug Safety, 9*(1), 177–188.

Matsumoto, M., Walton, N., Yamada, H., Kondo, Y., Marek, G., & Tajinda, K. (2017). The impact of genetics on future drug discovery in schizophrenia. *Expert Opinion on Drug Discovery, 12*(7), 673–686.

McCann, B., & Roy-Byrne, P. (2000). Attention-deficit/hyperactivity disorder and learning disabilities in adults. *Seminars in Clinical Neuropsychiatry, 5*(3), 191–197.

McCleane, G. (2008). Antidepressants as analgesics. *CNS Drugs, 22*(2), 139–156.

McElroy, S., Guerdjikova, A., Martens, B., Keck, P., Jr., Pope, H. G., & Hudson, J. I. (2009). Role of antiepileptic drugs in the management of eating disorders. *CNS Drugs, 23*(2), 139–156.

McIntyre, R., Muller, A., Mancini, D., & Silver, E. (2003). What to do if an antidepressant fails? *Canadian Family Physician, 49*, 449–457.

McKnight, R., & Park, R. (2010). Atypical antipsychotics and anorexia nervosa: A review. *European Eating Disorders Review, 18*(1), 10–21.

Mease, P. (2009). Further strategies for treating fibromyalgia: The role of serotonin and norepinephrine reuptake inhibitors. *American Journal of Medicine, 2*(12), 44–55.

Mehler, P. (2003). Clinical practice: Bulimia nervosa. *New England Journal of Medicine, 349*(9), 875–881.

Meijer, W., Faber, A., van den Ban, E., & Tobi, H. (2009). Current issues around the pharmacotherapy of ADHD in children and adults. *Pharmacy World and Science, 31*, 509–516.

Merikangas, K., Akiskal, H., Angst, J., Greenberg, P., Hirschfeld, R., Petukhova, M., & Kessler, R. (2007). Lifetime and 12-month prevalence of bipolar spectrum disorder in the national comorbidity survey replication. *Archives of General Psychiatry, 64*(5), 543–552.

Merskey, H. (1979). Pain terms: A list with definitions and notes on usage. Recommended by the International Association for the Study of Pain (IASP) Subcommittee on Taxonomy. *Pain, 6*, 249–252.

Meyer, J. (2016). Forgotten but not gone: New developments in the understanding and treatment of tardive dyskinesia. *CNS Spectrums, 21*, 16–23.

Milanlioglu, A., & Kilic, S. (2011). The efficiency of valproic acid in a child with trichotillomania. *Journal of Clinical and Experimental Investigations, 2*(2), 214–215.

Milkman, H., & Sunderwirth, S. (1987). *Craving for ecstasy.* Lexington, MA: Lexington Books.

Mitchell, J., de Zwaan, M., & Roerig, J. (2003). Drug therapy for patients with eating disorders. *Current Drug Targets: CNS and Neurological Disorders, 1*, 17–29.

Mitchell, J., Peterson, C., Myers, T., & Wonderlich, S. (2001). Combining pharmacotherapy and psychotherapy in the treatment of patients with eating disorders. *Psychiatric Clinics of North America, 24*, 315–323.

Moller, H., & Nasrallah, H. (2003). Treatment of bipolar disorder. *Journal of Clinical Psychiatry, 64*(Suppl. 6), 9–17.

Montgomery, S., & Moller, H. (2009). Is the significant superiority of escitalopram compared with other antidepressants clinically relevant? *International Clinical Psychopharmacology, 24*(3), 111–118.

Monti, J. M., & Jantos, H. (2014). The role of serotonin 5-HT7 receptor in regulating sleep and wakefulness. *Reviews in the Neurosciences, 25*(3), 429–437. http://doi.org/10.1515/revneuro-2014-0016

Montoya, I., & Vocci, F. (2008). Novel medications to treat addictive disorders. *Current Psychiatry Reports, 10*(5), 392–398.

Moore, C., & Bokor, B. (2017). *Anorexia nervosa.* StatPearls. https://www.ncbi.nlm.nih.gov/books/NBK459148

Moulin, D., Boulanger, A., Clark, A., Clarke, H., Dao, T., Finley, G., … Williamson, O. (2014). Pharmacological management of chronic neuropathic pain: Revised consensus statement from the Canadian Pain Society. *Pain Research and Management, 19*(6), 328–335.

Mufson, M. (1999). What is the role of psychiatry in the management of chronic pain? *Harvard Mental Health Letter, 16*(3), 8.

Muskin, P., Gerbard, P., & Brown, R. (2013). Complimentary and integrative therapies for psychiatric disorders. *Psychiatric Clinics of North America, 36*, 1.

Muzyk, A., Rivelli, S., & Gagliardi, J. (2012). Defining the role of baclofen for the treatment of alcohol dependence: A systematic review of the evidence. *CNS Drugs, 26*, 69–78.

Muzik, M., & Hamilton, S. (2016). Use of antidepressants during pregnancy? What to consider when weighing treatment with antidepressants against untreated depression. *Maternal and Child Health Journal, 20*, 2268–2279.

Myrseth, H., & Pallesen, S. (2010). Pharmacological treatments of impulse control disorders. In M. Hertzman & L. Adler (Eds.), *Clinical trials in psychopharmacology* (2nd. ed., pp. 289–308). Hoboken, NJ: Wiley and Sons.

Nair, R., & Moss, S. (2009). Management of attention-deficit hyperactivity disorder in adults: Focus on methylphenidate hydrochloride. *Neuropsychiatric Disease and Treatment, 5*, 421–432.

Nardi, A., Freire, R., Valença, A., Amrein, R., de Cerqueira, A., Lopes, F., … Versiani, M. (2010). Tapering clonazepam in patients with panic disorder after at least 3 years of treatment. *Journal of Clinical Psychopharmacology, 30*(3), 290–293. doi:10.1097/JCP.0b013e3181dcb2f3

National Institute of Aging. (2018). Alzheimer's disease facts and figures. Available at www.nia.nih.gov/Alzheimers

Nelson, J., Pikalov, A., & Berman, R. (2008). Augmentation treatment in major depressive disorder: Focus on aripiprazole. *Neuropsychiatric Disease and Treatment, 4*(5):937–948.

Neubauer, D. (2009). Current and new thinking in the management of comorbid insomnia. *American Journal of Managed Care, 15*(1), 24–30.

Nevels, R., Dehone, E., Alexander, K., & Gontkovsky, S. (2010). Psychopharmacology of aggression in children and adolescents with primary neuropsychiatric disorders: A review of current and potentially promising treatment options. *Experimental and Clinical Psychopharmacology, 18*(2), 184–201.

New, A., Triebwassar, J., & Goodman, M. (2009). The neurobiology of personality disorders. In D. Charney & E. Nestler (Eds.), *Neurobiology of Mental Illness* (3rd ed., 1286–1306), Oxford, UK: Oxford University Press.

Newport, D., Stowe, Z., Viguera, A., Calamaras, M., Juric, S., Knight, B., ... Baldessarini, R. (2008). Lamotrigine in bipolar disorder: Efficacy during pregnancy. *Bipolar Disorders, 10*(3), 432–436.

Ng, Q., Venkatanarayanan, N., & Ho, C. (2017). Clinical use of Hypericum perforatum (St. John's wort) in depression: A meta-analysis. *Journal of Affective Disorders, 210*, 211–221.

Nugent, N., Christopher, N., Crow, J., Browne, L., Ostrowski, S., & Delahanty, D. (2010). The efficacy of early propranolol administration at reducing PTSD symptoms in pediatric injury patients: A pilot study. *Journal of Traumatic Stress, 23*(2), 282–287.

Nutt, D., & Lingford-Hughes, A. (2008). Addiction: The clinical interface. *British Journal of Pharmacology, 154*, 397–405.

O'Connor, A. (2009). Neuropathic pain: A review of the quality of life impact, costs, and cost-effectiveness of therapy. *Pharmacoeconomics, 27*(2), 95–112.

O'Connor, M., & Irwin, M. (2010). Links between behavioral factors and inflammation. *Clinical Pharmacology & Therapeutics, 87*(4), 479–482.

Olive, M., Cleva, R., Kalivas, P., & Malcolm, R. (2012). Glutamatergic medications for the treatment of drug and behavioral addictions. *Pharmacology Biochemistry and Behavior, 100*(4): 801–810. doi: 10.1016/j.pbb.2011.04.015.

Olvera, R. (2002). Intermittent explosive disorder: Epidemiology, diagnosis and management. *CNS Drugs, 16*(8), 517–526.

Ondo, W. G., Simmons, J. H., Shahid, M. H., Hashem, V., Hunter, C., & Jankovic, J. (2018). Onabotulinum toxin-A injections for sleep bruxism: A double-blind, placebo-controlled study. *Neurology, 90*(7), e559–e564. http://doi.org/10.1212/WNL.0000000000004951

Opatrny, L., Delaney, J., & Suissa, S. (2008). Gastro-intestinal haemorrhage risks of selective serotonin receptor antagonist therapy: A new look. *British Journal of Clinical Pharmacology, 66*(1), 76–81.

Orman, S., & Keating, G. (2009). Spotlight on buprenorphine/naloxone in the treatment of opioid dependence. *CNS Drugs, 23*(10), 899–902.

Oxenkrug, G., & Requintina, P. (2003). Melatonin and jet lag syndrome: Experimental model and clinical implications. *CNS Spectrums, 8*(2), 139–148.

Pae, C., Wang, S., Han, C., Lee, S., Patkar, A., Masand, P., & Serretti, A. (2015). Vortioxetine, a multimodal antidepressant for generalized anxiety disorder: A systematic review and meta-analysis. *Journal of Psychiatric Research, 64*, 88–98.

Paolini, E., Mezzetti, F., Pierri, F., & Moretti, P. (2017). Pharmacological treatment of borderline personality disorder: A retrospective observational study at inpatient unit in Italy. *International Journal of Psychiatry in Clinical Practice, 21*(1), 75–79.

Paraskevaidi, M., Morais, C., Lima, K., Snowden, J., Saxon, J., Richardson, A., ... Martin, F. (2017). Differential diagnosis of Alzheimer's disease using spectrochemical analysis of blood. *Proceedings of the National Academy of Sciences, 114*(38), E7929–E7938. https://doi.org/10.1073/pnas.1701517114

Patel, K. V., Aspesi, A. V., & Evoy, K. E. (2015). Suvorexant. *Annals of Pharmacotherapy, 49*(4), 477–483. http://doi.org/10.1177/1060028015570467

Pederson, K., Roerig, J., & Mitchell J. (2003). Towards the pharmacotherapy of eating disorders. *Expert Opinion on Pharmacotherapy, 10*, 1659–1678.

Pettinati, H., Gastfriend, D., Dong, Q., Kranzler, H., & O'Malley, S. (2008). Effect of extended-release naltrexone (XR-NTX) on quality of life in alcohol-dependent patients. *Alcoholism: Clinical & Experimental Reviews, 33*(2), 350–356.

Philipsen, A., Richter, H., Peters, J., Alm, B., Sobanski, E., Colla, M., ... Hesslinger, B. (2007). Structured group psychotherapy in adults with attention deficit hyperactivity disorder: Results of an open multicentre study. *The Journal of Nervous and Mental Disease, 195*(12), 1013–1019.

Pinel, J. (2009). *Biopsychology* (7th ed.). Boston, MA: Allyn and Bacon.

Polanczyk, G., de Lima, M., Horta, B., Biederman, J., & Rohde, L. (2007). The worldwide prevalence of ADHD: A systematic review and metaregression analysis. *The American Journal of Psychiatry, 164*(6), 942–948. http://doi.org/10.1176/ajp.2007.164.6.942

Porsteinsson, A., Drye, L., Pollock, B., Devanand, D., Frangakis, C., Ismail, Z., ... Lyketsos, C. (2014). Effect of citalopram on agitation in Alzheimer disease: The CitAD randomized clinical trial. *JAMA, 311*(7), 682–691.

Pratt, L., & Brody, D. (2014). Depression in the U.S. household population, 2009–2012. *NCHS Data Brief*, No. 172.

Prudic, J., Fitzsimons, L., Nobler, M. S., & Sackeim, H. A. (1999). Naloxone in the prevention of the adverse cognitive effects of ECT: A within-subject, placebo controlled study. *Neuropsychopharmacology, 21*(2), 285–293.

Qureshi, N., & Al-Bedah, A. (2013). Mood disorders and complementary and alternative medicine: A literature review. *Neuropsychiatric Disease and Treatment, 9*, 639–658.

Raine, A. (2002). Biosocial studies of antisocial and violent behavior in children and adults: A review. *Journal of Abnormal Child Psychology, 30*(4), 311–326.

Rakel, R. (1999). Depression. *Mental Health, 26*(2), 211–224.

Rao, G. (2010). Office-based strategies for the management of obesity. *American Family Physician, 81*(12), 1406–1408.

Ravindran, A., da Silva, T., Ravindran, L., Richter, M., & Rector, N. (2009). Obsessive-compulsive spectrum disorders: A review of the evidence-based treatments. *Canadian Journal of Psychiatry, 54*(5), 331–43.

Ray, L., Bujarski, S., Courtney, K., Moallem, N., Lunny, K., Roche, D., ... Miotto, K. (2015). The effects of naltrexone on subjective response to methamphetamine in a clinical sample: A double-blind, placebo-controlled laboratory study. *Neuropsychopharmacology*, *40*(10), 2347–2356. doi:10.1038/npp.2015.83

Reardon, C., & Factor, R. (2008). Bizarre behavior in a patient treated with prazosin. *American Journal of Psychiatry*, *165*(6), 774–775.

Recupero, P. (2008). Forensic evaluation of problematic Internet use. *Journal of the American Academy of Psychiatry and the Law*, *36*, 505–514.

Reich, J. (2002). Drug treatment of personality disorder traits. *Psychiatric Annals*, *32*(10), 590–596.

Reich, J. (2003). The effect of Axis II disorders on the outcome of treatment of anxiety and unipolar depressive disorders: A review. *Journal of Personality Disorders*, *17*(5), 387–405.

Regier, D., Farmer, M., Rae, D., Locke, B., Keith, S., Judd, L., & Goodwin, F. (1990). Comorbidity of mental disorders with alcohol and other drugs of abuse. *Journal of the American Medical Association*, *264*, 2511–2518.

Rhein, V., Song, X., Wiesner, A., Ittner, L., Baysang, G., Meier, F., ... Eckert, A. (2009). Amyloid-beta and tau synergistically impair the oxidative phosphorylation system in triple transgenic Alzheimer's disease mice. *Proceedings of the National Academy of Science*, *106*, 20,057–20,062.

Richardson, G., & Wang-Weigand, S. (2009). Effects of long-term exposure to ramelteon, a melatonin receptor agonist, on endocrine function in adults with chronic insomnia. *Human Psychopharmacology*, *24*(2), 103–111.

Richardson, G., Zammit, G., Wang-Weigand, S., & Zhang, J. (2009). Safety and subjective sleep effects of ramelteon administration in adults and older adults with chronic primary insomnia: A 1-year, open-label study. *Journal of Clinical Psychiatry*, *70*(4), 467–476.

Richert, A., & Baran, A. (2003). A review of common sleep disorders. *CNS Spectrums*, *8*(2), 102–109.

Rogers, S. L., & Friedhoff, L. T. (1996). The efficacy and safety of donepezil in patients with Alzheimer's disease: Results of a U.S. multicenter, randomized, double-blind, placebo-controlled trial. The donepezil study group. *Dementia*, *7*(6), 293–303.

Rosa, A. R., Franco, C., Torrent, C., Comes, M., Cruz, N., Horga, G., ... Vieta, E. (2008). Ziprasidone in the treatment of affective disorders: A review. *CNS Neuroscience & Therapeutics*, *14*(4), 278–286.

Rothbaum, B., Kearns, M., Price, M., Malcoun, E., Davis, M., Ressler, K., ... Houry, D. (2012). Early intervention may prevent the development of posttraumatic stress disorder: A randomized pilot civilian study with modified prolonged exposure. *Biological Psychiatry*, *72*, 957–963.

Rothschild, A., Mahableshwarkar, A., Jacobsen, P., Yan, M., & Sheehan, D. (2012). Vortioxetine (LU AA 21004) 5 mg. in generalized anxiety disorder: Results of an 8-week randomized, double-blind, placebo controlled clinical study in the United States. *European Neuropsychopharmacology*, *22*, 12, 858–866.

Roy Chengappa, K., Kupfer, D., Parepally, H., John, V., Basu, R., Buttenfield, J., ... Gershon, S. (2007). A placebo-controlled, random-assignment, parallel-group pilot study of adjunctive topiramate for patients with schizoaffective disorder, bipolar type. *Bipolar Disorders*, *9*(6), 609–617.

Sabia, S., Dugravot, A., Dartigues, J., Abell, J., Elbaz, A., Kivimäki, M., & Singh-Manoux, A. (2017). Physical activity, cognitive decline, and risk of dementia: 28 year follow-up of Whitehall II cohort study. *British Medical Journal*, *357*, j2709. https://doi.org/10.1136/bmj.j2709

Sadock, B., Sadock, V. A., & Ruiz, P. (2015). *Kaplan & Sadock's Synopsis of Psychiatry* (11th ed.). Philadelphia, PA: Lippincott Williams & Wilkins.

Sadock, B., Sadock, V., & Ruiz, P. (2017). *Kaplan & Sadock's Comprehensive Textbook of Psychiatry* (10th ed.). Philadelphia, PA: Lippincott Williams & Wilkins.

Safren, S., Sprich, S., Mimiaga, M., Surman, C., Knouse, L., Groves, M., & Otto, M. (2010). Cognitive behavioral therapy vs relaxation with educational support for medication-treated adults with ADHD and persistent symptoms: A randomized controlled trial. *JAMA*, *304*(8), 875–880. http://doi.org/10.1001/jama.2010.1192

Saloheimo, H., Markowitz, J., Saloheimo, T., Laitinen, J., Sundell, J., Huttunen, M., ... Katila, H. (2016). Psychotherapy effectiveness for major depression: A randomized trial in a Finnish community. *BMC Psychiatry*, *16*, 131.

Sanacora, G., Frye, M., McDonald, W., Mathew, S., Turner, M., Schatzberg, A., ... Nemeroff, C. American Psychiatric Association (APA) Council of Research Task Force on Novel Biomarkers and Treatments. (2017). A consensus statement on the use of ketamine in the treatment of mood disorders. *JAMA Psychiatry*, *74*(4), 399–405. doi: 10.1001/jamapsychiatry.2017.0080

Sano, M. (2003). Noncholinergic treatment options for Alzheimer's disease. *Journal of Clinical Psychiatry*, *64*(Suppl. 9), 23–28.

Sano, M., Ernesto, C., Thomas, R., Klauber, M., Schafer, K., Grundman, M., ... Thal, L. (1997). A controlled trial of selegiline, alpha-tocopherol, or both as treatment for Alzheimer's disease. The Alzheimer's disease cooperative study. *New England Journal of Medicine*, *336*(17), 1216–1222.

Sansone, R., & Sansone, L. (2008). Pain, pain, go away: Antidepressants and pain management. *Psychiatry*, *5*(12), 16–19.

Sansone, R., & Sansone, L. (2010). Is seroquel developing an illicit reputation for misuse/abuse? *Psychiatry*, *7*(1), 13–16.

Sattar, S., & Bhatia, S. (2003). Benzodiazepines for substance users? *Current Psychiatry*, *2*(5), 25–32.

Saxena, A., Grace, J., Olympia, J. L., Trigoboff, E., Watson, T., Cushman, S., & Newcomer, D. (2008). Risperidone long-acting injections: Successful alternative deltoid muscle injections for refractory schizophrenia. *Psychiatry*, *5*(9), 40–42.

Scharf, M. (2001). Individualizing therapy for early, middle-of-the-night and late-night insomnia. *International Journal of Clinical Practice*, *116*, 20–24.

Schatzberg, A., Cole, J., & DeBattista, C. (1997). *Manual of clinical psychopharmacology* (3rd ed.). Washington, DC: American Psychiatric Press.

Schneider, J., & Irons, R. (2001). Assessment and treatment of addictive sexual disorders: Relevance for chemical dependency relapse. *Substance Use and Misuse*, *36*(13), 1795–1820.

Schreiber, L., Odlaug, B., & Grant, J. (2011). Impulse control disorders: Updated review of clinical characteristics and pharmacological management. *Frontiers in Psychiatry*, 2, 1–16.

Seeman, M. (2007). Symptoms of schizophrenia: Normal adaptations to inability. *Medical Hypotheses*, 69, 253–257.

Segal, Z., Kennedy, S., Cohen, N., & CANMAT Depression Work Group. (2000). Combining psychotherapy and pharmacotherapy. *Canadian Journal of Psychiatry*, 46(Suppl. 1), 59S–62S.

Sevigny, J., Chiao, P., Bussière, T., Weinreb, P., Williams, L., Maier, M., ... Sandrock, A. (2016). The antibody aducanumab reduces AB plaques in Alzheimer's disease. *Nature*, 537(7618), 50–56. doi:10.1038/nature19323

Sheehan, D. (1999). Venlafaxine extended release (XR) in the treatment of generalized anxiety disorder. *Journal of Clinical Psychiatry*, 60(Suppl. 22), 23–28.

Sheehan, D. (2002). The management of panic disorder. *Journal of Clinical Psychiatry*, 63(Suppl. 14), 17–21.

Sheehan, D., Croft, H., Gossen, R., Levitt, R., Brulle, C., Bouchard, S., & Rozova, A. (2009). Extended-release trazodone in major depressive disorder: A randomized, double-blind, placebo-controlled study. *Psychiatry*, 6(5), 20–33.

Sinacola, R. (1997). Clinical psychopharmacology: The basics for licensed professional counselors. *Michigan Journal of College Student Development*, 2(1), 15–22.

Sinacola, R. (1998). The use of therapeutic assistants in outpatient psychotherapy. *Psychotherapy in Private Practice*, 17(3), 35–44.

Sinacola, R. (2017). Spirituality and mental health. *Audio Digest Psychology*, 6, 15.

Sinha, A., Shariq, A., Said, K., Sharma, A., Newport, D., & Salloum, I. (2018). Medical comorbidities in bipolar disorder. *Current Psychiatry Reports*, 20(5), 36.

Smith, S., Wallace, E., O'Dowd, T., & Fortin, M. (2016). Interventions for improving outcomes in patients with multimorbidity in primary care and community settings. *Cochrane Database of Systematic Reviews*, 3. doi:10.1002/14651858.CD006560.pub3

Solanto, M., Marks, D., Wasserstein, J., Mitchell, K., Abikoff, H., Alvir, J., & Kofman, M. (2010). Efficacy of metacognitive therapy for adult ADHD. *The American Journal of Psychiatry*, 167(8), 958–968. http://doi.org/10.1176/appi.ajp.2009.09081123

Solberg, B. S., Halmøy, A., Engeland, A., Igland, J., Haavik, J., & Klungsøyr, K. (2018). Gender differences in psychiatric comorbidity: A population-based study of 40 000 adults with attention deficit hyperactivity disorder. *Acta Psychiatrica Scandinavica*, 137(3), 176–186. http://doi.org/10.1111/acps.12845

Sonawalla, S. B., & Fava, M. (2001). Severe depression: Is there a best approach? *CNS Drugs*, 15(10), 765–776.

Sondergard, L., Lopez, A., Andersen, P., & Kressing, L. (2008). Mood-stabilizing pharmacological treatment in bipolar disorders and risk of suicide. *Bipolar Disorders*, 10(1), 87–94.

Sowa-Kucma, M., Panczyszyn-Trzewik, P., Misztaka, P., Jaeschke, R., Sendek, K., Styczen, K., ... Koperny, M. (2017). Vortioxetine: A review of the pharmacology and clinical profile of the novel antidepressant. *Pharmacological Reports*, 69, 595–601.

Spada, M. (2014). An overview of problematic Internet use. *Addictive Behaviors*, 39, 3–6.

Spaeth, M., & Briley, M. (2009). Fibromyalgia: A complex syndrome requiring a multidisciplinary approach. *Human Psychopharmacology of Clinical Experience*, 24, 3–10.

Spencer, T., Biederman, J., Wilens, T., & Faraone, S. (2002). Overview and neurobiology of attention-deficit/hyperactivity disorder. *Journal of Clinical Psychiatry*, 63(Suppl. 12), 3–9.

Spencer, T. J., Greenbaum, M., Ginsberg, L. D., & Murphy, W. R. (2009). Safety and effectiveness of coadministration of guanfacine extended release and psychostimulants in children and adolescents with attention-deficit/hyperactivity disorder. *Journal of Child and Adolescent Psychopharmacology*, 19(5), 501–510. http://doi.org/10.1089/cap.2008.0152

Srivastava, G., & Apovian, C. (2018). Current pharmacotherapy for obesity. *Nature Reviews Endocrinology*, 14, 12–24.

Staner, C., Joly, F., Jacquot, N., Vlasova, I., Nehlin, M., Lundqvist, T., ... Staner, L. (2010). Sublingual zolpidem in early onset of sleep compared to oral zolpidem: Polysomnographic study in patients with primary insomnia. *Current Medical Research and Opinion*, 26(6), 1423–1431.

Starcevic, V. (2012). Benzodiazepines for anxiety disorders: Maximizing the benefits and minimizing the risks. *Advances in Psychiatric Treatment*, 18(4), 250–258. doi:10.1192/apt.bp.110.008631

Starcevic, V., & Janca, A. (2017). Pharmacotherapy of borderline personality disorder: Replacing confusion with prudent pragmatism. *Current Opinion in Psychiatry*, 31(1), 69–73.

Stewart, D. (2002). Hepatic adverse reactions associated with nefazodone. *Canadian Journal of Psychiatry*, 47(4), 375–377.

Strachey, J. (1953). On the physical mechanisms of hysterical phenomena (1893). *The standard edition of the complete psychological works of Sigmund Freud*, 3, 25–42.

Strange, B. (2008). Once-daily treatment of ADHD with guanfacine: Patient implications. *Neuropsychiatric Disease and Treatment*, 4(3), 499–506.

Sullivan, H. (1953). *Conceptions of modern psychiatry*. New York, NY: Norton.

Sun, E., Dixit, A., Humphreys, K., Darnall, B., Baker, L., & Mackey, S. (2017). Association between concurrent use of prescription opioids and benzodiazepines and overdose: Retrospective analysis. *British Medical Journal*. doi:10.1136/bmj.j760

Sutherland, J., Sutherland, S., & Hoehns, J. (2003). Achieving the best outcome in treatment of depression. *The Journal of Family Medicine*, 52(3), 201–209.

Szewczyk, B., Poleszak, E., Sowa-Kućma, M., Siwek, M., Dudek, D., Ryszewska-Pokraśniewicz, B., ... Nowak, G. (2008). Antidepressant activity of zinc and magnesium in view of the current hypotheses of antidepressant action. *Pharmacological Reports*, 60, 588–599.

Tandon, R., & Jibson, M. (2003). Efficacy of newer generation antipsychotics in the treatment of schizophrenia. *Psychoneuroendocrinology*, 28, 9–26.

Tariot, P. N., Farlow, M. R., Grossberg, G. T., Graham, S. M., McDonald, S., & Gergel, I. Memantine Study Group. (2004). Memantine treatment in patients with moderate to severe Alzheimer's disease already receiving donepezil: A randomized controlled trial. *Journal of the American Medical Association, 291*(3), 317–324.

Thase, M., Youakim, J., Skuban, A., Hobart, M., Augustine, C., Zhang, P., … Eriksson, H. (2015). Efficacy and safety of adjunctive brexpiprazole 2 mg in major depression. *Journal of Clinical Psychiatry, 76*(9), 1224–1231.

Thomas, J., Vartanian, L., & Brownell, K. (2009). The relationship between Eating Disorder Not Otherwise Specified (EDNOS) and officially recognized eating disorders: Meta-analysis and implications for DSM. *Psychological Bulletin, 135*(3), 407–433.

Tobin, M. (2007). Why choose varenicline (Chantix) for smoking cessation treatment? *Issues in Mental Health Nursing, 28*, 663–667.

Toda, N., Kaneko, T., & Kogen, H. (2010). Development of an efficient therapeutic agent for Alzheimer's disease: Design and synthesis of dual inhibitors of acetylcholinesterase and serotonin transporter. *Chemical and Pharmaceutical Bulletin, 58*(3), 273–287.

Topolov, M., & Getova, D. (2016). Cognitive impairment in schizophrenia, neurotransmitters and the new atypical antipsychotic aripiprazole. *Folia Medica, 58*(1), 12–18.

Tosini, G., Ferguson, I., & Tsubota, K. (2016). Effects of blue light on the circadian system and eye physiology. *Molecular Vision, 22*, 61–72.

Trebatická, J., & Duracková, Z. (2015). Psychiatric disorders and polyphenols: Can they be helpful in therapy? *Oxidative Medicine and Cellular Longevity, 2015*, 248529.

Treede, R., Jensen, T., Campbell, J., Cruccu, G., Dostrovsky, J., Griffin, J., … Serra, J. (2008). Neuropathic pain: Redefinition and a grading system for clinical research purposes. *Neurology, 70*(18), 1630–1635.

Triggs, W., McCoy K., Greer R., Rossi F., Bowers D., Kortenkamp S., … Goodman, W. (1999). Effects of left frontal transcranial magnetic stimulation on depressed mood, cognition, and corticomotor threshold. *Biological Psychiatry, 45*, 1440–1446.

Tyler, V. (1993). *The honest herbal* (3rd ed.). New York, NY: Pharmaceutical Products Press/Haworth Press.

Tziomalos, K., Krassas, G. E., & Tzotzas, T. (2009). Use of sibutramine in the management of obesity and related disorders: An update. *Journal of Vascular Health and Risk Management, 5*(1), 441–452.

van der Weide, J., Steijns, L. S., & van Weelden, M. J. (2003). The effect of smoking and cytochrome P450 CYP1A2 genetic polymorphism on clozapine clearance and dose requirement. *Pharmacogenetics, 13*(3), 169–172.

Van Harten, P., Hoek, H., Matroos, G., & Van Os, J. (2008). Evidence that lithium protects against tardive dyskinesia: The Curacao extrapyramidal syndromes study VI. *European Neuropsychopharmacology: The Journal of the European College of Neuropsychopharmacolgy, 18*(2), 152–155.

Van Veen, V., & Carter, C. S. (2002). The anterior cingulate as a conflict monitor: fMRI and ERP studies. *Physiology & Behavior, 77*(4), 477–482. http://doi.org/https://doi.org/10.1016/S0031-9384(02)00930-7

Vellas, B., Coley, N., Ousset, P., Berrut, G., Dartigues, J., Dubois, B., … Andrieu, S. GuidAge Study Group. (2012). Long-term use of standardized ginkgo biloba extract for the prevention of Alzheimer's disease: Outcomes from CATIE-AD. *American Jounrnal of Psychiatry, 168*, 831–839.

Vieta, E., Berk, M., Schulze, T., Carvalho, A., Suppes, T., Calabrese, J., … Grande, I. (2018). Bipolar disorders. *Nature Reviews Disease Primers, 4*.

Viguera, A., Cohen, L., Baldessarini, R., & Nonacs, R. (2002). Managing bipolar disorder during pregnancy: Weighing the risk and benefits. *Canadian Journal of Psychiatry, 47*(5), 426–436.

Volkow, N., Wang, G., Fowler, J., Tomasi, D., & Telang, F. (2011). Addiction: Beyond dopamine reward circuitry. *Proceedings of the Natural Academy of Science, 108*, 15,037–15,042.

Wadden, T., Sarwer, D., & Womble, L. (2001). Psychosocial aspects of obesity and obesity surgery. *Surgical Clinics of North America, 81*, 1004–1024.

Walsh, S., Comer, S., Lofwall, M., Vince, B., Levy-Cooperman, N., Kelsh, D., … Kim, S. (2017). Effect of buprenorphine weekly depot (CAM2038) and hydromorphone blockade in individuals with opioid use disorder: A randomized clinical trial. *JAMA Psychiatry, 74*(9), 894–902. doi:10.1001/jamapsychiatry.2017.1874

Wang, S., Han, C., Lee, S., Patkar, A., Masand, P., & Pae, C. (2016). Vilazodone for the treatment of depression: An update. *Chonnam Medical Journal, 52*, 91–100.

Warren, M. (2004). A comparative review of the risks and benefits of hormone replacement therapy regimens. *American Journal of Obstetrics and Gynecology, 190*(4), 1141–1167.

Weiss, M., & Murray, C. (2003). Assessment and management of attention-deficit hyperactivity disorder in adults. *Canadian Medical Association Journal, 168*(6), 715–722.

Welsh, C., Sherman, S., & Tobin, K. (2008). A case of heroin overdose reversed by sublingually administered buprenorphine/naloxone (suboxone). *Addiction, 103*, 1226–1228.

Wentrup, A., Oertel, W., & Dodel, R. (2008). Once-daily transdermal rivastigmine in the treatment of Alzheimer's disease. *Drug Design, Development and Therapy, 2*, 245–254.

Wilens, T., Haight, B., Horrigan, J., Hudziak, J., Rosenthal, N., Connor, D., … Modell, J. (2005). Bupropion XL in adults with attention-deficit/hyperactivity disorder: A randomized, placebo-controlled study. *Biological Psychiatry, 57*, 793–801.

Williams, J., & Hughes, J. (2003). Treatments for tobacco dependence among smokers with mental illness or addiction. *Psychiatric Annals, 33*(7), 457–466.

Wilson, J., & Levin, F. (2001). Attention deficit hyperactivity disorder (ADHD) and substance use disorders. *Current Psychiatry Reports, 3*, 497–506.

Zammit, G. (2009). Comparative tolerability of newer agents for insomnia. *Drug Safety, 32*(9), 735–748.

Zhang, A., Park, S., Sullivan, J., & Jing, S. (2018). The effectiveness of problem-solving therapy for primary care patients' depressive and/or anxiety disorders: A systematic review and meta-analysis. *Journal for the American Board of Family Medicine, 31*(1), 139–150.

Zimmerman, M. (2003). Attention-deficit hyperactivity disorders. *Nursing Clinics of North America, 38*, 55–66.

INDEX